OPERATIVE SURGERY

Fundamental International Techniques

Vascular Surgery

OPERATIVE SURGERY

Fundamental International Techniques

Third Edition

Under the General Editorship of

Charles Rob
M.C., M.D., M.Chir., F.R.C.S.

Professor and Chairman of the Department of Surgery,
University of Rochester School of Medicine and Dentistry,
Rochester, New York

and

Rodney Smith (Lord Smith of Marlow)
K.B.E., Hon.D.Sc., M.S., F.R.C.S., Hon.F.R.A.C.S.,
Hon.F.R.C.S.(Ed.), Hon.F.A.C.S., Hon.F.R.C.S. (Can.),
Hon.F.R.C.S.(I.), Hon.F.D.S.

Associate Editor

Hugh Dudley
Ch.M., F.R.C.S., F.R.C.S.(Ed.), F.R.A.C.S.

Professor of Surgery,
St. Mary's Hospital, London

OPERATIVE SURGERY

Fundamental International Techniques

Vascular Surgery

Edited by

Charles Rob
M.C., M.D., M.Chir., F.R.C.S.

Professor and Chairman of the Department of Surgery,
University of Rochester School of Medicine and Dentistry,
Rochester, New York

BUTTERWORTHS
LONDON · BOSTON
Sydney · Wellington · Durban · Toronto

THE BUTTERWORTH GROUP

ENGLAND

Butterworth & Co (Publishers) Ltd
London: 88 Kingsway, WC2B 6AB

AUSTRALIA

Butterworths Pty Ltd
Sydney: 586 Pacific Highway, Chatswood, NSW 2067
Also at Melbourne, Brisbane, Adelaide and Perth

SOUTH AFRICA

Butterworth & Co (South Africa) (Pty) Ltd
Durban: 152–154 Gale Street

NEW ZEALAND

Butterworths of New Zealand Ltd
Wellington: T & W Young Building,
77–85 Customhouse Quay 1, CPO Box 472

CANADA

Butterworth & Co (Canada) Ltd
Toronto: 2265 Midland Avenue, Scarborough, Ontario M1P 4S1

USA

Butterworths (Publishers) Inc
Boston: 19 Cummings Park, Woburn, Mass. 01801

First Edition Published in Eight Volumes, 1956–1958
Second Edition Published in Fourteen Volumes, 1968–1971
Third Edition Published in Eighteen Volumes, 1976–1978
This Volume First Published 1976
This Volume Reprinted 1979

© Butterworth & Co (Publishers) Ltd 1976

ISBN 0 407 00644 3

Library of Congress Cataloging in Publication Data
Main entry under title:

Operative Surgery.

    Vol. 3 issued under the general editorship of
C. Rob, Sir R. Smith, with associate editor, Hugh
Dudley.
    Includes indexes.
    CONTENTS: (1) Ear, edited by J. Ballantyne.–
(2) Nose throat, edited by J. Ballantyne.–(3) Eyes,
edited by S. J. H. Miller.–(4) Vascular Surgery,
edited by Charles Rob.
    1. Surgery, Operative. I. Rob, Charles. II. Smith,
Rodney, Sir. III. Dudley, Hugh Arnold Freeman.
[DNLM: 1. Eye–Surgery. W0500 061 v.3]

RD32.06   1976   617'.91   75-42330
ISBN 0-407-00644-3 (v.4)

Typeset by Butterworths Litho Preparation Department
Printed in England by The Whitefriars Press Ltd., London and Tonbridge
Bound by the Newdigate Press Ltd., Dorking, Surrey

OPERATIVE SURGERY

Volumes and Editors

ABDOMEN *120.⁰⁰*

Hugh Dudley, Ch.M., F.R.C.S., F.R.C.S.(Ed.), F.R.A.C.S.
Charles Rob, *M.C.,* M.D., M.Chir., F.R.C.S.
Rodney Smith (Lord Smith of Marlow), K.B.E., M.S., F.R.C.S.

ACCIDENT SURGERY *149.95*

P. S. London, M.B.E., F.R.C.S.

CARDIOTHORACIC
SURGERY *110.⁰⁰*

John W. Jackson, M.Ch., F.R.C.S.

COLON, RECTUM AND
ANUS *79.95*

Ian P. Todd, M.S., M.D.(Tor.), F.R.C.S.

EAR *39.95*

John Ballantyne, F.R.C.S., Hon.F.R.C.S.(I.)

EYES *44.95*

Stephen J. H. Miller, M.D., F.R.C.S.

GENERAL PRINCIPLES,
BREAST AND HERNIA
149.95

Hugh Dudley, Ch.M., F.R.C.S., F.R.C.S.(Ed.), F.R.A.C.S.
Charles Rob, *M.C.,* M.D., M.Chir., F.R.C.S.
Rodney Smith (Lord Smith of Marlow), K.B.E., M.S., F.R.C.S.

GYNAECOLOGY AND
OBSTETRICS *45.95*

D. W. T. Roberts, M.Chir., F.R.C.S., F.R.C.O.G.

THE HAND
64.95

R. Guy Pulvertaft, C.B.E., Hon.M.D., M.Chir., F.R.C.S.

VOLUMES AND EDITORS

Butterworth's have doesn't have our est. price on this yet

✓ HEAD AND NECK   John S. P. Wilson, F.R.C.S.(Eng.), F.R.C.S.(Ed.)
Oct '80

NEUROSURGERY *have*   Lindsay Symon, T.D., F.R.C.S.

✓ NOSE AND THROAT *67.00*   John Ballantyne, F.R.C.S., Hon.F.R.C.S.(I.)

✗ ✓ ORTHOPAEDICS *225.00*
[in 2 volumes]   George Bentley, Ch.M., F.R.C.S.

✓ PAEDIATRIC *110.00*
SURGERY   H. H. Nixon, F.R.C.S., Hon.F.A.A.P.

PLASTIC SURGERY   Robert M. McCormack, M.D.
120.00   John Watson, F.R.C.S.

✓ UROLOGY *79.95*   D. Innes Williams, M.D., M.Chir., F.R.C.S.

VASCULAR SURGERY *have*   Charles Rob, *M.C.*, M.D., M.Chir., F.R.C.S.

OPERATIVE SURGERY

Contributors to this Volume

CARL H. ANDRUS
M.D.

Assistant Professor of Surgery, University of Rochester Medical Centre and Strong Memorial Hospital, Rochester, New York

The Late
HAROLD W. BALES
M.D.

Associate Professor of Plastic Surgery, University of Rochester School of Medicine and Dentistry, Rochester, New York

F. B. COCKETT
B.Sc.(Lond.), M.S.(Lond.),
F.R.C.S.(Eng.)

Teacher and Examiner in Surgery, The University of London; and Consultant Surgeon, St. Thomas's Hospital, London

JAMES A. DEWEESE
M.D., F.A.C.S.

Chairman of the Division of Cardiothoracic Surgery, University of Rochester Medical Centre, and Professor and Surgeon, Strong Memorial Hospital, Rochester, New York

H. H. G. EASTCOTT
M.S., F.R.C.S.

Senior Surgeon, St. Mary's Hospital, London

W. G. FEGAN
M.Ch., F.R.C.S.(I.)

Research Professor of Surgery, University College of Dublin, Trinity College at Sir Patrick Dun's Hospital, Dublin

ALASTAIR J. GILLIES
M.D.

Professor and Chairman, Department of Anesthesiology, Professor of Pharmacology and Toxicology, University of Rochester School of Medicine and Dentistry, Rochester, New York

R. P. JEPSON
F.R.C.S.

Honorary Consultant Surgeon, The Royal Adelaide Hospital, South Australia

ELLIOT O. LIPCHIK
M.D.

Professor of Radiology, Head Cardiovascular Section, Department of Radiology, University of Rochester Medical Centre, Rochester, New York

JERE W. LORD, JR.
M.D., F.A.C.S.

Clinical Professor of Surgery, New York University School of Medicine

J. S. P. LUMLEY
F.R.C.S.

Assistant Director, Surgical Professorial Unit, St. Bartholomew's Hospital, London

ALLYN G. MAY
M.D.

Associate Professor of Surgery, University of Rochester and Strong Memorial Hospital, Rochester, New York

KENNETH OWEN
M.S., F.R.C.S.

Consultant Urologist, St. Mary's Hospital, St. Peter's Hospital and King Edward VII Hospital for Officers, London

JEFFERSON RAY, III
M.D., F.A.C.S.

Attending, Thoracic Surgery, St. Joseph's Hospital, Marshfield, Wisconsin

CHARLES ROB
M.C., M.D., M.Chir., F.R.C.S.

Professor and Chairman of the Department of Surgery, University of Rochester School of Medicine and Dentistry, Rochester, New York

CONTRIBUTORS TO THIS VOLUME

EDWIN D. SAVLOV
M.D.

Associate Professor of Surgery, University of Rochester School of Medicine and Dentistry, and Director of Surgical Oncology, Highland Hospital, Rochester, New York

ROBERT D. SCHROCK, JR.
M.D.

Clinical Assistant Professor of Orthopaedic Surgery, University of Rochester School of Medicine and Dentistry, Rochester, New York

SEYMOUR I. SCHWARTZ
M.D.

Professor of Surgery, University of Rochester School of Medicine and Dentistry, Rochester, New York

CHARLES D. SHERMAN,
M.D.   JR.

Clinical Professor of Surgery, University of Rochester School of Medicine and Dentistry, Rochester, New York

G. W. TAYLOR
M.S., F.R.C.S.

Professor of Surgery and Director, Surgical Professorial Unit, St. Bartholomew's Hospital, London

A. E. THOMPSON
M.S., F.R.C.S.

Consultant Surgeon, St. Thomas's Hospital, London

OPERATIVE SURGERY

Contents of this Volume

CONTENTS OF THIS VOLUME

CONTENTS OF THIS VOLUME

Introduction

Vascular surgery may be defined as the surgery of the arteries, the veins and the lymphatics, together with certain related procedures such as amputations for ischaemia and fasciotomy for acute vascular occlusion. For convenience most cardiac operations have been placed in the **Cardiothoracic Surgery** volume. There is also a close association between vascular surgery and organ transplantation, because the success or failure of an organ transplant procedure depends in no small measure upon the vascular anastomoses between the host and the transplanted organ.

A brief history of the development of vascular surgery is now given because a note of this type is a useful introduction to any subject.

The first permanent union of two blood vessels either in the laboratory or clinical practice appears to have been accomplished in 1897 by Eck, a Russian surgeon. Before this there were occasional reports of lateral suture of blood vessels, but in 1900 Dörfler reviewed this subject and he concluded that the literature contained reports of only nine patients with a successful arterial repair by direct suture. In 1906 Carrel and Guthrie began experimenting with the anastomosis of blood vessels in the Hull Physiological Laboratory of the University of Chicago, and the techniques they developed have, except for minor variations, remained unchanged to the present time.

In the field of operative surgery some events stand out as milestones where a genuinely new clinical procedure was performed for the first time. Murphy in 1897 reported the first successful end-to-end arterial anastomosis using an invagination technique of the proximal into the distal artery. In 1906 Jose Goyanes used an autogenous vein graft for the first time to replace a peripheral aneurysm, this procedure was repeated in 1907 by Lexer, and in 1913 Pringle was the first English-speaking surgeon to report the insertion of a vein graft into the human arterial system. In 1947 Dos Santos was the first to perform the procedure of thrombo-endarterectomy in the way we use this technique today. In 1949 Kunlin introduced the procedure of femoropopliteal bypass grafting using an autogenous vein, and in 1951 Dubost, Allery and Oeconomos reported for the first time the successful resection of an aneurysm of the abdominal aorta and its replacement by an arterial homograft. In 1952 Voorhees, Jaretzki and Blakemore were the first to report the use of porous plastic cloth tubes to bridge arterial defects, a procedure which DeBakey and others have developed and improved. In 1963 Fogarty introduced the balloon embolectomy catheter which bears his name.

We must not forget sympathectomy and the surgery of the venous system. In 1890 Trendelenburg reported ligature of the long saphenous vein for lower limb varices and admitted a recurrence rate of 22 per cent after a four-year follow-up. This led to the improved techniques used today. Sympathectomy was performed as a peri-arterial procedure by Jaboulay in 1899 and it appears that Jonnesco in 1923 was the first to resect the sympathetic ganglia.

Finally, we should remember the debt that vascular surgeons owe to those who developed arteriography and phlebography. In 1923 Berberich and Hirsch performed phlebograms in humans and in 1924 Brooks injected sodium iodide into a patient's femoral artery producing the first arteriogram. These techniques were improved and developed by Moniz and Dos Santos in Portugal together with many of our Swedish colleagues.

CHARLES ROB

Exposure of Major Blood Vessels

H. H. G. Eastcott, M.S., F.R.C.S.
Senior Surgeon, St. Mary's Hospital, London

and

A. E. Thompson, M.S., F.R.C.S.
Consultant Surgeon, St. Thomas's Hospital, London

PRE-OPERATIVE

Indications

The exposure of blood vessels is indicated under emergency circumstances for local injury and control of bleeding, or for the relief of occlusion. It is also required for very rapid blood transfusion, for the intra-arterial injection of radio-opaque contrast media, extracorporeal circulation and regional perfusion.

The major vessels are most often exposed for the elective surgical treatment of aneurysms, arterio-venous fistulae and arteriosclerotic obstruction.

Contra-indications

No major blood vessel should be exposed if the surgeon's purpose can be adequately achieved in any other way, such as by pressure in local injury for control of bleeding, or percutaneous injection for radiology. An overlying layer of infected or densely adherent tissue should not be disturbed; an alternative normal adjacent site should be chosen for the approach.

Special pre-operative treatment

Some patients will have been receiving anticoagulant drugs. It is wise to counteract these by giving the appropriate antidote: for heparin, the appropriate amount of 10 per cent protamine sulphate (2 mg protamine for 1 mg heparin); and for the pro-thrombin depressor group, such as warfarin, 20 mg of vitamin K_1.

Compatible blood transfusion should be available in adequate quantity to replace blood losses.

Anaesthesia

General anaesthesia is preferable for most patients, although local infiltration with 1 per cent Xylocaine is very suitable for limb embolectomy in patients with severe heart disease. Hypotension should be avoided in the presence of coronary or cerebrovascular disease.

Heparin

Total heparinization may be used if protracted clamping is anticipated (1·5 mg/kg body weight). Alternatively, heparin—saline solution (1:200,000) may be instilled into the arterial tree distal to the site of operation. A vasodilator (e.g. thymoxamine 30 mg) may be added to this solution to reduce vasospasm.

Exposure

'The use of wide approach for dealing thoroughly with nerves and vessels needs no defence' (Henry, 1946). When reconstructive surgery is necessary flexures may be crossed, muscles and tendons divided and the abdomen opened to its fullest extent.

1

THE OPERATIONS

EXPOSURE OF ASCENDING AORTA

1

The incision

This is in the mid-line extending from the suprasternal notch to just beyond the xiphisternum. The extent is dictated by the need for extracorporeal circulation. A transverse component at the upper end improves the cosmetic result.

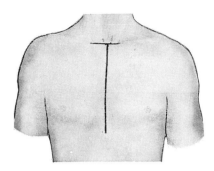

1

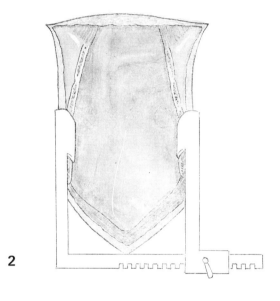

2

2

Entering the mediastinum

The sternum is divided with a counter-rotating power-driven saw or a Gigli saw. The line of division deviates slightly to the left in its lower half to avoid entering the right pleural cavity.

3

Deep dissection

The thymic remnant is divided and the innominate vein identified. Final access to the ascending aorta is obtained by opening the pericardium longitudinally.

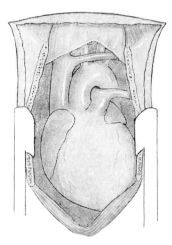

3

**EXPOSURE OF INNOMINATE ARTERY AND
THORACIC PART OF RIGHT SUBCLAVIAN
ARTERY**

4

The incision

The shoulder girdle is displaced backwards by placing a sandbag between the patient's shoulders. The incision is centred over the right sternoclavicular joint, exposing the medial third of the clavicle, the manubrium and the first two intercostal spaces.

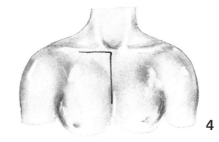

5

Splitting the manubrium

The manubrium is divided in the mid line with Sauerbruch's shears or a Gigli saw. The two halves are separated with a Tuffier's retractor. Further exposure can then be obtained by transecting the sternum below the manubrium or dividing the clavicle and anterior ends of the first and second ribs.

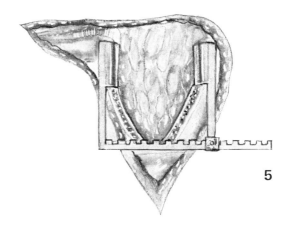

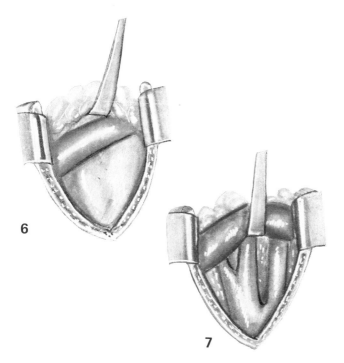

6

Deep dissection

The thymic remnant and anterior mediastinal fat are cleared to expose the innominate vein. The anterior borders of the pleural cavities are swept away laterally.

7

Exposure of great vessels

Mobilization of the innominate vein permits it to be retracted upwards, revealing the origins of the great vessels.

EXPOSURE OF THORACIC PART OF LEFT SUBCLAVIAN ARTERY

This can be exposed by modifying the approach for the innominate and right subclavian arteries (above), or by lateral approach through the fourth left intercostal space.

8

The incision

With the patient in the right lateral position a curved incision skirts the angle of the left scapula.

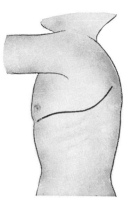

8

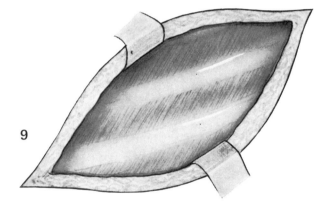

9

9

Deep dissection

The trapezius and serratus anterior muscles are divided and the chest is entered through an incision along the upper border of the fifth rib. Adequate exposure requires division of the fifth rib (and fourth if necessary) at the posterior end.

10

Intrathoracic exposure

The intrathoracic segment of the left subclavian artery can be exposed by incision of the overlying mediastinal pleura. The vagus nerve, the left superior intercostal vein and the thoracic duct lie close to the vessel.

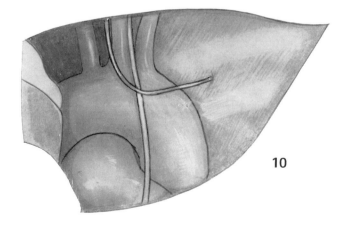

10

**EXPOSURE OF CERVICAL PART OF
SUBCLAVIAN ARTERY AND ORIGIN OF
VERTEBRAL ARTERY**

11

The incision

The patient's neck is extended and turned to the opposite side. A skin crease incision is made one finger's breadth above the middle third of the clavicle. The platysma and the clavicular head of the sterno-mastoid are divided.

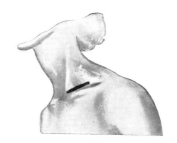

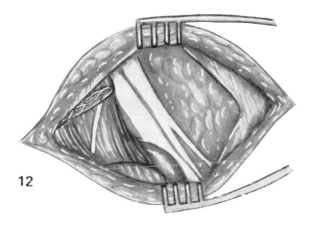

12

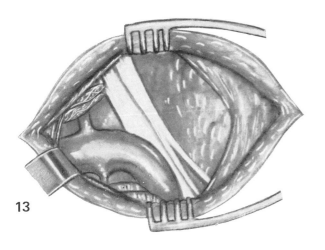

13

12 & 13

Deep dissection

The omohyoid fascia is incised and the scalenus anterior muscle exposed with the phrenic nerve on its surface. The internal jugular vein and the termination of the thoracic duct (on the left side) lie in the medial end of the field. The phrenic nerve is delicately mobilized and retracted medially, before the scalenus anterior muscle is divided piecemeal to avoid damage to the underlying vessel and its branches. The artery is finally exposed by incision of its sheath. The lower trunks of the brachial plexus lie above and lateral to the vessel.

More extensive exposure of the distal part of the vessel and the axillary artery is obtained by sub-periosteal excision of the appropriate part of the clavicle.

ANOTHER EXPOSURE OF LOWER PART OF VERTEBRAL ARTERY

14

The incision

The patient's neck is extended and the head turned to the opposite side. An incision, 8 cm in length, is made over the lower third of the sternomastoid in the groove between its sternal and clavicular heads, in line with the muscle fibres. The two heads of the muscle are separated.

15

Deep dissection

The internal jugular vein is retracted medially. The triangular space between the scalenus anterior laterally and the longus colli medially is cleared to expose the artery. Division of the scalenus anterior may be required; if so, the phrenic nerve has to be preserved. Branches of the thyrocervical trunk are divided. The thoracic duct is avoided on the left side.

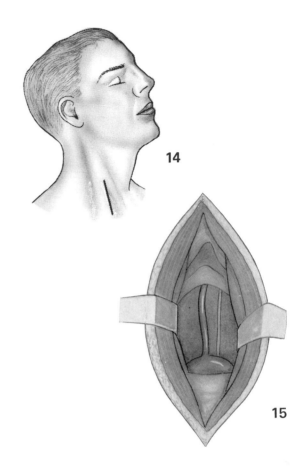

14

15

EXPOSURE OF VERTEBRAL ARTERY IN ITS CANAL

16

The incision

An incision, 8 cm in length, is made along the anterior border of the sternomastoid muscle, similar to that made for the common carotid artery.

17

Deep dissection

The sternomastoid muscle is retracted laterally and the carotid sheath medially. The scalenus anterior muscle is detached from its origin from the transverse processes of the cervical vertebra. The vessel is exposed by removal of the anterior margins of the foramina in the transverse processes. Branches of the thyrocervical trunk are ligated and the sympathetic and vagus nerves preserved.

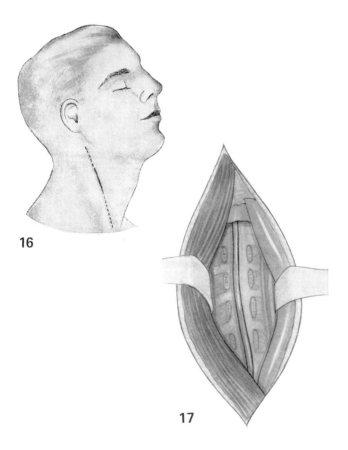

16

17

EXPOSURE OF AXILLARY ARTERY (FIRST PART)

18

The incision

With the arm abducted to a right angle, the incision is made just below the clavicle and parallel to it.

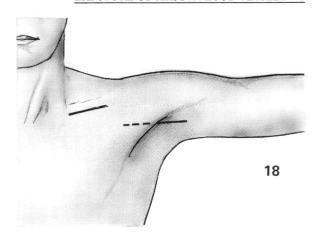

18

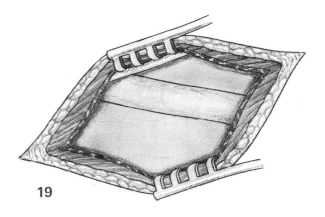

19

19

Dissection

The pectoral fascia is divided along the line of the muscle fibres of the clavicular head of the pectoralis major, which are then split to expose the vascular sheath. The pectoral branch of the acromiothoracic axis may require division.

20

Division of sheath

The pulsations of the artery are palpated and the vascular sheath is divided along the line thus indicated. Here the only other important structure is the axillary vein which lies below and medial to the artery from which it is then carefully separated. This is the site for axillofemoral bypass.

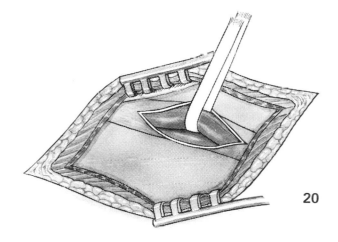

20

EXPOSURE OF AXILLARY ARTERY
(SECOND AND THIRD PARTS)

21

The incision

With the arm abducted to a right angle the incision is made along the line of the pulsating artery up to the lower border of the pectoralis major muscle. If the artery is pulseless the groove between the coraco-brachialis and triceps is the guide.

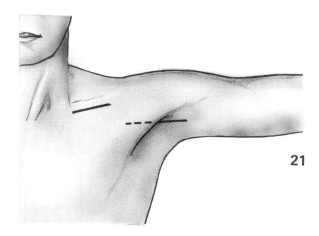

21

22

Dissection

The pectorals are retracted upwards and medially to expose the distal two thirds of the axillary artery. If necessary both muscles are divided and a portion of the clavicle resected to gain exposure of the whole subclavian–axillary axis. Sections of bone should not be replaced (Elkin, 1946; DeBakey, 1955).

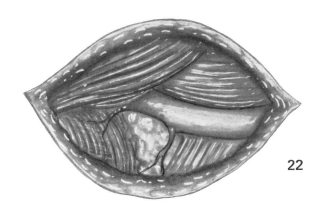

22

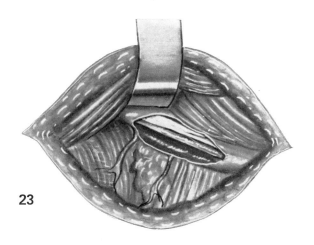

23

23

Exposure of artery

The axillary sheath is opened to reveal the vein medially and the brachial plexus laterally. Between these two structures the artery will be found. It can also be identified by following the subscapular artery to its origin.

EXPOSURE OF BRACHIAL ARTERY IN THE ARM

24

The incision

The incision is made along the line of the pulsating artery or in the line of the sulcus separating the biceps muscle from the triceps muscle. The length of the incision is governed by the procedure to be performed. A sandbag placed to support the elbow in extension facilitates exposure.

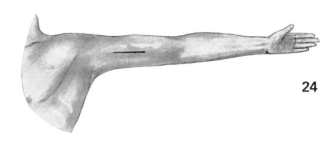

24

25

Dissection

The neurovascular sheath is opened. The veins, and the median nerve which crosses the artery from the lateral to the medial side, are separated from the artery. Care must be taken to recognize a high bifurcation of the vessel. The ulnar collateral artery and medial cutaneous nerve of the forearm lie close to the brachial artery and must not be included in clamps. The dissection is further complicated by the basilic vein which perforates the deep fascia and joins the brachial vein in this region.

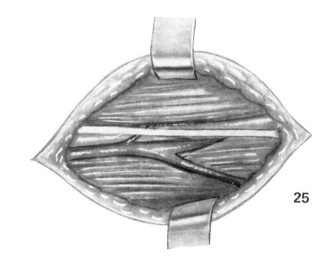

25

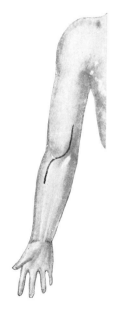

26

EXPOSURE OF BRACHIAL ARTERY AT THE ELBOW

26

The incision

A skin crease incision is made at the elbow with longitudinal extensions along the line of the brachial artery medially, and down the brachioradialis laterally. The skin should be marked to allow an accurate closure.

27

Superficial dissection

The artery is obscured by the cubital veins, the deep fascia and the bicipital aponeurosis. The two cutaneous nerves to the forearm lie deep to the veins at the medial and lateral ends of this plane of the incision and should be avoided.

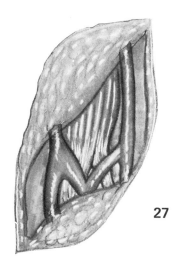

27

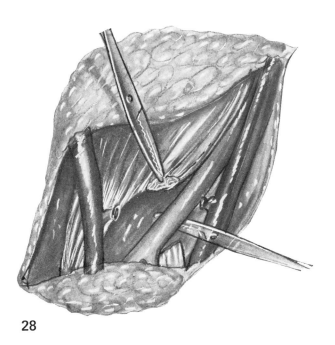

28

28

Deep dissection

The overlying superficial veins and the bicipital aponeurosis are divided; this exposes the artery, with its accompanying deep veins, just above the bifurcation which is close to the medial side of the biceps tendon. Opening the sheath allows the vessel to be lifted away from its venae comites and the median nerve which lies on its medial side. This exposure is most commonly indicated when the brachial artery has been damaged in a supracondylar fracture. Spasm in the intact vessel can be overcome by the injection of saline into the lumen of the affected segment between arterial clamps (Mustard and Bull, 1962).

EXPOSURE OF THE RADIAL ARTERY AT THE WRIST

29

The incision

A longitudinal or transverse incision centred 3–4 cm above the radial styloid is used.

30

Dissection

The origin of the cephalic vein is found in the superficial tissues and the artery beneath the deep fascia on the ulnar side of the brachioradialis tendon. The vessels can be mobilized to allow side-to-side approximation for the construction of a fistula for dialysis.

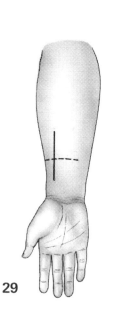

29

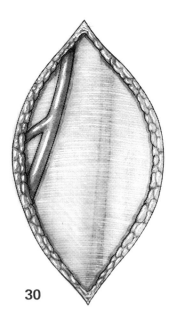

30

EXPOSURE OF COMMON CAROTID ARTERY

31

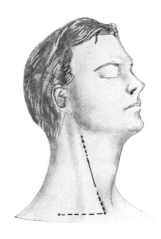

31

The incision

With the neck slightly extended, and the head turned to the opposite side, a 6 cm incision is made along the anterior edge of the sternomastoid with its centre three fingers' breadth above the clavicle.

For a wider exposure of the common carotid artery and internal jugular vein the incision is extended along the dotted lines, dividing the origin of the sternomastoid.

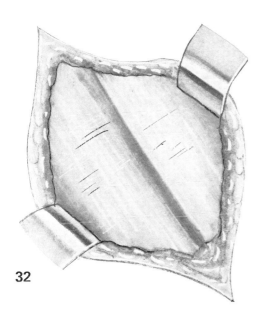

32

32

Dissection

The deep fascia is opened in the same line and the sternomastoid and infrahyoid muscles are separated from the underlying vascular sheath. This plane of dissection is bloodless except for a sternomastoid branch of the superior thyroid artery.

33

Exposure

The sheath is opened above the omohyoid. The jugular vein is dissected free and retracted laterally to isolate the artery. The vagus lies well back between the vessels, and the sympathetic trunk farther still and more medially. Lower in the neck the inferior thyroid artery crosses behind the carotid artery.

Note: Ligation produces hemiplegia in some subjects owing to defective anastomosis of the cerebral vessels through the circle of Willis. The operation should be performed under local anaesthesia and a temporary ligature applied for 5–15 min, or longer if there is any doubt.

In elderly women the common carotid artery is often dilated and tortuous, resembling an aneurysm.

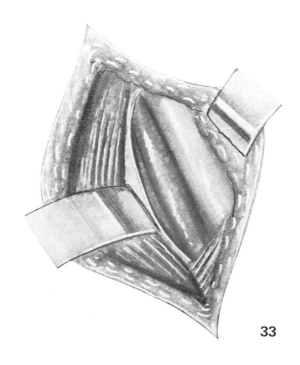

33

EXPOSURE OF INTERNAL AND EXTERNAL CAROTID ARTERIES

34

The incision

An incision is made along the anterior border of the sternomastoid from just above the angle of the jaw, passing downwards for 7—9 cm. For simple ligation a shorter skin crease incision may be preferred.

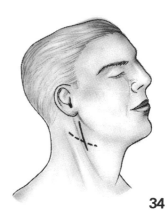

34

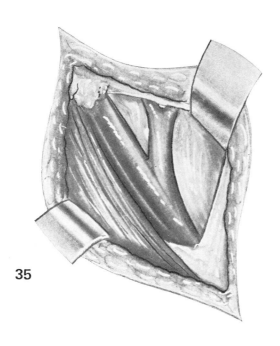

35

35

Dissection

The platysma is divided and the sternomastoid defined and retracted posteriorly. The common facial vein is divided at the upper end of the incision and the vascular sheath opened.

36

Exposure

The common carotid bifurcation usually lies much higher in the neck than is supposed. The two arteries lie close together beneath the angle of the jaw. Branches identify the external carotid, which is anterior and deeper. The hypoglossal nerve must be avoided as it crosses the vessels, and the vagus, superior laryngeal and sympathetic nerves which lie behind the bifurcation. The upper part of the internal carotid artery is difficult to expose; it runs deeply and is covered for the most part by the ascending ramus of the mandible. The sternomastoid can be detached from the mastoid process, which may itself be partly removed. The digastric muscle, the occipital artery and the styloid process are divided. This exposes the superficial aspect of the artery to some extent.
Note: The internal carotid artery may be tied for intracranial aneurysm. Hemiplegia often follows. The external carotid is ligated preliminary to radical pharyngolaryngeal or faciomaxillary operations.

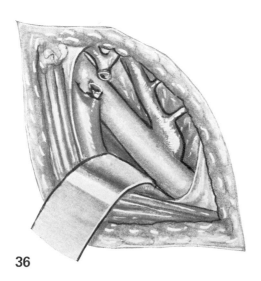

36

EXPOSURE OF AORTIC ARCH

37

The incision

With the patient in the right lateral position the chest is opened through a long curved incision skirting the angle of the left scapula. The lateral chest wall muscles are divided in the same line.

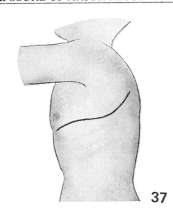

37

38

Dissection

The thorax is entered through the fourth intercostal space. Adequate exposure is obtained by division of the fifth rib (and fourth if required) posteriorly, or by division of the sternum anteriorly.

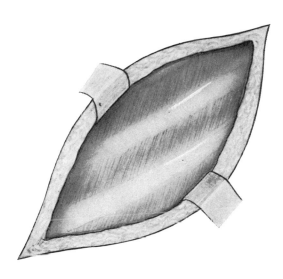

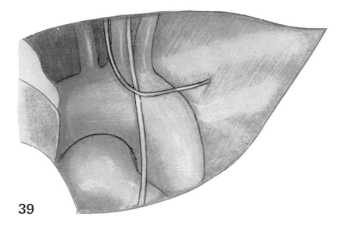

39

39

Exposure

The lung is retracted downwards and the arch of the aorta is seen beneath the mediastinal pleura. It is crossed on its left side by the phrenic nerve, the vagus nerve and the left superior intercostal vein. The left main bronchus and left pulmonary artery lie beneath the arch and the oesophagus and thoracic duct on the deep aspect.

EXPOSURE OF DESCENDING THORACIC AORTA

40

The incision

The site of the incision and the position of the patient depend upon the level of the lesion. A posterolateral incision is made over the appropriate rib space, with the patient rotated slightly backwards from the right lateral position. The chest wall muscles are incised in the same line.

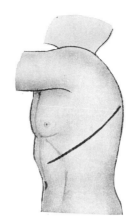

40

41

Dissection

The thorax is entered through the appropriate rib space. The incision can be extended across the costal margin into the abdomen and the diaphragm divided peripherally if necessary. The lung is emptied and retracted forwards to reveal the descending aorta beneath the mediastinal pleura. The oesophagus must be carefully avoided in mobilizing the aorta.
Note: The main blood supply to the spinal cord comes from the branches of the thoracic and upper abdominal aorta.

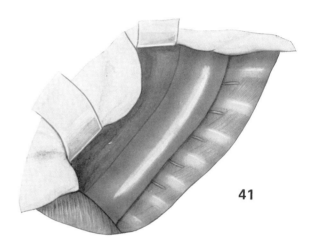

41

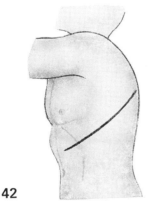

42

EXPOSURE OF AORTA ABOVE RENAL VESSELS

42

The incision

A thoraco-abdominal incision is made along the line of the eighth rib and continued into the abdomen, with the patient inclined backwards from the right lateral position. If temporary control of the upper abdominal aorta is all that is required during an operation on the distal vessel, a very long paramedian incision will suffice.

43

Deep dissection

The latissimus dorsi is divided. The chest is opened along the upper border of the eighth rib and the costal cartilage divided. The diaphragm is divided peripherally until the incision sweeps up to the aorta. The stomach, spleen and pancreas are swept forwards from the posterior abdominal wall to expose the aorta, the left kidney and the suprarenal gland. The visceral branches can be identified and controlled. Care must be taken in dividing intercostal vessels from which the spinal cord derives its blood supply. Temporary occlusion and hypothermia minimize the risk.

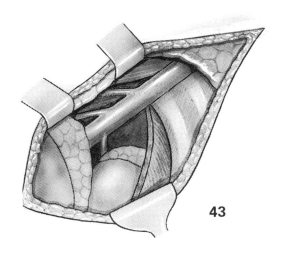

43

EXPOSURE OF RENAL ARTERIES

44

The incision

Either a mid-line upper abdominal (Morris *et al.*, 1962) or a transverse incision 1 inch (2·5 cm) above the umbilicus (Owen, 1964) gives adequate exposure.

44

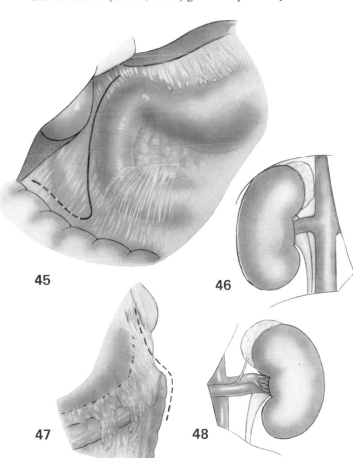

45

46

47   48

45–48

Deep dissection

On the right side, the peritoneum around the hepatic flexure of the colon is incised and the colon displaced downwards. The peritoneum on the right side of the duodenum is incised up to the free border of the lesser omentum. The duodenum can be displaced forwards and to the left, exposing the renal vessels, the vena cava and the aorta.

The left renal vessels are exposed by dividing the peritoneum lateral to the splenic flexure, continuing upwards behind the spleen. The spleen and colon can be displaced forwards and to the right to expose the left kidney and its vessels. The arteries lie behind the larger, more superficial, renal veins.

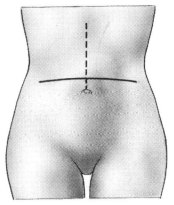

EXPOSURE OF SUPERIOR MESENTERIC ARTERY

49

The incision

A high left paramedian incision is made and the peritoneal cavity opened.

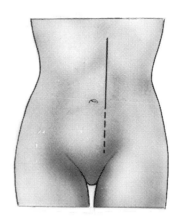

49

50

Deep dissection

The omentum and transverse colon are elevated and the posterior peritoneum incised. The superior mesenteric artery is seen where it emerges below the pancreas. The superior mesenteric vein lies on its right side. The origin of the vessel is exposed by upward dissection and retraction of the pancreas.

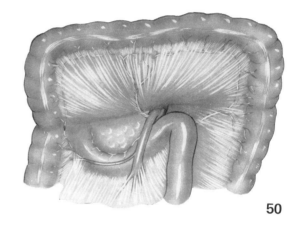

50

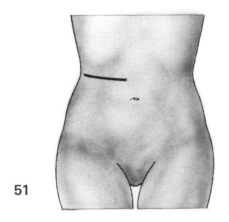

51

EXPOSURE OF THE INFRARENAL INFERIOR VENA CAVA

51

The incision

A transverse incision is made in the upper part of the right lumbar region.

52

Deep dissection

The oblique abdominal muscles and transversus are divided in line with the skin incision. The extra-peritoneal space is entered and the peritoneum pushed to the left, to expose the inferior vena cava.

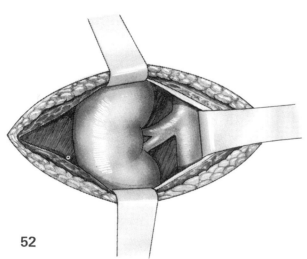

52

EXPOSURE OF ABDOMINAL AORTA BELOW RENAL VESSELS (TRANSPERITONEAL)

53

The incision

A long left paramedian or a median para-umbilical incision runs from the xiphisternum to just above the symphysis pubis. This will provide good access for most abdominal aortic grafts. Complete muscle relaxation is essential. The operator stands on the patient's left.

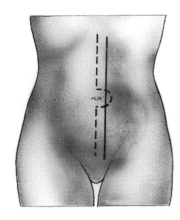

53

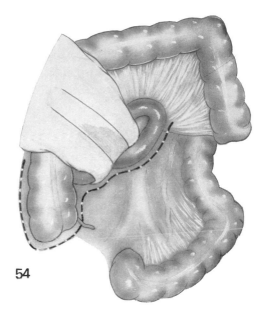

54

54

Dissection

Often it is sufficient to turn the small bowel across to the right side of the abdomen and to hold it there under a large abdominal pack with deep retraction. In very obese subjects, or where the aortic lesion is juxtarenal, it is better to mobilize the whole mid-gut loop by dividing the peritoneal reflection lateral to the right colon and round across the base of the small bowel mesentery. The intestines are then drawn up out of the abdomen and a plastic bag is placed over them.

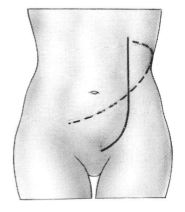

55

EXPOSURE OF ABDOMINAL AORTA BELOW RENAL VESSELS (EXTRAPERITONEAL)

55

The incision

A long J-shaped incision runs along the left linea semilunaris, and lateral to its upper half (Helsby and Moossa, 1975). The patient's left side is lifted up on a sandbag. Alternatively a more oblique incision as recommended by Rob (1963) may be preferred, running from the tip of the left twelfth rib downwards and across the lower abdomen.

56

Dissection

The oblique and transversus muscles are divided in the same line over most of the central part of the incision. They are kept intact with their nerve supply at its two ends. The peritoneal sac is then wiped off the muscles. The aortic bifurcation and iliacs are exposed. Difficulty is most likely with the lower right iliac and the upper aorta. The inferior mesenteric artery retracts with the peritoneum across the aorta to the right.

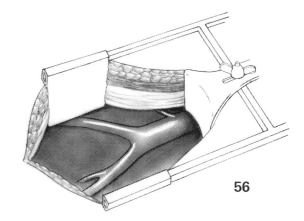

56

EXPOSURE OF THE ABDOMINAL AORTA BELOW RENAL VESSELS (BOTH ROUTES)

57

Exposure of the aorta

Whichever route has been used the deep dissection after displacing the abdominal contents consists in reflecting the duodenum over to the right. Intraperitoneally the aorta can now be isolated as far as the renal vein above. The inferior mesenteric vessels are retracted to the left, as in this diagram. With the extraperitoneal exposure the inferior mesenteric vessels are retracted up with the peritoneum across to the right as shown in *Illustration 56*. A Goligher's retractor with deep blades is valuable for both routes.

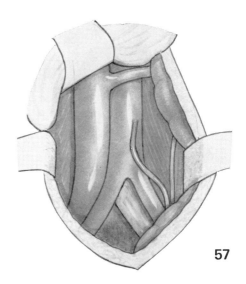

57

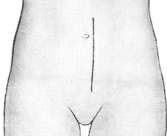

58

EXPOSURE OF THE COMMON ILIAC ARTERY (INTRAPERITONEAL)

58

The incision

A long lower left paramedian incision is required for adequate control of this vessel.

59

Dissection

If the need is for a good view of the lower end and bifurcation the left colon is mobilized and retracted across to the right. Similarly on the right side the caecum is lifted up and over to the left. The ureter is seen crossing the bifurcation and can be identified by its peristalsis. The internal iliac disappears on the deep surface of the bifurcation and is closely related to the pelvic veins.

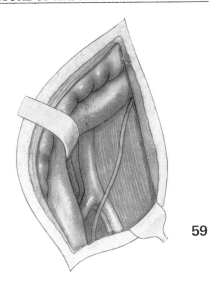

59

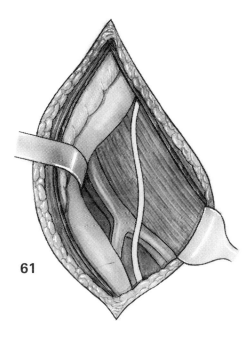

60

EXPOSURE OF THE COMMON ILIAC ARTERY (EXTRAPERITONEAL)

60

The incision

An oblique incision crosses the spino umbilical line in its upper third.

61

Dissection

The oblique and transversus muscles are divided in the same line. The peritoneum is carefully separated from beneath the transversus aponeurosis and the plane developed so as to displace the peritoneal sac medially. A good view is obtained of the lower part of the artery.

61

EXTRAPERITONEAL EXPOSURE OF EXTERNAL ILIAC ARTERY

62

The incision

The classical muscle-cutting in the iliac fossa remains the best. The deep epigastric artery at its inner end should be preserved.

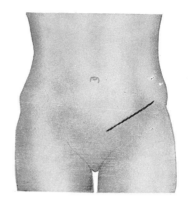

62

63

Deep dissection

The posterior parietal peritoneum is pushed up under the medial edge of the incision. The external iliac vessels are found lying on the pelvic brim on the medial side of the psoas muscle. The obturator nerve lies under the vein in its upper part and the genito-femoral nerve on the muscle lateral to the artery. The ureter is seen crossing its origin. This incision is suitable for renal transplantation.

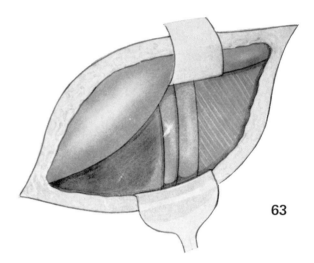

63

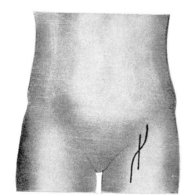

64

EXPOSURE OF COMMON FEMORAL ARTERY

64

The incision

A longitudinal incision allows adequate exposure of the common femoral artery, particularly of its deep branch, and can be extended if necessary.

65

Superficial dissection

The termination of the long saphenous vein is exposed and retracted medially, dividing such tributaries as required. The main vein should be preserved for grafting purposes. The superficial external pudendal artery is ligated.

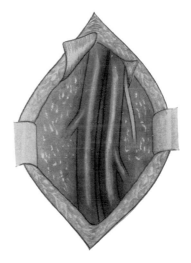

65

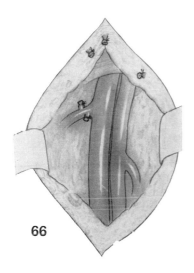

66

66

Deep dissection

The femoral sheath is opened to expose the common femoral vessels. The femoral nerve lies on the lateral side. The profunda femoris artery must be located with care. It arises from the posterior and lateral aspect of the common femoral artery. Its origin is closely related to the termination of the profunda femoris vein. A multiple origin or early branching of the vessel may cause difficulty.

67

Iliofemoral junction

This can be exposed by an upward extension of the above dissection, dividing the inguinal ligament. The deep epigastric vessels are preserved. If this manoeuvre is anticipated, the S-shaped incision shown in *Illustration 64* is preferred.

67

**EXPOSURE OF SUPERFICIAL FEMORAL
ARTERY IN HUNTER'S CANAL**

68

The incision

This is made along the line of the anterior border of
the sartorius muscle. The limb is slightly flexed and
abducted, with a sandbag beneath the knee.

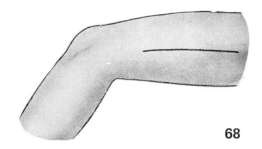

68

69

Superficial dissection

The saphenous vein is carefully preserved in the
posterior flap. The fascia over the sartorius muscle is
incised.

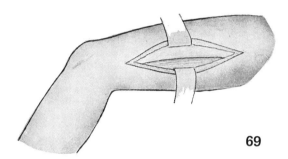

69

70

Deep dissection

The sartorius muscle is retracted backwards. The
fascial roof of Hunter's canal is exposed and incised.
The saphenous nerve is separated from the artery
which is then dissected from the underlying vein.
Care is taken to preserve as many collateral vessels
as possible.

70

EXPOSURE OF THE POPLITEAL ARTERY

The medial approach is used for most bypass operations, but the posterior approach is better for direct procedures such as the repair of arterial cysts or entrapment.

Medial approach (upper)

71

The incision

The patient is placed supine with the knee flexed over a sandbag. The line of the incision should run from four fingers' breadth above the adductor opening downwards and backwards to a little behind the medial femoral condyle, avoiding the long saphenous vein.

72

Dissection

The deep fascia is incised and the anterior border of the sartorius is defined. The muscle is displaced backwards to reveal the thicker aponeurosis of the adductor canal, running into the tendon of the adductor opening. The saphenous nerve leads the dissection to the artery; the fascia is incised to free it and the artery which can then be followed downwards into the popliteal fat.

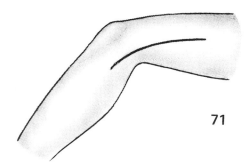

71

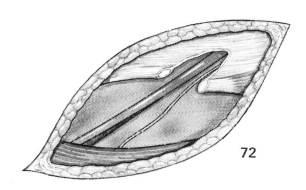

72

Medial approach (lower)

73

The incision

This is along the posterior tibial border from the lower aspect of the medial condyle, avoiding the long saphenous vein.

74

Dissection

The deep fascia, here very thick, is incised and the medial head of the gastrocnemius is displaced backwards. The loose popliteal fat is stroked free from the vascular bundle to reveal the vein, with the artery beneath it. Care should be taken not to damage the medial popliteal nerve. The bifurcation is obscured by the soleus arch and muscular veins but by division of these the posterior tibial artery can be exposed.

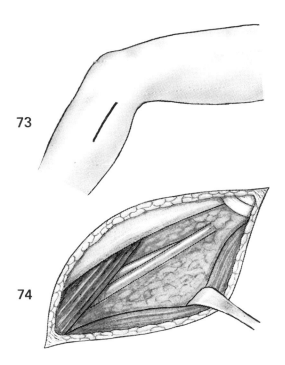

73

74

Posterior approach

75

The incision

Recurrent ulceration and contraction often complicate the vertical incision which crosses the flexure at right angles. An S-shaped incision, with its upper limit medial, avoids this. The middle portion should run in the skin crease. A vertical incision is satisfactory, however, for exposing the lower portion of the popliteal vessels. Placed between the two heads of the gastrocnemius, it commences below the flexure, and can be extended downwards to expose as much of the upper course of the posterior tibial vessels as may be necessary.

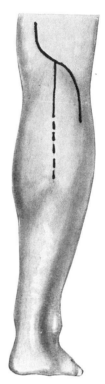

75

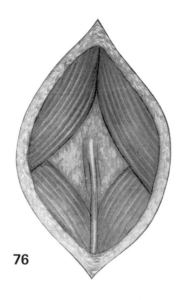

76

76

Superficial dissection

The short saphenous vein is followed through the popliteal fascia and the posterior cutaneous nerve dissected aside. The fascia, whose fibres run transversely, is split longitudinally to reveal the popliteal fat.

77

Deep dissection

The fat is cleared from the two popliteal nerves. The popliteal vein is next found, usually via one of its deep tributaries, or perhaps the short saphenous vein. The artery lies deeper still. It is crossed by a very constant leash of vessels, mainly some large veins from the medial head of the gastrocnemius; they must be divided. The short saphenous vein is preserved if possible.

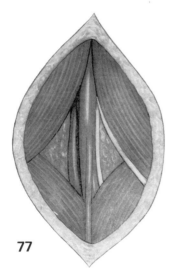

77

Extension of exposure

Upward

To reach the femoral vessels, the semimembranosus belly and tendon of semitendinosus are retracted, or divided, along the line of the artery. The tight hiatus in the adductor magnus is also cut through.

Downward

The posterior tibial artery is readily exposed by splitting the gastrocnemius and soleus fibres in its line, also the fascia which covers the vessels as they lie on the long deep flexors.

Note: These extensions of the posterior approach are limited and can be difficult. If long exposure is required the medial approach should be chosen.

THE ARTERIOVENOUS SHUNT

78

The incision

To construct a shunt for access in haemodialysis the incision is centred 4–6 cm above the medial malleolous, 0·5 cm behind the posterior border of the tibia.

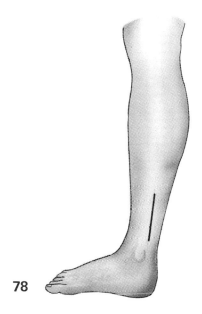

78

79

Dissection

The origin of the long saphenous vein lies in the superficial tissue in the anterior flap and the posterior tibial artery beneath the deep fascia directly under the incision. Limited mobilization of the vessels permits insertion of the silastic cannulae.

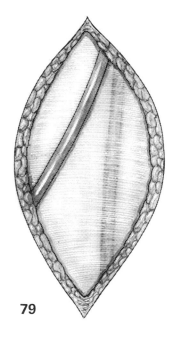

79

POSTOPERATIVE CARE

This depends upon the regular, detailed and careful observation of local and general signs. There must be continuity of responsibility to ensure accurate interpretation of the local and general circulation.

In the surgery of atherosclerosis it must be remembered that the disease is generalized. Hypovolaemia and hypotension must be stringently avoided. In all cases of major arterial surgery, postoperative monitoring of central venous pressure and a continuous electrocardiogram are recommended, in addition to the usual observations on pulse, blood pressure and respirations. Oxygen administration by mask or catheter maintains maximal saturation. The urine output is best collected by catheter drainage over the first 24–48 hr.

Posture

The cerebral and coronary circulations take precedence over the peripheral circulation. If postoperative shock is present or the patient has not regained consciousness, head-down tilt is required. When the central circulation is adequate, dependency of an operated extremity promotes the local arterial circulation.

Local signs

Immediately after operation, the state of the distal circulation must be established. In the extremities, the colour of the limb, the skin temperature, filling of the superficial veins and the pulses are all guides to adequate circulation.

Pulses

The distal pulses may not be felt immediately after an operation in which a limb artery is clamped. They return following improvement in the general circulation and progressive local vasodilatation. The latter can be encouraged before the closure of the arteriotomy by the injection of a vasodilator (tolazoline 25 mg, or thymoxamine 10 mg in heparinized saline) into the distal arterial tree (Hall, 1964). Intravenous infusion of low molecular weight dextran promotes capillary circulation in the operated limb.

Skin temperature

After clamping the arterial supply, the distal part of the limb becomes pale and cold. The peripheral veins are collapsed. As recovery progresses the level of transition from warm to cold skin becomes more distal, with improvement in the colour and filling of the peripheral veins.

Sensory impairment

Numbness of the skin is a serious sign, though some skin sensation will often persist in parts of a limb which are on the same level as patches of established necrosis.

Complications

Haemorrhage

The use of heparin during operation, and the presence of arterial suture lines, requires close observation of the operative site. The use of a vacuum drainage system gives early indication of undue blood loss. The effect of heparin can be reversed at the end of the operation if necessary by the injection of protamine sulphate (2 mg protamine neutralizes 1 mg heparin). If excessive haemorrhage occurs, re-exploration of the site of operation is required.

Ischaemic muscle necrosis

The musculature of a limb is more sensitive to ischaemia than most other tissues. Prolonged ischaemia of the leg may cause necrosis of muscle, particularly in the anterior tibial compartment, where the muscles are firmly enclosed by osseous and fascial boundaries. The presence of tenderness over this area and loss of dorsiflexion of the ankle demand early decompression. Delay in diagnosis or deferring active treatment will jeopardize recovery and lead to gangrene, ischaemic muscle contracture and an equinovarus deformity.

Swelling of leg

Mild oedema of the foot and leg frequently follows operations on the femoral and popliteal vessels even in the presence of normal deep veins (Husni, 1967). This disappears with increasing activity and early mobilization should be practised whenever possible.

References

Elkin, D. C. (1946). *J. Am. med. Ass.* **132,** 421
Elkin, D. C. and DeBakey, M. E. (1955). *Vascular Surgery in World War II.* Office of the Surgeon General
Hall, K. V. (1964). *Acta chir. scand.* **128,** 365
Helsby and Moossa (1975). *Br. J. Surg.* **62,** 596
Henry, A. K. (1946). *Extensile Exposure as Applied to Limb Surgery.* Edinburgh: Livingstone
Husni, E. A. (1967). *Circulation* **35,** Suppl. 1, 169
Morris, G. C., DeBakey, M. F., Cooley, D. A. and Crawford, E. S. (1962). *Surgery* **51,** 62
Mustard, W. T. and Bull, C. (1962). *Ann. Surg.* **155,** 339
Owen, K. (1964). *Br. J. Urol.* **36,** 7
Rob, C. (1963). *Surgery* **53,** 87

[*The illustrations for this Chapter on Exposure of Major Blood Vessels were drawn by Mr. G. Lyth and Mr. F. Price.*]

Arterial Suture and Anastomosis

H. H. G. Eastcott, M.S., F.R.C.S.
Senior Surgeon, St. Mary's Hospital, London

and

A. E. Thompson, M.S., F.R.C.S.
Consultant Surgeon, St. Thomas's Hospital, London

PRE-OPERATIVE

Indications

Repair of a divided or injured major artery is usually preferable to tying its ends. This applies particularly in the lower limb. Trauma, surgical accident and the radical surgery of cancer, as well as the elective treatment of arterial lesions, require the surgeon to be familiar with methods of arterial suture. The methods illustrated will meet the requirements of the arterial operations shown in other sections.

Increasing surgical expertise has allowed anastomosis of very small vessels. The technique for this microsurgery is learned by experience and constant practice. Although under emergency circumstances, a surgeon may be required to attempt small vessel surgery, the techniques are believed to be outside the scope of this chapter (O'Brien, 1976).

Contra-indications

Arteries should never be sutured in the presence of infection. Severe compound or crushing injury with loss of the main artery are indications for amputation, not arterial repair. Simpler procedures are similarly necessary in treating battle casualties when tactical considerations demand early evacuation. Some viscera regularly survive arterial ligation (for example, the left colon). Arterial reconstruction under such circumstances is superfluous.

Suture materials

Fine sutures on atraumatic needles are most frequently used for arterial anastomosis. A number of mechanical devices have been developed for the same purpose. These are very useful for the anastomosis of small vessels, making them valuable in experimental surgery. They have not been widely adopted in clinical surgery. Similarly, adhesives (epoxy resins) have been tried but not found satisfactory in normal clinical practice.

Silk has been used extensively in arterial surgery. It can be obtained in varying sizes (2/0–7/0) with appropriate sized and shaped needles, depending upon the type of tissue to be sutured. It is now being replaced by man-made fibres, which are less traumatic to the arterial wall than silk. Both braided and monofilament sutures in a wide range of sizes are available. These sutures have the advantage that the anastomosis can be tightened more easily by longitudinal tension than with silk. Monofilament fibres are crushed and weakened if grasped by instruments. Extra care is required when tying these materials to avoid loosening of knots and the ends must be cut long. Polypropylene (Prolene) is the most widely used synthetic monofilament suture for vessels. Though less easy to handle than silk or man-made multifilamentous sutures such as Dacron it passes more easily through the tissues and engenders no reaction in them.

THE OPERATIONS

LATERAL SUTURE

1

This is a simple method of closing a longitudinal incision in the artery wall, as after embolectomy or thrombo-endarterectomy. Some narrowing of the vessel is always produced and the blood pressure tends to open the repair instead of tightening it, unlike the circumferential suture of an anastomosis. Where there is loss of substance of the arterial wall, resection and anastomosis or grafting is preferable.

A simple continuous stitch is used, rather than an everting stitch which would narrow the artery even more. A patch graft will sometimes be required.

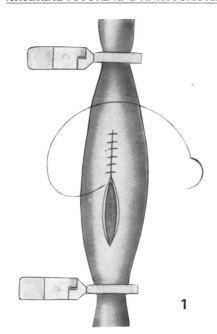

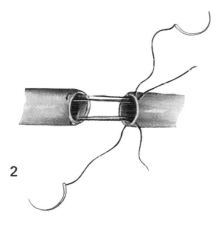

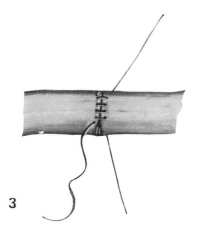

END-TO-END ANASTOMOSIS BY MODIFIED CARREL METHOD

2

Stay sutures

The ends of the vessels to be anastomosed are carefully cleared of excess adventitia. Inclusion of adventitia or other extraneous tissue in the suture line may promote thrombus formation. Stay sutures are placed to define the anterior and posterior aspects of the anastomosis. Everting horizontal mattress sutures are used for this purpose.

3

Continuous suture of anterior aspect

A simple continuous suture is placed along the anterior aspect at intervals of 1–2 mm, according to the size of the artery, and a similar distance from the edges which, if the wall is normal, will have already been everted by the stay sutures. These are held apart with sufficient tension to equalize the diameter of the ends of the vessels.

4

Rotation of anastomosis

The clamps and stay sutures are then used to rotate the anastomosis so that the posterior half can be seen and sutured in the same way. It is often possible to place the clamps in such a position that the anastomosis can be rotated without releasing them.

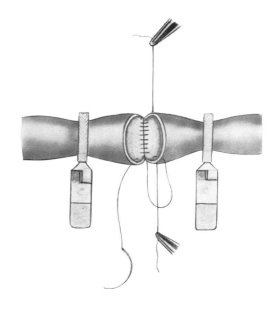

5

Single stitch method

If difficulty is anticipated in rotating the ends of the artery—near a large bifurcation, for example—a single continuous stitch is used. One supporting suture is placed nearest the operator and this is continued forwards from within the lumen, then back along the front of the anastomosis until the starting point is reached in an accessible position.

This method is particularly useful in diseased arteries which will not allow the smooth pull-up of the Blalock suture.

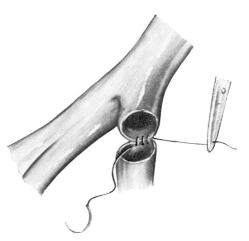

EVERTING MATTRESS SUTURE

This method still has some place in arterial surgery. It does evert the edges of the vessel and may therefore be chosen in circumstances where a second continuous suture is intended for haemostasis, for example in a healthy aorta. It is also useful in large arteries for ensuring haemostasis and a firm repair when suturing normal to diseased arteries.

6

Insertion of stay sutures

Two everting mattress sutures are placed as shown with the loop on the adventitia. Traction is exerted on them to equalize the diameter of the two ends.

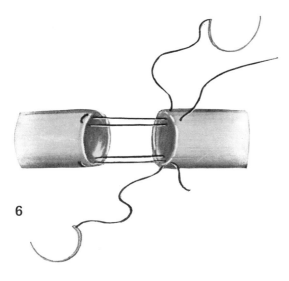

6

7

Continuous everting suture

A continuous everting suture is then placed, first anteriorly, then posteriorly by rotating the anastomosis. One stay suture is passed behind the anastomosis and the ends pulled in opposite directions.

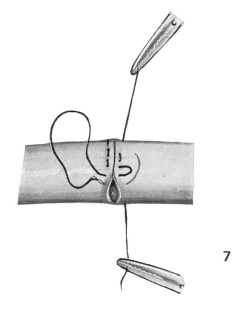

7

8

Use of interrupted sutures

Where growth of the anastomosis must be allowed for, as in coarctation of the aorta in children, interrupted everting mattress sutures may be used.

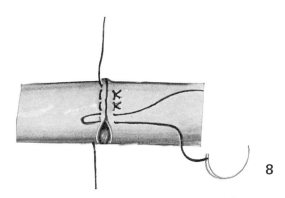

8

BLALOCK SUTURE

This is a valuable method of anastomosing normal or thin-walled arteries or veins when access to the posterior aspect of the anastomosis cannot be obtained by rotation. It is used in coarctation, Blalock's and Pott's operations, portacaval anastomoses, and in the bypass type of arterial graft.

9

Continuous everting suture

A continuous everting suture of polypropylene fibre is placed in the posterior half of the anastomosis with the loops on the adventitia. The ends are not tied.

9

10

Completion of suture

When this suture line is complete the ends are drawn together with steady traction and the edges are everted. It is then completed as a normal continuous everting stitch, maintaining the tension in the stitch throughout. The suture is finally tied to the free end.

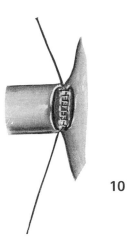

10

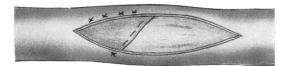

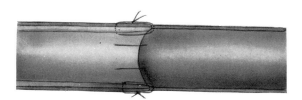

11

SUTURING THE DISEASED ARTERY

Stronger material (2/0) may be used for suturing densely sclerotic or calcified vessels. Care must be taken that the suture is not cut by a sharp plaque. A second, finer suture is recommended to ensure haemostasis.

11

Fixation of plaque

If possible the lower limit of a resected artery or an arteriotomy should be firmly sutured by several longitudinal sutures to the vessel wall, with the ligations on the outer aspect. Unsecured plaques are liable to be dissected free by the subsequent blood flow and to cause thrombosis.

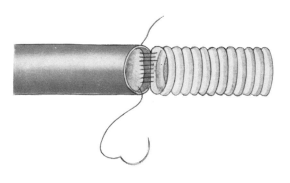

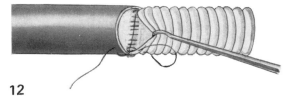

12

12

Including plaques in end-to-end suture

The anastomosis can sometimes be made to include these plaques in the suture line. The needle should be passed through the plaque from within outwards to avoid loosening the plaques.

13

Including plaques in lateral suture

Often it is necessary to suture a synthetic graft to the side of a diseased artery, e.g. the femoral. It is here particularly important to secure the plaque at its distal end where it may easily become loose. Interrupted silk sutures hold it well.

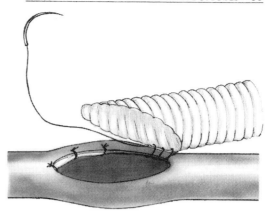

13

14

Completing lateral anastomosis to include plaques

Beginning at the proximal corner of the anastomosis a continuous suture of polypropylene is inserted from within the lumen. This effectively completes the approximation of the plaque to the arterial wall and the graft.

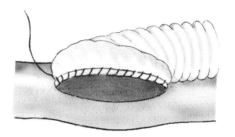

14

INVAGINATION OF GRAFT

A cloth graft or vein graft also may be sutured within the lumen of a diseased vessel using a continuous everting mattress suture. The blood flow then tends to dilate the diseased vessel, reducing the tendency to strip plaques by longitudinal pressure.

RELEASE OF CLAMPS

While the artery is clamped the peripheral vessels are constricted. Early recovery of the circulation can be promoted by instillation of a vasodilator (tolazoline 25 mg or thymoxamine 10 mg, in heparin saline) into the distal vessel before completing the anastomosis. The lower clamp is released first. This allows the air in the vessel to be expelled and the suture to take up the slack gently. It is customary to have some initial bleeding from the suture lines and the needle holes. This stops after applying steady pressure for 5–6 min over 'Surgicel' absorbable gauze. An inclination to add supplementary sutures should be resisted until an adequate period of pressure has been tried, as further stitch holes often increase rather than decrease the haemorrhage.

If haemorrhage is persistent, the possibility of the persistence of circulating heparin must be considered. The common practice is to reverse half the dose of heparin originally used with the appropriate amount of protamine sulphate (2 mg protamine sulphate neutralizes 1 mg heparin). Rarely, a second continuous suture or reinforcement of a suture line with fascia, muscle or a cloth graft may be necessary.

After prolonged arterial procedures with massive blood transfusion, an excess of fibrinolysis in the blood may cause persistent haemorrhage from the operative wounds. If this is confirmed by laboratory investigations, the effect of the increased fibrinolysis can be reversed by intravenous epsilonaminocaproic acid (0·1 g/kg body weight every 4 hr) (Nilsson, Sjoerdsma and Waldenström, 1960).

POSTOPERATIVE CARE

The measures enumerated in the Chapter on 'Exposure of Major Blood Vessels', page 26 are equally applicable under these circumstances. Both the general condition of the patient and the state of the local circulation must be carefully watched.

Local circulation

Improving colour and increasing temperature of the extremity, filling of the superficial veins and peripheral pulses are indicative of satisfactory circulation.

Haemorrhage

The use of vacuum suction to drain the site of an arterial anastomosis gives early warning of excessive blood loss. There is an increased risk of haemorrhage when a grossly atherosclerotic or calcified artery is sutured. Under such circumstances it is imperative to neutralize the heparin used at operation.

Postoperative anticoagulants

It is rarely necessary to use anticoagulants post-operatively, except after embolectomy when it is wise to prevent the re-formation of propagated thrombus. Some bleeding from the suture line in a relatively healthy vessel is preferable to re-thrombosis of the peripheral arterial tree. Heparin (500 mg/24 hr) in a low molecular weight dextran by intravenous infusion is recommended. One litre of the latter is the maximum in 24 hr. Also the subcutaneous injection of 50 mg 12-hourly over the first postoperative week, or longer in poor risk subjects.

References

Carrel, A. (1905). *Ann. Med.* **10,** 284
Jahnke, E. J. and Howard, I. M. (1953). *Archs Surg.* **66,** 646
Nilsson, I. M., Sjoerdsma, A. and Waldenström, J. (1960). *Lancet* **1,** 1322
O'Brien, B. McC. (1976). *Ann. R. Coll. Surg.* **58,** 87, 171

[*The illustrations for this Chapter on Arterial Suture and Anastomosis were drawn by Mr. G. Lyth and Mr. F. Price.*]

Arterial Embolectomy

James A. DeWeese, M.D., F.A.C.S.
Chairman of the Division of Cardiothoracic Surgery,
University of Rochester Medical Centre, and
Professor and Surgeon, Strong Memorial Hospital,
Rochester, New York

and

Charles Rob, *M.C.,* M.D., M. Chir., F.R.C.S.
Professor and Chairman of the Department of Surgery,
University of Rochester School of Medicine and
Dentistry, Rochester, New York

PRE-OPERATIVE

Indications

With rare exception surgical intervention is indicated whenever the diagnosis of arterial embolism to the upper or lower extremity is suspected. At the present time the risk of the operation itself is practically nil and there is an excellent chance of improving distal circulation in all but the most advanced cases. This more aggressive approach to the problem of arterial embolism is warranted for the following reasons.

(*1*) The increased familiarity of surgeons with the mobilization of major arteries and with the making of and proper closure of an arteriotomy. (*2*) The Fogarty balloon catheter which allows removal of almost all emboli and thrombi from the arteries of the aorta and lower extremity through an arteriotomy in the femoral artery in the groin made under local anaesthesia. The procedure is also indicated in many patients with embolic obstruction of visceral arteries such as the carotid, renal or mesenteric vessels.

Classically, arterial emboli occur in patients with rheumatic heart disease and atrial fibrillation, or in patients with arteriosclerotic heart disease and atrial fibrillation, or in the patient with a recent myocardial infarction. Patients may embolize for other reasons, and any patient with sudden onset of severe limb-threatening ischaemia should not be denied a groin exploration under local anaesthetic because of age, senility or chronic illness. A patient with a viable limb is always happier and easier to manage even if he is bedridden.

The symptoms of arterial embolus in order of increasing severity include sudden onset of claudication, numbness, coldness, rest pain and inability to move the extremity. Similarly, the signs include loss of pulse, coldness, pallor, anaesthesia, paralysis, hard and tender muscles and mottled cyanosis.

The time from onset of symptoms should not determine whether or not an operation should be performed. A patient with an embolus without significant propagation of thrombosis and with good collateral circulation may be seen several days after onset of symptoms and still have a localized problem that can be treated successfully with extraction of the embolus.

Pre-operative preparation

A rapid cardiac evaluation should be obtained and appropriate treatment should be started before surgery. The operation should not be delayed, however, for lengthy evaluations and treatment that can be performed following the operation.

A pre-operative trial of conservative care is rarely, if ever, indicated today. But heparin may be commenced as soon as the diagnosis has been made.

The groins are prepared and draped. Local anaesthesia is used. Almost all emboli of the lower extremity including those at the aortic bifurcation can now be removed through an arteriotomy in the common femoral artery with the use of the Fogarty catheter.

THE OPERATION

EXPOSURE OF COMMON FEMORAL ARTERY

1

The incision

The incision begins one finger's breadth lateral to the pubic tubercle and passes laterally in the inguinal crease. In an obese patient the incision should actually be made above the inguinal crease.

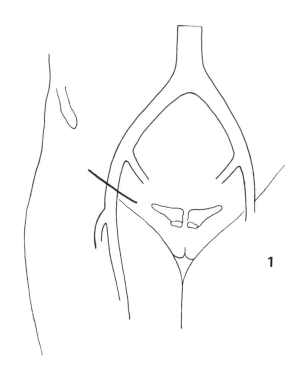

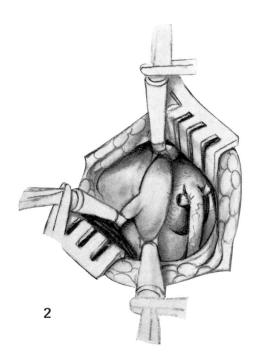

2

Exposure of vessels

The incision is carried down to the lower edge of the inguinal ligament. Medially, the saphenous vein is seen but only its superior and lateral branches need be divided and ligated. The common femoral artery is mobilized from just distal to the inguinal ligament to its bifurcation into the deep and superficial femoral artery. Tapes are passed around the common, deep and superficial femoral arteries. Small pieces of rubber are placed over the tape so that the vessel can be occluded over a catheter.

COMMON FEMORAL EMBOLUS

The iliac and femoral pulse above the embolus may be bounding, but distal pulses are absent and the temperature and colour changes occur at knee level.

Embolectomy

A short arteriotomy is made and stay sutures placed in the edges to avoid repeated handling of the vessel with forceps. The arteriotomy incision may be longitudinal (*illustrated*) or transverse. The embolus may be quite easily removed with forceps and flushing. Completeness of the embolectomy cannot be judged by antegrade or retrograde blood flow alone. Non-obstructing thrombi may still be present at the iliac or popliteal level. Fogarty catheters should be passed upward and downward as will be described.

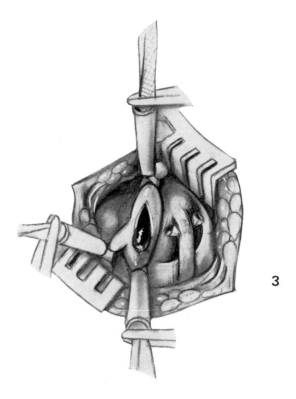

3

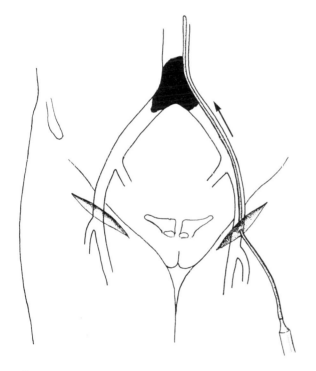

4

AORTIC EMBOLECTOMY

Patients present with no pulses palpable below the aorta. Colour and temperature changes occur in the mid-thigh.

Bilateral incisions

It is important to expose the common femoral artery in both groins. Both common femoral arteries are occluded and a Fogarty catheter with the balloon collapsed is passed up one iliac artery.

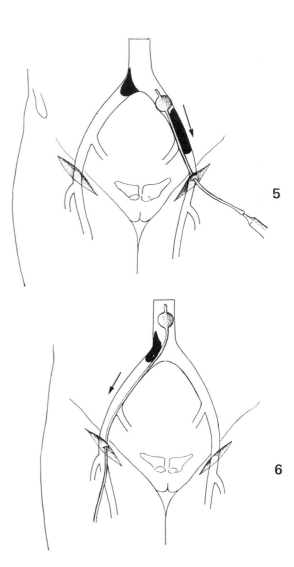

5

6

5 & 6

Embolectomy

The balloon is distended and the catheter removed. Usually the saddle embolus will break into smaller pieces during this manoeuvre and becomes extruded through the arteriotomy incision.

The catheter is now passed up the opposite iliac artery and further embolus removed. The catheters should be repeatedly passed until no further clot is found. Excessive blood loss is prevented by occluding the vessel around the catheter with the tape when the catheter is being passed.

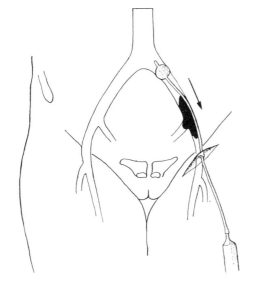

7

ILIAC EMBOLECTOMY

No femoral pulse is present and temperature changes occur at mid-thigh level.

7

The incision

Exposure of the opposite groin is advisable since it is possible to push portions of the embolus into the aorta from whence it could embolize to the opposite leg. The Fogarty catheter is inserted to the common iliac artery, the balloon distended and the catheter removed.

POPLITEAL EMBOLUS

The popliteal pulse may be bounding above the embolus. The temperature changes occur at mid-calf level.

8

Embolectomy

The Fogarty catheter is passed well down the posterior tibial artery, the balloon distended, and the catheter removed. The balloon must not be disturbed too much in smaller vessels since plaques may be cracked or the vessel ruptured. The person blowing up the balloon should be the one to remove the catheter, since he can best judge whether the balloon is under-distended or over-distended.

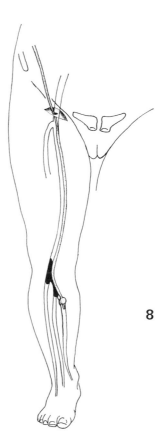

8

POSTOPERATIVE CARE

Anticoagulation with coumarin drugs is begun the day of surgery and if the patient's cardiac state permits 500 ml of dextran may be given twice a day for the first 2 days. A continued search for the source of the embolus is made. Angiographic studies of the left atrium should be performed in patients with rheumatic heart disease and atrial fibrillation, since thrombi can and should be removed. Similarly, a careful search for a ventricular aneurysm should be made in patients who have had myocardial infarctions, since the aneurysms are resectable.

References

Darling, R.C., Austen, W.G. and Linton, R.R. (1967). 'Arterial embolism.' *Surgery Gynec. Obstet.* **124**, 106
Fogarty, T.J. and Cranley, J.J. (1965). 'Catheter technique for arterial embolectomy.' *Ann. Surg.* **161**, 325
Green, R.M., DeWeese, J.A. and Rob, C.G. (1975). 'Arterial embolectomy: before and after the Fogarty catheter.' *Surgery* **77**, 24

[*The illustrations for this Chapter on Arterial Embolectomy were drawn by Miss D. Elliott.*]

Arteriography

Elliot O. Lipchik, M.D.
Professor of Radiology, Head, Cardiovascular Section,
Department of Radiology, University of Rochester
Medical Centre, Rochester, New York

INTRODUCTION

The roentgen demonstration of the cardiovascular system probably has been the most notable advance in radiology in the last 20 years. Improvements in contrast material, new techniques of vessel catheterization, and ever-increasing equipment sophistication have led to the widespread and routine use of arteriography. It has become easy, safe, efficient and accurate. Arteriography is a special radiographic procedure, requiring training, experience and skill. It is not to be dealt with casually. Arteriography is not only a useful diagnostic tool, but has also become important in the *treatment* of certain disorders such as massive bleeding from the gastro-intestinal tract. The mechanics of the examination can easily be learned, but in order to obtain the proper information on film with little risk to the patient, a thorough knowledge of the technique and the tools required is mandatory.

ESSENTIAL EQUIPMENT

X-ray unit and film changers

There are many x-ray units, tables, films, screens and film changers of varying design and cost. Rapid serial film changers capable of at least two films per second are essential for areas of high velocity blood flow—for example in the thoracic and abdominal aorta and their branches. A manually-operated serial changer capable of three films, spanning any desired length of time, may be sufficient for peripheral limb arteriography or venography where the contrast or blood flow has a decidedly slower course. However, apparatus of this sort is not considered optimal. Single plane units are sufficient for most arteriographic procedures. Since 70–85 kV give the best diagnostic quality films, high milli-amperage generators of a 1000 or more are recommended for arteriographic work.

Image intensification for adequate fluoroscopic control at lower dose rates is essential. Television monitors are desirable, but not essential. The dynamics of blood flow may best be evaluated by cineroentgenography, rather than static films, but at the risk of sacrificing anatomic detail and shrinking the field size recorded. The shortest possible exposure times, proper coning, and the smallest practicable focal spot, all help to improve detail. Magnification radiography is a refinement, luxurious, but not essential in a routine practice. A relatively long series of films may be necessary to encompass the complete circulation of contrast material from the arteries to the veins—for example in visceral arteriography the veins may maximally opacify from 8 to 20 sec after the start of the injection.

Pressure injectors

A pressure injector is necessary for catheter aorto-graphy and in most areas of non-selective arterio-graphy, where a large bolus of contrast material has to be injected in a relatively short period of time. Most units have systems to control the volume and rate of injection of contrast; some simply have adjustable pressure systems. The majority of injectors also automatically 'trigger' the x-ray exposure at a predetermined time. The newer ones are reliable, easily manoeuvred, and warm the contrast material to body temperature before injection. The units of pressure indicated for the different makes do not correspond, i.e. the same 'dial' pressure produces different effective pressure and flow rates with different injectors. Each apparatus should therefore be tested prior to clinical use to determine the pressures and times needed to inject a given amount of contrast material through selected catheters. In any event, the radiologist is the specialist who should be fully conversant with the problems of apparatus and its use. He must know the capabilities and characteristics of the entire injection system which includes the injector, connecting tubes, connectors, catheters and contrast material.

Contrast material

The newer and safer contrast materials are all water-soluble organic molecules with bound iodine. There are literally hundreds of brand names, different in every country. All the contrast materials are hyper-tonic, viscid solutions, some with high sodium as well as iodine content, all are expensive. In proper dosage they are quite safe, but they are toxic in overdosage, and when stasis allows longer periods of tissue contact. The toxic effects of contrast material vary, depending on the region or organ examined. No one contrast agent necessarily qualifies as best for all regional circulations. For example, pure methylglucamine salts of low or *no* sodium content are least toxic in the cerebral circulation, whereas methylglucamine–sodium diatrizoate mixtures—are recommended for the heart, aorta and its branches.

The trade names and numbers of various agents are confusing. For example, the iodine content of Renografin 60 (meglumine diatrizoate) and Hypaque 50 (sodium diatrizoate) are almost identical. It is the iodine content which determines the radiodensity of the material. The exact concentration of the iodine is listed on the label, not in the trademark.

In all aspects of arteriography, the examination has to be tailored and modified to suit the individual and the specific problem. Thus, the amount and the site of injection of contrast cannot be rigidly applied to every patient. Non-selective aortography may require from 30 to 50 ml of the more concentrated materials at a rate of at least 20 ml/sec. Selective arterial injections, directly into a carotid artery for example, usually need about 10 ml. From 8 to 15 ml are recommended for selective renal arteriograms, whereas 25–60 ml are used for selective superior mesenteric or coeliac artery injection at a rate of 8–12 ml/sec. Less concentrated opaque material is recommended for the selective studies. The *flow rate* of the contrast material into the vessel is the determining factor in the quality of the opacification of that vessel. Repeat injections may safely be made after 10–15 min intervals. In the demonstration of peripheral arteriosclerosis, relatively slow rates and larger volumes is the usual successful combination. With a slower injection rate of 8–10 ml/sec, the distal aorta and iliac vessels are usually fully opacified by the first exposure just before the end of the injection (4–6 sec). The popliteal and trifurcation vessels in the calf are usually opacified from within 7–12 sec after the *beginning* of the injection. Vessels in the ankle and foot begin to fill after 12–18 sec.

Catheter, needles and cannulae

New catheter materials are continually appearing on the market. Selective catheterization of vessels often requires specially designed, preformed catheters. The Ödman catheters are excellent for beginners and experts in the field. They are visible under the fluoro-scope, easily fashioned into proper length and curve, and relatively inexpensive. These radiopaque poly-ethylene catheters are still among the safest and least thrombogenic.

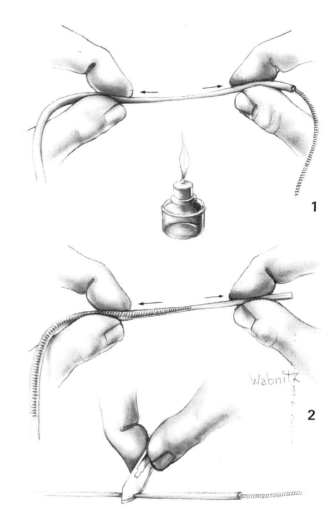

1

2

1 & 2

In order to mould a tapered tip on to an Ödman catheter, it has to be heated in almost boiling water, or over a flame with a guide wire inside. When the catheter softens it can be gently drawn over the guide wire into an even taper, cooled in sterile water or saline, and cut at its narrow point with a scalpel blade.

A blunt-ended, non-tapered catheter is difficult to force into a vessel, and can cause a haematoma or haemorrhage. Catheters with multiple side-holes are recommended for non-selective aortograms. Selective catheterization of branch vessels whether into the head, heart or viscera, should be attempted only by experienced workers in the field. All catheters should be frequently or continuously flushed with normal saline.

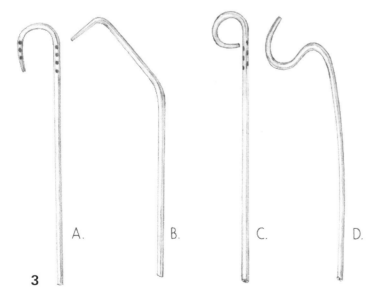

A.   B.   C.   D.

3

3

This illustration shows four catheters each shaped for a specific purpose: (A) aortography catheter; (B) selective visceral; (C) left ventricular; and (D) selective cerebral.

Many different needle-cannula assemblies are also available. In general, smaller needle and catheters are safer, 18-gauge needles and No. 7–8 F catheters being large enough for most purposes.

The *Stille–Seldinger* needle consists of an innermost obturator which is within a sharp pointed needle, and an external cannula with a blunt, tapered end. There are many modifications that accomplish the same purpose. The most useful sizes are 16–18-gauge or a No. 160 Stille. The guide wires also come in various diameters and lengths which have to correspond with the internal diameter and length of the catheter used. A very useful guide wire is one with a 'floppy' curve at the end which facilitates the negotiation of tortuous, arteriosclerotic vessels.

PERCUTANEOUS CATHETERIZATION

The percutaneous catheter placement of Seldinger allows easy entrance into almost any vessel system in the body. The transfemoral route is the method of choice for most patients except those with advanced aorto-iliac atherosclerosis and obstruction. Via this route one may easily study the entire aorta and its branches, including the head as well as the lower limbs, depending on the position of the tip of the catheter. It is recommended to study the intracranial circulation by manoeuvring a properly shaped catheter into the desired brachiocephalic vessel. If bilateral femoral arteriography is requested, the catheter tip should be placed above the aortic bifurcation.

The patient may feel pain only at the time of needle insertion for induction of local anaesthesia. Pain at any other time during the catheter manipulation is abnormal, and most often due to intramural placement of catheter or wire (or improper anaesthesia). The rapid injection of contrast may cause the patient to feel intense heat, bordering on pain, in the region of perfusion.

Under fluoroscopic control the catheter may be inserted to any level of the aorta or selectively into almost any vessel depending on the shape of the catheter tip. A test injection of several millilitres of contrast material to determine catheter position prior to injection of the main bolus is mandatory.

TECHNIQUE

The patient should not eat solids but should be allowed, and in certain instances encouraged, to drink fluids starting approximately 6–8 hr prior to the examination. For *all* selective abdominal angiography, including renal angiography, a bowel preparation with laxatives starting 24–36 hr before is highly recommended. Light sedation with tranquillizing agents is acceptable. The author does not generally use barbiturates or antihistamines; pethidine (Demerol) is contra-indicated in all angiographic procedures as it may act as a vasoplegic with resultant hypotension. Atropine is occasionally indicated. We are now anticoagulating selected patients, just prior to insertion of the catheter, with 75–100 units/kg heparin intravenously. Routine shave and sterile skin preparation are done with the patient on the x-ray table.

4

Identification of femoral artery

The femoral artery pulsation is identified in either groin, below the inguinal ligament in the inguinal crease. A needle puncture above this ligament makes haemostasis difficult during and after the examination. The surgeon also has easier access to a damaged or thrombosed artery below the inguinal ligament. The skin and subcutaneous tissues are infiltrated with locally-acting anaesthetics, down to the arterial wall. The pulsations of the artery are transmitted by the needle and can easily be felt by the operator. Proper anaesthesia ensures a painless procedure. A tiny slit puncture is made through the skin by a No. 11 scalpel blade, followed by insertion of a small haemostat to spread the subcutaneous tissues. This allows free passage of catheter and guide wire through the skin layers into the artery.

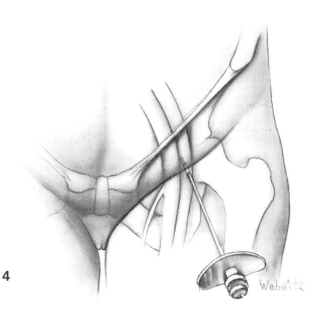

4

5

Insertion of needle-cannula

The needle-cannula is then inserted until the pulsations of the vessel are felt at its tip. The needle is inserted quickly at an approximate angle of 45–60°, with fixation of the tissues and vessel by the left index and middle fingers. At first, it may be wise to transfix both walls of the vessel. With practice, puncture of only the anterior wall may be accomplished, but the added danger of subintimal placement of wire and catheter may offset the gain in haemostasis.

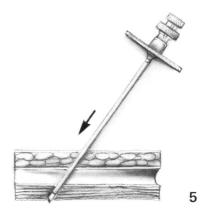

5

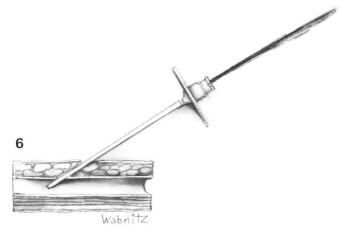

6

Wabnitz

6

Withdrawal of cannula

After withdrawal of the inner needle and obturator, the cannula is gently and slowly withdrawn until blood spurts forcefully from the open end. The cannula should then be lowered to almost 20° to the horizontal and slightly advanced to assure intraluminal position.

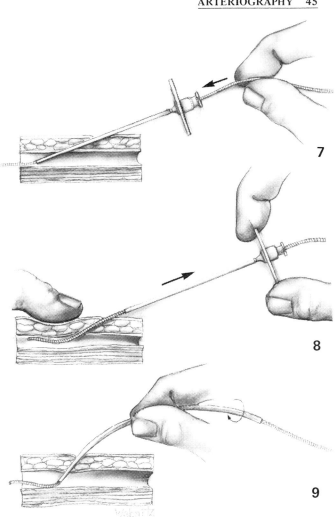

7

8

9

7, 8 & 9

Removal of cannula

The guide wire is then inserted through the cannula at least 10 cm past the tip into the artery. It should pass through the needle into the vessel without any resistance. With the guide wire remaining in the vessel, the cannula is removed. Compression is applied over the puncture site since the guide wire has a narrower diameter than the cannula. The catheter is threaded over the spring guide wire and advanced to the skin. Obviously, the guide has to be longer than the catheter so that it protrudes outside and can be grasped for removal. Wire guides have various shapes and flexible tip configurations.

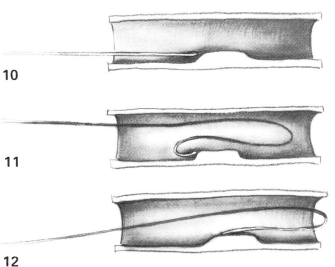

10

11

12

10, 11 & 12

Illustrations 10–12 show the use of a very flexible guide wire as it overcomes an atherosclerotic plaque.

Insertion of guide and catheter

Both guide and catheter are inserted into the vessel by firm pressure and rotation. The catheter is positioned at its proper level under fluoroscopic control. The digital pressure is released, the guide withdrawn, and the catheter flushed with normal saline. A drip infusion provides reliable, continuous flushing of an end-hole catheter, but catheters with multiple side-holes require frequent, continual, forceful manual flushes. When the arteriogram is completed, the catheter is withdrawn from the vessel. Firm, but not occlusive, manual pressure must be maintained on, and slightly proximal to the puncture site for at least 10 min. The patient is advised to remain on bedrest for at least 6 hr, most often till the next morning.

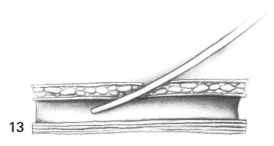

13

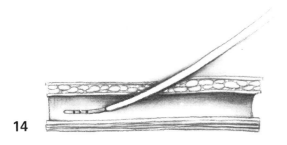

14

13 & 14

A closed tip side-hole catheter, even a balloon-tipped catheter may be inserted into a vessel by the same technique. A wide bore sheath is slipped into the vessel over a guide wire and tapered catheter. The catheter and wire are removed, and the special catheter inserted through the short sheath. The balloon-tipped catheters may be used for pressure monitoring, removal of clots, or purposeful occlusion of smaller branch vessels.

15

Catheterization of axillary artery

Either axillary artery is also easily catheterized. This route provides easy access, with some extra manipulation required in the elderly, to the aorta and vessels below the diaphragm. The patient should be supine with the appropriate arm abducted and the hand resting under the patient's head. The artery may be palpated in the axilla, preferably just distal to the fold of the pectoralis muscle, but frequently the artery is more easily fixated and catheterized several centimetres distal to the axilla. The arterial puncture is the same as described above for the femoral artery except that the needle has to be inserted almost at right angles to the axillary artery. Extra care has to be taken to prevent brachial plexus injury. When using the left axillary artery approach, the catheter usually enters the descending aorta in patients under 40 years of age.

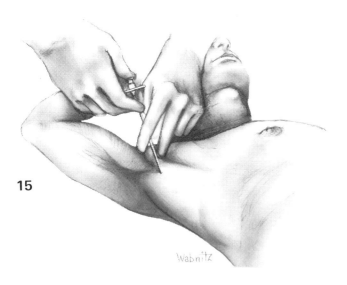

15

Wabnitz

Other vessel punctures

Other vessels which can be percutaneously punctured for catheterization are the subclavian arteries, either by infra- or supraclavicular approaches; the carotid arteries; and the brachial arteries. Surgical arteriotomy is preferred for brachial artery catheterization since this vessel is highly prone to spasm and resultant thrombosis.

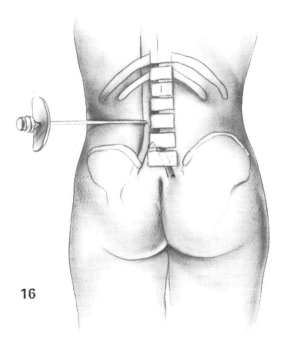

16

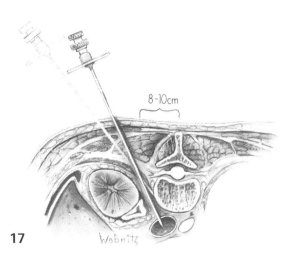

8-10cm

17

TRANSLUMBAR AORTOGRAPHY

TECHNIQUE

If there is severe occlusive disease of the aorto-iliac system and arteriograms of this system are needed, translumbar puncture of the aorta may be necessary. If fluoroscopy is available, and if there is good circulation to the upper extremities, the percutaneous axillary approach is recommended.

16 & 17

Insertion of needle

An 18-gauge, 8-inch (20-cm) long, aortographic needle or a Teflon sleeve needle catheter may be used. After sterile preparation and local anaesthesia, the needle is inserted between the twelfth rib and the iliac crest, 8–10 cm (4–5 fingers' breadth) to the left of the mid-line, with the patient prone. The tip of the needle is directed medially and cranially towards the anterior portion of the twelfth vertebral body if a 'higher' aortogram is needed. The author prefers to begin with a 'low' aortogram (*below* the renal arteries) by directing the needle medially only, towards L3. Fluoroscopic control of the site and direction of the needle can lead to a shortening of the procedure time and to a more accurate placement.

Withdrawal of needle

After striking the vertebral body, the needle is then withdrawn somewhat and redirected a little more vertically. After puncturing the aorta, a test film is exposed with an injection of 5–10 ml of contrast material to judge the position of the needle tip. It is hazardous to do multiple punctures of the aorta at the same site.

This method makes it more difficult to inject the contrast selectively at a particular level. There is no control or possibility, short of major surgery, to apply haemostasis. Manipulation of the needle is impossible, and selective injection of contrast into other vessels is also not feasible. Movement of the patient to either oblique may be hazardous. Very flexible guide wires can be inserted into the aorta for catheter placement via this translumbar route, but this technique is advised for those experienced in the technique of translumbar aortography as well as catheter manipulation.

It should be emphasized that translumbar aortography when properly performed is about as safe as other aortographic procedures, but at times is more discomforting to the patient.

CAROTID ARTERIOGRAPHY

18

Carotid arteriography ought to be accomplished by percutaneous transfemoral catheterization, as described. However, in many centres direct puncture of the carotid artery is still performed. To avoid most of the complications of direct carotid angiography, the author recommends a short bevel 19- or 20-gauge needle, at least 3 inches (7·5 cm) in length, snugly fit inside a flexible Teflon or polyethylene sleeve or cannula of gauge 18 (*see Illustration 18, inset*). When the arterial puncture is made, the sharp needle may be withdrawn, leaving the blunt but flexible cannula in the lumen of the vessel. This flexible atraumatic cannula may easily be inserted further into the vessel, without causing intimal damage. There is also less danger of vessel wall damage if the patient has to be moved, or moves inadvertently.

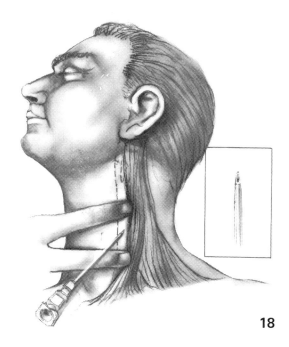

18

TECHNIQUE

The head should be mildly extended (a soft support under the shoulders helps). Sterile preparation and local anaesthesia are carried out. The common carotid artery is fixed with the second and third fingers of the left hand. The sternocleidomastoid muscle is displaced posterolaterally by these fingers. The bifurcation of the common carotid artery is usually above the level of the superior margin of the thyroid cartilage, just below the angle of the jaw. A nearly right angle approach of the needle, using exactly the technique of arterial puncture described above, should be employed. Both walls of the vessel may be transfixed. Slow, gentle withdrawal of the inner needle is advised so that as the posterior wall 'pops' away, the cannula tip remains within the vessel lumen. The cannula hub should then be lowered to a more horizontal position and eased inwards. Control of the intraluminal position is maintained and secured by the pulsatile jet of blood. Ten millilitres of lower concentration, low sodium pure methylglucamine contrast material gives adequate detail of the intracranial vessel system. Several repeat injections of contrast may safely be given. The normal intracranial circulation may be successfully mapped if rapid, serial films are exposed to span at least a 6-sec period. The author recommends x-ray texts for a proper discussion of head positioning and programming for intracranial arteriography.

COMPLICATIONS

PERCUTANEOUS CATHETERIZATION

A relatively simple examination can lead to a catastrophe if measures are not instituted to prevent and treat emergencies. Total complication rates should be below 2 per cent.

(*1*) Fatal allergic reactions to contrast material are unusually rare. Subcutaneous, conjunctival and even small intravenous tests of contrast material have proved unreliable in eliciting allergic reactions. The best safeguard against any serious reaction is its immediate recognition and treatment. A history of serious reaction to previous injections of contrast is a contra-indication to further studies. Antihistamines may be useful for minor allergic phenomena, for example, itching and urticaria. Adrenaline (1 : 1000) and steroids may be necessary to treat life-threatening allergic complications such as laryngeal oedema.

(*2*) Contrary to popular belief, contrast materials do not cause vasospasm; in fact, they are potent vasodilators. Most of the haemodynamic effects of contrast media injection such as increased stroke volume, heart rate and cardiac output as well as expansion of the circulatory blood volume, fall of the haematocrit, and hypotension, are due to the hypertonicity of the injectate and the introduction of large volumes of fluid. Adequate hydration of the patient and electrolyte balance should be assured before attempting arteriography. Cardiovascular collapse and shock are rarely seen with routine arteriographic procedures, but oxygen, airways and emergency drugs to maintain blood pressure and cardiac output have to be within easy reach.

(*3*) The majority of complications of percutaneous catheterization are local, that is at the site of arterial puncture. Serious complications should be less than 0·5 per cent.

(*a*) *Haemorrhage* usually occurs during two phases of the procedure. First, just after puncture of the artery with the guide wire *in situ*, as the catheter is being slipped on; second, when the catheter is removed at the end of the examination. Digital pressure at both times prevents this complication. Hypertensive patients bleed more readily.

(*b*) *Thrombosis* of the punctured artery can be recognized as soon as it occurs. The typical signs are a cool, blanched, painful lower limb, with no peripheral pulse. This complication is usually due to excessive manipulation of the catheter, prolonged duration of the catheter in the vessel, low cardiac output, hypotension, or a catheter which was too large for the blood vessel. Acute anticoagulation with heparin during the examination is recommended particularly in patients who have small vessels or low cardiac output.

(*c*) *Spasm* of the artery is more often seen in younger individuals, and may lead to stasis and thrombus formation. Spasm may be caused by multiple traumatic punctures and excessive, prolonged catheterization time. The brachial artery is much more prone to spasm than the femoral or the axillary artery and ought *not* to be percutaneously catheterized.

(*d*) *Other complications.* False aneurysms, intravascular breakage of the guide wire tip, haematomas, arteriovenous fistulas and intramural injections have all been reported and may usually be avoided by meticulous, correct technique.

References

Allen, J. H., Parera, C. and Potts, D. G. (1965). 'The relation of arterial trauma and complications of cerebral angiography.' *Am. J. Roentg.* **95**, 845
Baum, S., Nusbaum, M., Blakemore, W. S. and Finkelstein, A. K. (1965). 'The preoperative radiographic demonstration of intra-abdominal bleeding.' *Surgery* **58**, 797
Baum, S. and Nusbaum, M. (1971). 'Control of g.i. bleeding by pharmacologic means.' *Radiology* **98**, 497
Curry, J. T. and Howland, W. T. (1966). *Arteriography: Principles and Techniques.* London: Saunders
Fischer, H. W. (1972). 'Some factors in selection of intravascular and urographic contrast agents.' *Current Concepts in Radiology,* Ed. by E. J. Potchen, p. 210. St. Louis: C. V. Mosby
Lang, E. K. (1963). 'A survey of the complication of percutaneous retrograde arteriography.' *Radiology* **81**, 257
McAfee, J. G. and Willson, J. K. V. (1956). 'A review of the complications of translumbar aortography.' *Am. J. Roentg.* **75**, 956
Newton, T. H. (1963). 'The axillary artery approach to arteriography of the aorta and its branches.' *Am. J. Roentg.* **89**, 275
Ödman, P. (1959). 'The radiopaque polythene catheter.' *Acta Radiol.* **52**, 52
Rogoff, S. M. and Lipchik, E. O. (1971). 'Lumbar aortography: background, technique, and indications.' In *Angiography,* Ed. by H. L. Abrams, Vol. 2, 2nd Edn., p. 707. Boston: Little, Brown & Co.
Seldinger, S. I. (1953). 'Catheter replacement of the needle in percutaneous arteriography: a new technique.' *Acta Radiol.* **39**, 368
Strain, W. H. and Rogoff, S. M. (1971). 'The radiopaque media: nomenclature and chemical formulas.' In *Angiography,* Ed. by H. L. Abrams, Vol. 1, 2nd Edn, p. 35. Boston: Little, Brown & Co.

[The illustrations for this Chapter on Arteriography were drawn by Mr. R. Wabnitz.]

Operative Angiography

Allyn G. May, M.D.
Associate Professor of Surgery,
University of Rochester and
Strong Memorial Hospital,
Rochester, New York

Operative angiography is a useful diagnostic tool for two reasons: (*1*) it may afford arteriographic information when a non-operative, percutaneous approach is impossible; and (*2*) it allows the surgeon to detect potentially troublesome technical lesions at the time of reconstruction when they can best be corrected. The study is too often omitted. The ease of its performance in the operating room compared to its difficulty after wound closure should encourage operative angiography as a routine procedure after each vascular reconstruction. In order to obtain the best films with the least trouble, preparation for the study should be started before surgery. If available, an operating table with a radiolucent surface and spaces for film encachement can be used to advantage. However, operative angiography can be done without such an operating table.

When the percutaneous approach is not possible

Sometimes, especially in acute arterial occlusions, a percutaneous femoral arteriogram will not be possible because of the absence of a palpable femoral pulse or because of lack of development of adequate collateral circulation to permit demonstration of reconstitution of the arterial system. In these circumstances the femoral or popliteal artery can be explored and, if a patent segment is found, arteriography can be done.

1

An x-ray film casette is placed in a sterile drape, e.g. a Mayo stand cover, and placed beneath the extremity so as to encompass the pertinent part of the arterial tree. A sterile 20-ml syringe is filled with contrast medium (Hypaque) and connected to a sterile venotube armed with a No. 20 hypodermic needle. The venotube is clamped and the needle inserted into the arterial lumen. The contrast is injected rapidly into the artery and the x-ray exposure is made just as the last 5 ml of contrast is being injected. The venotube can then be clamped and the needle left *in situ* until the film has been developed and studied.

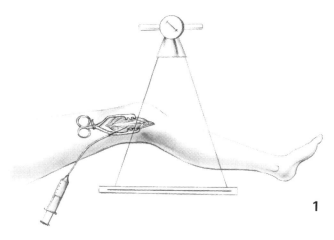

1

ANGIOGRAPHY AFTER RECONSTRUCTIVE ARTERIAL SURGERY

Before the skin incisions are closed, arteriography can be done to ascertain patency of all distal arteries, to detect unrecognized twists in grafts, stenoses, intimal flaps, thrombi, when these lesions are most easily and successfully corrected.

2

In the case of arterial reconstruction, such as by means of a vein graft, a No. 20 hypodermic needle assembly is introduced through the wall of the proximal parent vessel after the film has been properly positioned. Just before the contrast injection is made, the vessel proximal to the needle is clamped and 20 ml of Hypaque is injected rapidly. As the final 5 ml of dye is being injected, the film is exposed. As soon as the exposure has been completed, the proximal clamp is removed so as not to interrupt blood flow too long and the needle left in position until the films are seen.

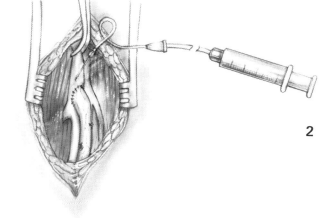

2

ANGIOGRAPHY AFTER RECONSTRUCTIVE VENOUS SURGERY

In patients with iliofemoral venous thrombosis, thrombectomy is accomplished most successfully in cases operated early. The most effective approach is by means of a venotomy in the common femoral vein. Thrombus inferior to the venotomy can frequently be expressed by wrapping the extremity very tightly with an Esmarch bandage from toes to the groin inci-

sion. Thrombus from the iliac system can best be removed by means of the Fogarty venous thrombectomy catheter introduced proximally through the femoral venotomy. However, if a venous valve is present in the clotted iliac vein, thrombectomy may be incomplete and may be followed by rethrombosis. It is helpful, therefore, to perform operative venography to determine whether additional passages of the catheter or direct exposure of the iliac vein is necessary to remove the thrombus completely.

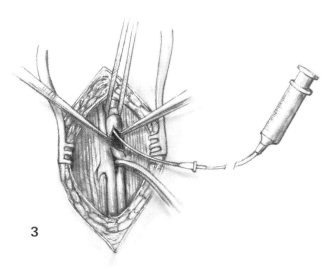

3

3

Technique

It is wise to heparinize the patient because it is helpful to occlude the vein temporarily distal to the site of injection of contrast. The venogram can be obtained by injection of 30–60 ml of 25–50 per cent Hypaque through a No. 16 plastic needle directed proximally through the open venotomy. The vein can be fitted closely about the plastic needle by means of an encircling tape. After the films have been read, the needle is withdrawn, the venotomy closed with standard suture technique, the occluding clamps are removed, and the heparin reversed with protamine.

References

Engelman, R. M., Clements, J. M. and Herrmann, J. B. (1969). 'Routine operative arteriography following vascular reconstruction.'
    Surgery Gynec. Obstet. **128**, 745
Mavor, G. E., Walker, M. G. and Dhall, D. P. (1972). 'Routine operative arteriography in arterial embolectomy.' *Br. J. Surg.* **59**,
    482

[*The illustrations for this Chapter on Operative Angiography were drawn by Mr. R. Wabnitz.*]

Occlusions of the Carotid and Vertebral Arteries

Charles Rob, *M.C.* M.D., M.Chir., F.R.C.S.
Professor and Chairman of the Department of Surgery,
University of Rochester School of Medicine and
Dentistry, Rochester, New York

and

James A. DeWeese, M. D., F.A.C.S.
Chairman of the Division of Cardiothoracic Surgery,
University of Rochester Medical Centre, and
Professor and Surgeon, Strong Memorial Hospital,
Rochester, New York

PRE-OPERATIVE

A high proportion of cerebral vascular accidents are due to occlusions of the cervical portions of the internal carotid and vertebral arteries (Rob, 1972). In nearly every patient the cause of this occlusion is atherosclerosis, and it is a remarkable fact that in many of these patients the arterial disease is much more pronounced in the extracranial than in the intracranial portions of these arteries (Hutchinson and Yates, 1956, 1957).

Occlusions of the carotid and vertebral arteries may be partial or complete, that is an arterial stenosis or a thrombosis. To date the results of arterial surgery in patients with complete occlusions have been poor because the thrombosis rapidly spreads up into the skull as far as the origin of the first branch from the internal carotid artery, and an arterial reconstruction operation fails because the surgeon is unable to obtain a satisfactory back-flow except when the occlusion is recent. On the other hand, it is technically possible to restore a normal lumen in nearly every patient with a stenosis or incomplete occlusion of the internal carotid artery and in some patients with stenosis of the vertebral artery near to its origin from the subclavian.

Type of operation

The best operation is a thrombo-endarterectomy with or without a venous patch graft, and in the case of stenosis of these arteries both the early and late results have been good (DeWeese *et al.*, 1973). We believe that this has largely been due to the localized nature of the arterial disease in many of these patients (Rob, 1959). Occasionally it is possible to excise the abnormal segment and restore continuity by a direct end-to-end anastomosis (Eastcott, Pickering and Rob, 1954); even less frequently it is necessary to insert an arterial substitute and in patients with fibromuscular hyperplasia, intraluminal dilatation may be of value (Stanley *et al.*, 1974).

Anaesthesia

Anaesthesia may be either local or general—we prefer general anaesthesia with an endotracheal tube. There is some evidence that this reduces the metabolism of the brain and this, combined with better control of oxygenation and blood pressure, particularly during the period of arterial clamping, is the probable reason why our results with general anaesthesia have been better than with local anaesthesia.

Special instruments

The instruments and material used for this operation include arterial clamps and 5/0 arterial sutures. It is also wise to have a silastic tube slightly smaller than the lumen of the internal carotid artery for use as an indwelling shunt if necessary.

THE OPERATIONS

1

The usual sites of arterial occlusion

This diagram, modified from one produced by Hutchinson and Yates (1956, 1957) shows the two main sites at which atherosclerosis causes stenosis or thrombosis of the extracranial portions of the internal carotid and vertebral arteries. In each case the plaque of atheroma lies close to the origin of these vessels from the common carotid and subclavian arteries respectively. It is a remarkable fact that the portions of the main stems of the internal carotid and vertebral arteries distal immediately to the atheromatous plaques are usually relatively normal, although there is often considerable involvement of the circle of Willis and its branches.

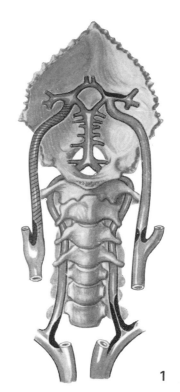

1

THROMBO-ENDARTERECTOMY OF INTERNAL CAROTID ARTERY

2

Exposure of carotid bifurcation

The incision, which follows the skin folds of the neck, is about 4 inches (10 cm) long and is placed over the carotid pulse at the level of the upper border of the body of the thyroid cartilage. The skin and platysma are divided; in the posterior part of the incision the great auricular nerve should be identified and preserved if possible. The dissection is then continued down to the carotid sheath, and the common facial vein identified as it crosses the carotid arteries to join the internal jugular vein; this vein is then divided between ligatures. The carotid sheath is now opened and the common, internal and external carotid arteries identified and mobilized throughout the operation field. In particular the internal carotid artery must be freed to as high a level as possible.

It is important to identify and preserve the XIIth cranial nerve as it crosses the carotid vessels. The carotid sinus nerve is identified and divided early in the operation. This prevents or corrects the brady-cardia and hypotension which may follow stimula-tion of this nerve. We have not seen permanent complications follow bilateral division of these nerves after staged operations, although there may be an immediate rise in blood pressure which returns to the pre-operative level in a few hours.

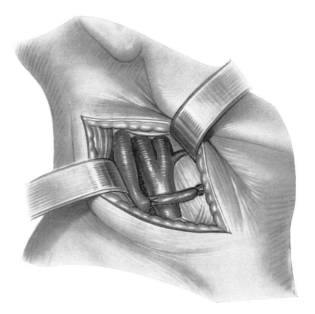

2

3

Determination of extent of arterial disease

The plaque of atheroma usually lies at the origin of the internal carotid artery and extends proximally for a short distance down the common carotid artery; it can be located either by inspection or palpation. It is important to palpate the artery gently because small emboli may be dislodged, and in our opinion such emboli are a very important cause of intra-operative cerebral deficits. The disease rarely involves more than the first 2 cm of the internal carotid artery. Beyond this point, when the occlusion is partial, the internal carotid is soft and compressible; after a complete thrombosis this portion of the artery rapidly becomes incompressible as the blood in it clots. Proximally the wall of the common carotid artery is often thickened but is rarely grossly diseased or stenosed.

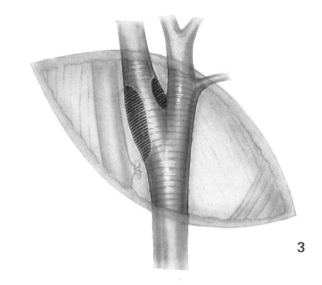

3

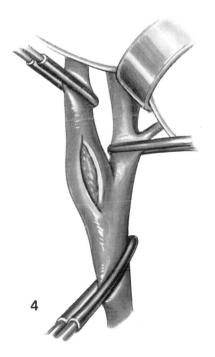

4

4

The arterial incision

The common carotid, external carotid and internal carotid arteries are now clamped; 5000 units (50 mg) of heparin are injected by the anaesthesiologist into a peripheral vein. In some patients it may be necessary to clamp the superior thyroid artery separately; bulldog clamps are satisfactory. A longitudinal incision is now made through the adventitia and outer part of the media; this incision begins on the distal 0·5 cm of the common carotid artery to the upper limit of the main atheromatous plaque. In the upper part of the operation site the hypoglossal nerve crosses the internal and external carotid arteries from the lateral to the medial side; this nerve should be identified and carefully retracted upwards and medially.

5

Indwelling arterial shunt

In many patients with stenosis of the internal carotid artery a thrombo-endarterectomy can be performed without the aid of a shunt. A shunt should always be used in operations for an acute occlusion and in other patients when the retrograde flow from the internal carotid artery is slow or cyanosed, a shunt should be inserted. A silastic tube just smaller than the lumen of the internal carotid artery is threaded up this vessel for about 6 cm, and down the common carotid artery for a similar distance. Tapes are then placed around the artery proximally and distally and these are closed tightly around the vessel with rubber tubes and the artery forceps to hold the rubber in position. A better way is illustrated with Javid clamps and a Javid type of shunt. An additional 50 mg of heparin is injected systemically making a total of 100 mg. This shunt permits a satisfactory flow to the intracranial portion of the internal carotid artery whilst the surgeon performs the thrombo-endarterectomy around the silastic tube.

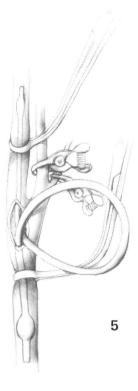

5

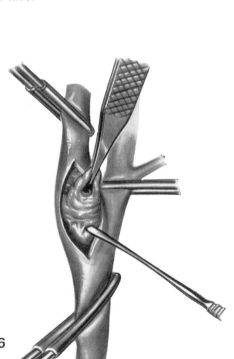

6

6

Establishing the plane of cleavage—the thrombo-endarterectomy

After incising the outer layers of the arterial wall, a blunt dissector is used to develop the well-marked plane of cleavage which lies in the media. Externally lie the adventitia, the external elastic lamina, the tunica intima and the atheromatous plaques; the surgeon removes the inner portion. The inner layers are cleanly divided circumferentially about 0·5 cm proximal to the carotid bifurcation. Distally the inner layers are divided just distal to the end of plaque of atheroma, and the surgeon then carefully cuts the intima on the internal carotid artery in such a way that no flaps remain.

7

The complete occlusion

The problem here is to establish a satisfactory back-flow. The thrombo-endarterectomy proceeds as just described. Proximally there is a satisfactory blood flow through the common and external carotid arteries; but distally, when the occlusion is complete, the clot extends rapidly up the internal carotid artery as far as its first major branch which lies within the skull. In a recent thrombosis it may be possible to obtain a satisfactory back-flow by applying gentle suction. A polyethylene tube only slightly smaller than the lumen of the internal carotid artery is attached to the suction apparatus and passed up the vessel. The blood clot is then removed, and when this clot is recent and non-adherent, it is possible to establish a satisfactory back-flow. Heparin (5000 units, 50 mg) is then injected into the lumen of this vessel and an indwelling silastic shunt inserted. Occasionally in long-standing lesions the injection of saline around the thrombosis may make possible the complete removal of the whole obstructing lesion. If a Fogarty catheter is used to remove a thrombus in this region, great care is necessary because of the risk of perforation of an intracranial artery.

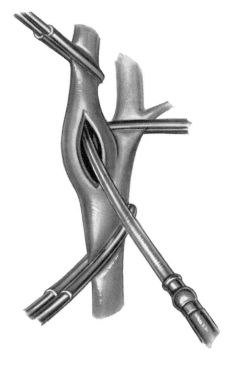

7

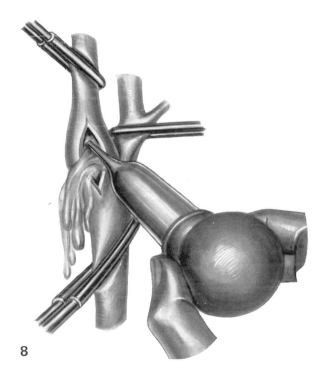

8

8

Removal of all debris

After completion of the thrombo-endarterectomy it is important to remove all debris and loose tags from the lumen of the vessel. This is achieved by washing thoroughly with saline solution from a glass syringe and picking out any loose fragments which remain. The next step is to remove temporarily the distal clamp so that the stagnant column of blood in this segment of the internal carotid artery is flushed out. This clamp is then re-applied and after a final wash with saline solution, the proximal clamp removed in a similar fashion; the vessel is ready for suture.

9

The arterial suture

We prefer to start the insertion of the arterial suture distally and to use 5/0 silk or polypropylene on a fine atraumatic needle. The first stitch is most important; it must anchor the intima to the arterial wall. This suture is, therefore, placed distal to the end of the arterial incision and it should pass through all the layers of the arterial wall. The distal intima, if cut so that there is not a loose flap, need not be anchored throughout the whole circumference of the artery. But if the surgeon thinks that distal stripping of dissection of the intima is possible, further interrupted sutures may be inserted to anchor this intima. The arterial closure is completed by an over-and-over suture. When this is completed, protamine sulphate is given intravenously and the distal clamp from the internal carotid artery is removed first and interrupted sutures placed at any large bleeding points; the proximal clamp and the clamp on the external carotid artery are then removed and firm pressure applied with a gauze swab for 5 min. This is usually sufficient to produce haemostasis; but occasionally extra sutures will be required. The total period of arterial occlusion need not exceed 15–20 min.

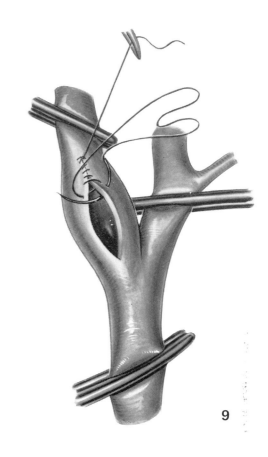

9

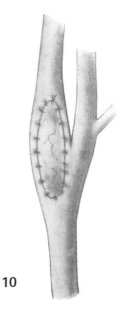

10

10

Venous patch graft

In many patients a satisfactory closure can be achieved by simple arterial suture, but if it appears that such a closure will constrict the lumen of the artery, then a patch graft should be inserted. A short length of the long saphenous from the lower leg (or another vein if this is not available) is isolated, laid open, and sutured in position. If a shunt is in use, the patch is sutured in position and the shunt removed just before the suture line has been completed. In our opinion Dacron patches are less satisfactory than are autogenous venous patches.

11

Removal of arterial shunt

Just before completion of the arterial closure the shunt is removed. The shunt is grasped with a clamp. The distal tape or Javid clamp is loosened and this portion of the shunt is removed, a bulldog clamp being applied to the distal carotid artery to control the retrograde flow. The proximal tape or clamp is then loosened, the shunt removed, and the proximal artery clamped. The whole area is then flushed with saline and the arterial closure completed, after which the heparin is neutralized and the clamps removed in the manner described (*see Illustration 9*).

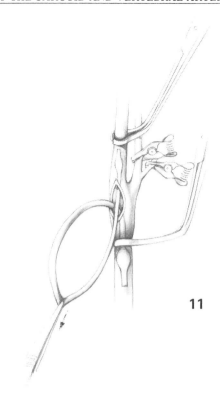

11

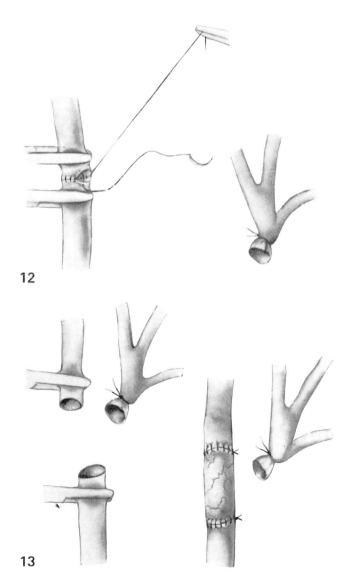

12

13

OTHER PROCEDURES

12

End-to-end anastomosis

In the case of well localized lesions and patients with tortous arteries or small aneurysms, resection and end-to-end anastomosis is a satisfactory procedure. It is usually necessary to divide and ligature the external carotid artery, after which the common and internal carotid arteries are united by an end-to-end anastomosis. The disparity in size between the arteries is not sufficient to cause a problem.

13

Graft replacement

If an end-to-end anastomosis is not possible because of insufficient length, a vein graft should be inserted. The long saphenous vein is preferred and after it has been removed and reversed, end-to-end anastomoses are performed. In both these procedures an indwelling shunt can be used if necessary. It is removed just before completion of the second anastomosis.

Reconstruction of the external carotid artery

When the internal carotid artery is thrombosed, the external carotid artery via the ophthalmic artery may become an important collateral to the brain. In these patients thrombo-endarterectomy of a stenosed external carotid artery may be a worthwhile procedure, particularly if the stenosis is tight and post-stenotic dilatation is present.

14

Exposure of the external carotid artery

The exposure is similar to that of the internal carotid. A first step is to confirm that the internal carotid artery is completely occluded and that reconstruction is not possible. The external carotid is then isolated to beyond the point of disease the proximal branches being carefully mobilized and preserved. Heparin is then given by the anaesthesiologist and clamps applied to the common and external carotid arteries and those branches which arise from the involved vessel.

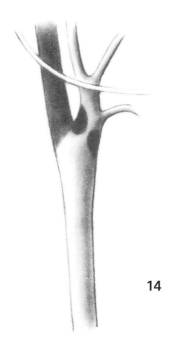

14

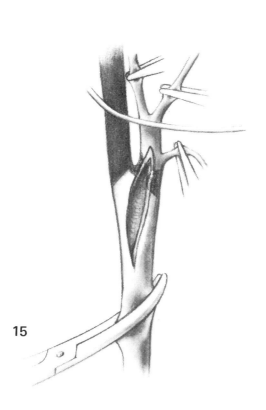

15

15

Thrombo-endarterectomy of the external carotid artery

The distal common and proximal external carotid arteries are opened by an incision which is usually slightly curved and about 2 cm long. It passes up the external carotid artery to the end of the diseased segment. The thrombo-endarterectomy is then performed in the way described in *Illustration 6* and after all debris has been removed and the retrograde flow confirmed, it is closed in the manner shown in *Illustration 9*.

THROMBO-ENDARTERECTOMY OF VERTEBRAL ARTERY

16

Incision for exposure of origin of vertebral artery

The vertebral artery can usually be exposed through a supraclavicular incision, but occasionally a better exposure may be needed than this: an additional sternal splitting incision is then satisfactory. The incision is placed 1 cm above the clavicle, starts medially at the mid-line and follows the line of the skin folds of the neck for a distance of about 7 cm. When the surgeon decides to split the sternum, this incision is continued into the mid-line and then down over the manubrium and upper part of the body of the sternum.

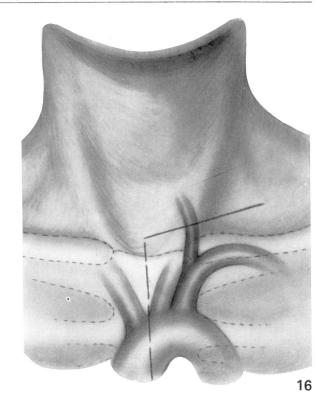

16

17

Exposure of the origin of vertebral artery

The cervical incision is taken through the platysma, the sternomastoid and infrahyoid muscles. The surgeon identifies the common carotid artery and retracts it medially. The internal jugular vein is retracted laterally. He can now identify the verte-bral artery as it arises from the subclavian artery. This vessel is then isolated as far as the point where it enters the vertebral foramen in the fifth or sixth cervical vertebra. It is stressed that the anterior scalene muscle is not divided. If further exposure is needed, the anterolateral portions of the transverse processes of the fifth or sixth cervical vertebra can be removed. The subclavian artery is also isolated for a short distance proximal and distal to the point of origin of the vertebral artery. Should this exposure be unsatisfactory or should there be evidence that the arterial disease extends more proximally, then the sternum is split in the mid-line and the whole length of the subclavian arteries, together with the innominate artery on the right and adjacent part of the aortic arch is exposed. The thrombo-end-arterectomy is then performed in the way already described; it is wise to remove in every case a ring of the inner layer from the wall of the subclavian artery around the origin of the vertebral artery. Closure is best performed with a venous patch graft angioplasty.

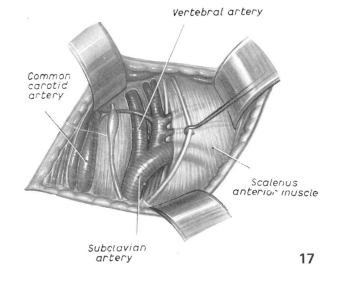

Vertebral artery

Common carotid artery

Scalenus anterior muscle

Subclavian artery

17

SPECIAL POSTOPERATIVE CARE

After 12–14 hr the patient should be allowed to get up if his neurological abnormality permits, and the majority of patients can leave the hospital by the fourth or fifth postoperative day. If the patient has a neurological defect, the treatment of this should be continued during convalescence from the operation.

Postoperative neurological deficits

This is a complicated subject with an incidence of severe problems which varies from 1 to 7 per cent depending on the type of patient, the indications for the operation, and the experience of the surgical team. It cannot be fully discussed here in the space available and the reader is referred to our article (DeWeese et al., 1973) and a chapter we have recently written (Rob, 1973).

Tranquillizer drugs

Many patients develop transient nervousness, anxiety and tension after revascularization of the brain. If this develops, a period of about 2 months on a tranquillizer drug such as Librium (10 mg twice or three times a day) is satisfactory.

Pain in the head and neck

The position of the head during endotracheal intubation and afterwards during the operation may cause pain in the neck and back of the head for 3 or 4 days after the operation. This is frequent in patients with degenerative arthritis of the cervical spine. Treatment with mild analgesic drugs is sufficient.

Anticoagulants

The use of anticoagulants in the postoperative period is of special importance. We find these drugs very difficult to control during the first 4 days. After this we may prescribe long-term anticoagulant drugs, usually using Coumadin. The value of this measure in these patients is still not proven. It may prevent further arterial occlusions but it is dangerous if there is any possibility of cerebral haemorrhage, and particularly in patients with arterial hypertension and over 65 years of age with occlusions of these arteries. A study is now proceeding to assess the value of aspirin in these patients, this is based on the work of many authors including Harrison, Marshall and Meadows (1971).

Re-operation

If there is any doubt about the adequacy of the thrombo-endarterectomy, an arteriogram should be performed before the patient leaves the operating room and any imperfections immediately corrected. After this rethrombosis is extremely unusual. But if it is suspected because the patient develops a hemiplegia, the diagnosis should be confirmed by ophthalmodynometry and the patient immediately explored. An indwelling shunt is placed in the vessel to restore the cerebral flow and a second reconstruction performed around this shunt. The usual reason for rethrombosis is incomplete removal of the distal atheroma; completion of the thrombo-endarterectomy is all that is required.

References

DeWeese, J. A., Rob, C. G., Satran, R., Marsh, D. G., Joynt, R. J., Summers, D. and Nichols, C. (1973). 'Results of carotid endarterectomies for transient ischemic attacks five years later.' *Ann. Surg.* **178**, 258

Eastcott, H. G., Pickering, G. W. and Rob, C. G. (1954). 'Reconstruction of internal carotid artery.' *Lancet* **2**, 994

Harrison, M. J. G., Marshall, J. and Meadows, J. C. (1971). 'Effect of aspirin on amaurosis fugax.' *Lancet* **2**, 743

Hutchinson, E. C. and Yates, P. O. (1956). 'The cervical portion of the vertebral artery.' *Brain* **79**, 319

Hutchinson, E. C. and Yates, P. O. (1957). *Lancet* **1**, 2

Rob, C. G. (1959). 'The surgical treatment of stenosis and thrombosis of internal carotid, cerebral and common carotid arteries.' *Proc. R. Soc. Med.* **52**, 549

Rob, C. G. (1972). 'The origin and development of surgery for occlusive disease of the carotid arteries.' *Rev. Surg.* **29**, 1

Rob, C. G. (1973). *Complications of Vascular Surgery*. Philadelphia: Beebe and Lippincott

Stanley, J. C., Fry, W. J., Seeger, J. F., Hoffman, G. L. and Gabrielson, T. G. (1974). 'Extracranial internal carotid and vertebral artery fibrodysplasia.' *Archs Surg.* **109**, 215

[The illustrations for this Chapter on Occlusions of the Carotid and Vertebral Arteries were drawn by Mr. R. N. Lane and Mr. R. Wabnitz.]

Cervical exposure of the origin of left common carotid artery

The muscles are divided in the same way as has been described in *Illustration 2*. The left common carotid artery is then identified and followed behind the sternum to the arch of the aorta. The accompanying veins are displaced forwards and care must be taken to avoid injury to the thoracic duct as it curves forwards to join the left internal jugular vein. In most patients the innominate and left common carotid artery can be exposed through their length without splitting the sternum. This applies only to patients with occlusions of these vessels; if they are aneurysmal the larger size of the vessel usually makes such a cervical exposure unsafe and the sternum must be split.

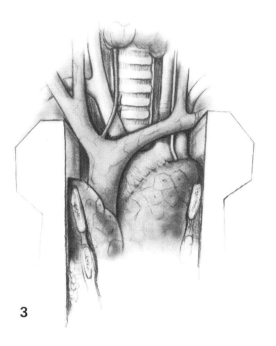

3

3

Trans-sternal exposure

If necessary the sternum is split to the level of the fourth intercostal space. The surgeon now identifies and isolates the innominate veins and the superior vena cava; the innominate and the left common carotid artery are now isolated to their origin from the aortic arch and an area about 2 cm in diameter is cleared on the aortic arch around the origin of each vessel. As stated, this incision does not provide a satisfactory exposure of the origin of the left sub-clavian artery in many patients.

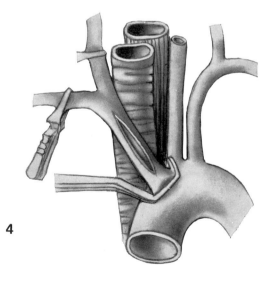

4

4

Thrombo-endarterectomy of innominate artery and its branches

A half circle arterial clamp is applied to the side of the aorta around the origin of the innominate artery. Distally, bulldog clamps are applied to the common carotid, subclavian and vertebral arteries. The innominate artery is then opened with a longitudinal incision. This incision must stop about 1 cm from the half circle clamp around the origin of the innominate artery; if it is continued too near to the clamp, closure is difficult. A thrombo-endarterectomy of the vessel and of the adjacent aorta is then performed (*see* pages 118–123). It is important to remove the inner layers of the artery and all plaques of atheroma down to the edge of the proximal clamp. The vessel is then carefully flushed with saline to remove all debris.

5

Closure of thrombo-endarterectomy incision

The first step is temporarily to remove the distal clamps to confirm that there is a good retrograde flow. We do not temporarily remove the proximal clamp because it may be difficult to re-apply before the vessel has been sutured. The incision in the artery is then closed with a continuous over-and-over suture of 4/0 silk. For a vessel of this size a patch graft angioplasty is rarely, if ever, used. The distal clamps are then removed and any major defects in the suture line closed with interrupted sutures. The proximal clamp is then removed and a pulsatile blood flow restored, pressure being applied until haemostasis is complete or extra sutures are required.

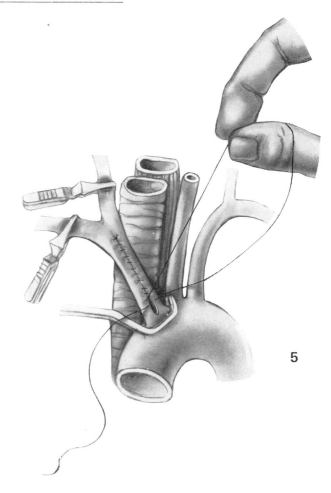

5

6

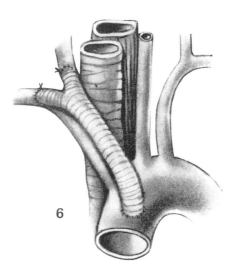

6

Bypass for occlusion of the innominate artery

A Dacron bifurcation graft of the type used for replacement of the aortic bifurcation is preferred. An anterior thoracotomy in the second right inter-costal space is used to expose the right side of the ascending aorta and the aortic arch. The main stem of the bifurcation graft is anastomosed to the side of the aorta at this point. The limbs of the graft are then passed behind the sternum into the neck where through a cervical incision they are anastomosed to the sides of the right common carotid and subclavian arteries respectively. If necessary a further side limb may be attached to the graft and anastomosed to the left common carotid artery, the anastomosis being performed with a 4/0 suture of polyester.

THROMBO-ENDARTERECTOMY OF LEFT COMMON CAROTID ARTERY

7

A thrombo-endarterectomy of the left common carotid artery requires exposure of the whole length of this artery. This is best achieved with an incision which follows the anterior border of the left sternomastoid muscle combined with a sternal split if necessary. The artery is then exposed from the aortic arch to its bifurcation. A half circle clamp is applied around its origin from the aorta and also to the internal and external carotid arteries. A longitudinal incision is then made in the vessel and a thrombo-endarterectomy carried out, great care being taken to include in the tissue removed a ring of the inner layers of the vessel from around its origin from the aorta. The incision is then closed with a continuous suture of 4/0 silk.

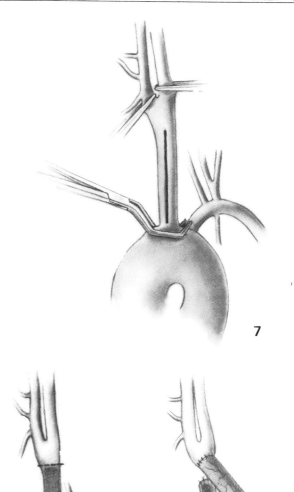

7

8a & b

Bypass-subclavian to internal carotid artery

In many patients this procedure is superior to a thrombo-endarterectomy of the common carotid artery. To ensure success the connection between the external and internal carotid arteries at the carotid bifurcation must be patent. The carotid bifurcation and origin of the internal carotid artery are exposed as is the second part of the subclavian artery. A saphenous vein graft is then anastomosed to the side of the second part of the subclavian artery, passed up the neck behind the sternomastoid muscle and anastomosed end-to-end to the distal common carotid artery. If necessary a thrombo-endarterectomy of this part of the common carotid artery is performed first to assure a good lumen at this point.

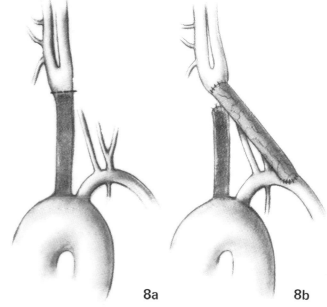

8a   8b

Exposure of first part of left subclavian artery

The origin of this vessel cannot be exposed satisfactorily through either a cervical or trans-sternal incision. A left anterolateral thoracotomy through the fourth intercostal space is preferred. The left subclavian and left common carotid arteries are identified at their origin from the aorta. The left

recurrent laryngeal nerve is carefully preserved. The left subclavian artery is fully mobilized from its origin to beyond the vertebral branch. This can be achieved from the thorax. A separate cervical incision is rarely necessary. The aortic arch for a distance of 1·5 cm around the origin of the left subclavian artery is carefully freed. If the operation is for ischaemic symptoms in the left upper limb, an upper dorsal sympathectomy can also be performed.

BYPASS FROM LEFT COMMON CAROTID TO LEFT SUBCLAVIAN ARTERIES

9

This procedure is valuable in patients with thrombosis of the first part of the left subclavian artery because it is a minor procedure compared with restoration of flow through the occluded vessel. It does not appear to reduce the flow through the left internal carotid artery. A side clamp is applied to the left common carotid artery at the base of the neck and a short length of the long saphenous vein or occasionally a Dacron graft (8 mm) is passed behind the sterno-mastoid muscle. The scalenus anterior muscle must be divided to obtain adequate exposure of the left subclavian artery. The cervical and internal mammary branches of the left subclavian artery are carefully preserved and the graft anastomosed to the sides of the common carotid and subclavian arteries.

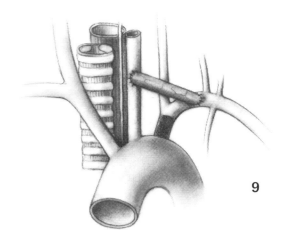

9

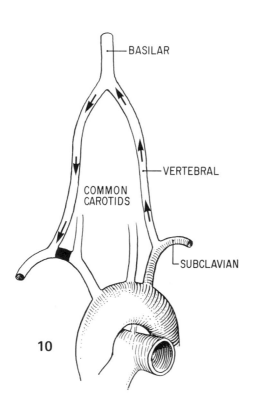

10

THE SUBCLAVIAN STEAL SYNDROME

Operation for subclavian steal syndrome

The first step is to correct any associated stenosis of the internal carotid arteries. The subclavian steal syndrome is then treated by a thrombo-endarterectomy of the right subclavian artery if this is the occluded vessel. If the left subclavian artery is occluded, a bypass graft from the left common carotid to the left subclavian artery is the preferred procedure. And in poor risk patients it may be sufficient to ligature the vertebral artery on the side of the subclavian thrombosis (Resnicoff, DeWeese and Rob, 1970).

10

The subclavian steal

Note that the two vertebral arteries and the basilar artery provide a U-shaped loop. Occlusion of the first part of either subclavian artery proximal to the origin of the vertebral artery provides the conditions for the subclavian steal syndrome. The vertebral–basilar U-shaped loop provides a collateral circulation for the ischaemic limb. This may be a radiological finding only, or the patient may develop symptoms due to cerebral ischaemia when the ischaemia area is excised. In many of these patients there is an associated stenosis of one or both of the internal carotid arteries.

POSTOPERATIVE CARE

These patients may have a cervical, a trans-sternal or a thoracotomy incision. A chest x-ray will be required after a thoracotomy and if the pleura has been opened in the case of the cervical or the trans-sternal approach to confirm that the lung has fully expanded. After operations the pulsations of the arteries in the neck and upper limbs should be checked regularly to confirm that the reconstructed vessels are patent. It is also important to monitor the blood pressure and correct any fall with a blood transfusion if necessary.

References

Broadbent, W. H. (1875). *Trans. clin. Soc. Lond.* 8, 165
DeBakey, M. E., Morris, G. C., Morgan, R. O., Crawford, E. S. and Cooley, D. A. (1964). *Ann. Surg.* **149**, 690
Resnicoff, S. A., DeWeese, J. A. and Rob, C. G. (1970). *Circulation* Suppl. II, **41**, and **42**.
Savory, D. S. (1856). *Med. Chir. Trans.* **39**, 205
Sen, P. K., Kinare, S. G., Kelkar, M. D. and Parulkar, G. B. (1973). *Non-specific Aorto-arteritis.* Bombay: Tata, McGraw-Hill
Takayusu, M. (1908). *Acta. Soc. ophthal. jap.* **12**, 554

[*The illustrations for this Chapter on Treatment of the Aortic Arch and Subclavian Steal Syndromes were drawn by Mr. R. Wabnitz and Miss D. Elliott.*]

Treatment of Arterial Aneurysms

Charles Rob, *M.C.*, M.D., M.Chir., F.R.C.S.
Professor and Chairman of the Department of Surgery,
University of Rochester School of Medicine
and Dentistry, Rochester, New York

and

James A. DeWeese, M.D., F.A.C.S.
Chairman of the Division of Cardiothoracic Surgery,
University of Rochester Medical Centre, and
Professor and Surgeon, Strong Memorial Hospital,
Rochester, New York

PRE-OPERATIVE

Operative procedures

Arterial aneurysms have been treated surgically for at least a thousand years. Many of the procedures used in the past have been abandoned but others, such as proximal ligation, still have a place in the management of arterial aneurysms. The following operations are in use today: (*1*) arterial ligation with or without an arterial bypass; (*2*) reinforcing procedures; (*3*) endo-aneurysmorrhaphy; (*4*) excision; and (*5*) excision followed by reconstruction.

Arterial ligation

Through the centuries an extensive literature has accumulated on this subject and surgeons have placed the ligature in a variety of positions relative to the aneurysm. Today proximal ligation is used in the treatment of intracranial aneurysms and combined with a sympathetic ganglionectomy in the treatment of some peripheral aneurysms, but where the aneurysm is on a major artery it is better to employ an operation which restores the arterial flow. This may take the form of an endo-aneurysmorrhaphy, but a better procedure is to use a venous or plastic graft. The insertion of this arterial graft may follow removal of the aneurysm or the surgeon may ligate the artery immediately proximal and distal to the sac and insert the arterial substitute as a bypass around the sac which is not disturbed.

Reinforcing procedures

These have included wrapping in polythene Cellophane sheeting, the injection of substances around the aneurysm and the introduction of various materials into the aneurysm to promote thrombosis. Wrapping in polythene Cellophane has not worked well in practice although other plastics have recently been employed again as a method of reinforcing intracranial aneurysms. Wiring, on the other hand, is still a worthwhile procedure, particularly in elderly and poor risk patients with an aneurysm so situated that operative excision carries an unduly high mortality, such as a leaking aneurysm in a patient with a recent myocardial infarction.

Endo-aneurysmorrhaphy

This operation may be performed in one of three ways: restorative, reconstructive, and obliterative endo-aneurysmorrhaphy. In the restorative operation the sac is opened after the circulation through it has been controlled, and sutures are inserted in such a way that the opening into the vessel is tightly sewn up without occluding the lumen of the artery; the sac is then obliterated by sutures. Reconstructive endo-aneurysmorrhaphy is a similar operation except that a new lumen is formed for the artery from the sac wall, and in the case of obliterative endo-aneurysmorrhaphy both the sac and the artery are completely occluded. The disadvantages of both the restorative and reconstructive operations have been the high recurrence rate and the fact that they are technically as difficult as inserting an arterial graft or transplant.

Excision

This is the treatment of choice for aneurysms on small and unimportant arteries and for saccular aneurysms of major vessels such as the thoracic aorta or the arteries which make up the circle of Willis. When the anatomical conditions allow, a saccular aneurysm on one of these vessels should be excised and the defect in the host artery closed by lateral suture.

Excision with reconstruction

This was performed by Lexer in 1907 and by Pringle in 1918. The aneurysm is either excised and the artery replaced by a plastic implant or an autogenous vein graft, or the artery is ligated above and below the aneurysms and an arterial transplant or vein graft is placed as a bypass around the occluded segment.

Indications

Most arterial aneurysms should be treated surgically. The reasons for this are that medical measures are without effect, that the aneurysm itself often produces severe symptoms, and that a variety of complications may arise. Amongst these may be listed rupture, thrombosis, peripheral embolization, dissection and pressure on surrounding structures. While many patients may live for years after an aneurysm has been diagnosed, Colt in 1927 studied 624 aneurysms of the aorta; of these 121 were of the abdominal aorta and the average duration of life was less than 2 years from the date of diagnosis. The usual cause of death was rupture of the aneurysms.

Special pre-operative preparation

Some aneurysms have a treatable cause, such as infection; when possible this should be controlled before the operation. In most patients blood transfusion will be required and arrangements should be made for this in adequate amounts. All patients with aneurysms of major arteries should have a full pre-operative assessment of their cardiovascular system, including an electrocardiogram. Prophylactic antibiotics are administered if a plastic graft is to be inserted. The patient should enter the operating room well hydrated. This can be accomplished by giving 1–2 litres of intravenous fluids during the 12 hr prior to operation.

Special contra-indications

Ischaemic heart diseases if severe may be a contra-indication to major surgery of this type. Another contra-indication is gross multiplicity of the aneurysms and arterial reconstruction operations are only possible when there is an adequate lumen to the arterial tree distal to the aneurysm.

Anaesthesia

General anaesthesia with an endotracheal tube is usually satisfactory. However, when an abdominal aneurysm has leaked recently or ruptures, the anaesthetic presents a special problem because there is a grave risk of further severe haemorrhage when the muscles of the abdominal wall are relaxed by the anaesthetic. Some surgeons have advocated the control of the lower thoracic aorta as a first step in these patients, but we have not found this satisfactory and prefer to take the following steps. Anaesthesia is induced without relaxants, the surgeon makes the abdominal incision down to the peritoneum, relaxants are given and the surgeon immediately opens the peritoneum and rapidly gains control of the aorta proximal to the sac of the aneurysm.

When the aneurysm is on an artery supplying the brain, the spinal cord or essential organs such as the kidneys, it is wise to take special precautions to protect these structures from the effects of ischaemia during the period of temporary arterial occlusion. In such patients the maintenance of the blood flow by a temporary indwelling arterial shunt, a shunt graft or perfusion with a total or partial cardiac bypass can maintain the viability of these organs.

THE OPERATIONS

THE INFRARENAL ABDOMINAL AORTA

1

Incision

For most aneurysms a long mid-line incision is made. The incision begins at the base of and to the left of the xiphoid process. It is carried downward and around the umbilicus and ends at the symphysis pubis. Care is taken to make the incision exactly in the mid-line by following the decussations of the fibres of the rectus sheath.

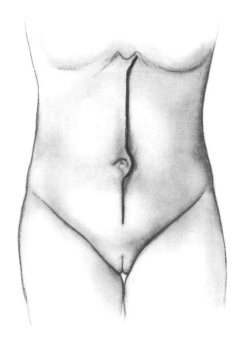

1

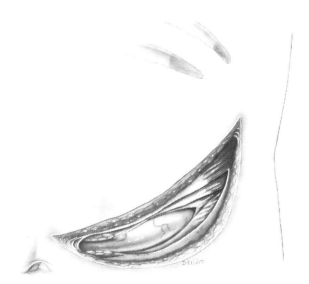

2

2

Incision (extraperitoneal)

This is useful for medium- and small-sized aneurysms (Rob, 1963). The incision follows the line of the segmental nerves and starts at the tip of the last large rib, usually the eleventh rib. It extends to the mid-line just above or just below the umbilicus. The rectus muscles and the oblique and transverse abdominal muscles are divided within the line of the incision. Care should be taken to avoid injury to the segmental nerves. The posterior sheath of the rectus muscle is also divided and the peritoneum stripped and retracted medially to expose the aorta and iliac arteries. If an opening is made in the peritoneum, it can be closed at once with sutures and the stripping continued or closed after completion of the graft replacement.

3

Exposure (transperitoneal)

The patient is hyperextended. The small intestine is mobilized superiorly and to the patient's right side and protected by moist pads or within a plastic bag. Moist pads and retractors are used to pack away the duodenum and large bowel. A self-retaining chest retractor with long blades is quite useful. The posterior peritoneum is incised beginning at the ligament of Treitz, carried distally to the right of the mid-line to avoid the mesenteric artery and vein, and over the sacral promontory in the mid-line.

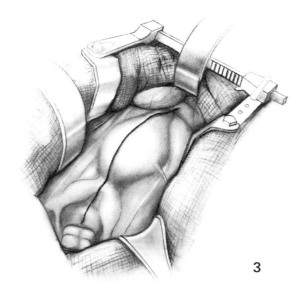

3

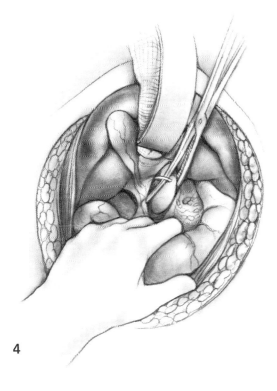

4

4

High proximal control of aorta

If the aneurysm extends to the renal arteries or if the aneurysm has ruptured, proximal control must be obtained above the level of the renal arteries. The transverse colon and stomach are retracted downward, the lesser omentum incised and the aorta exposed by bluntly separating the right and left crus of the diaphragm. A large vascular clamp is applied taking care not to injure the coeliac artery.

5

Infrarenal control of aorta

The duodenum is retracted superiorly and the left renal vein exposed. Using sharp and blunt dissection, the aorta is mobilized just distal to the left renal artery. The aorta can be encircled with a tape taking care not to injure lumbar veins or arteries posteriorly. In most instances encirclement is not necessary. The inferior mesenteric artery is divided between two ligatures. It is important that a second suture ligature is placed distally to avoid later bleeding.

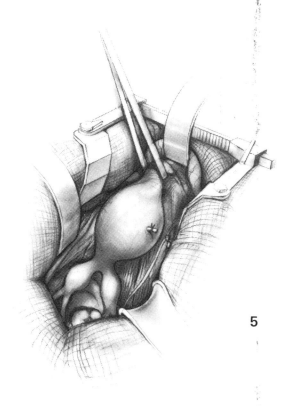

5

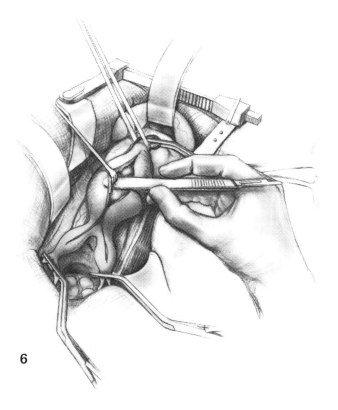

6

6

Clamping of aorta and aortotomy

Heparin sodium in 5000—7500 unit amounts is administered intravenously. After 2 min vascular clamps are applied to the aorta just distal to the renal arteries and also across both iliac arteries. It is important not to try to separate the iliac arteries from the veins at this point. An aortotomy is made through the wall of the aneurysm from its origin to the bifurcation and then down both iliac arteries. If possible a plane of dissection is established either between the media and intima or between the intima and the old thrombus, which is almost always found within the aneurysm.

7

Removal of aneurysm contents and control of lumbar arteries

The thrombus and, if possible, the atherosclerotic intima is removed from within the aneurysm. Most of the lumbar arteries are usually thrombosed. Bleeding from the patent vessels is controlled with mattress or figure-of-8 stitches of 2/0 sutures. Atherosclerotic plaques must be debrided away before attempting to suture these vessels.

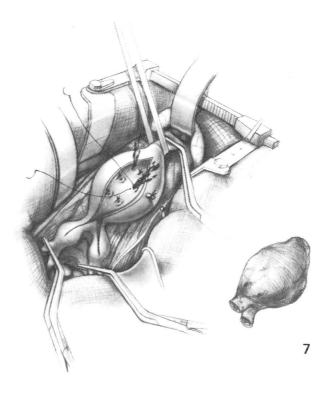

7

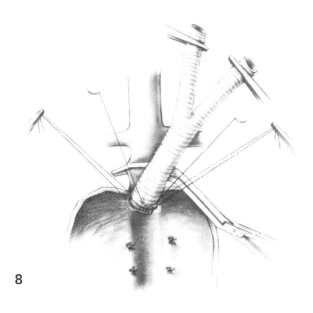

8

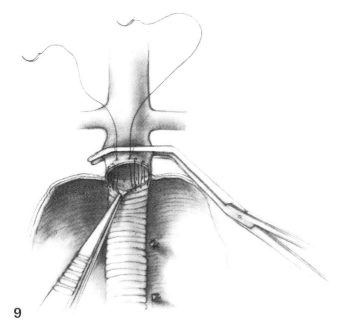

9

8

Proximal anastomosis—suturing posterior half

To avoid extensive mobilization of the aorta the posterior half of the proximal anastomosis can be performed from within the aneurysm. The body of the graft is usually much longer than needed and must be cut prior to beginning the anastomosis. Usually a distinct ridge can be identified at the point where the aorta becomes aneurysmal. A deep mattress stitch is placed through this ridge and carried through the mid-point of the posterior edge of the graft as an everting stitch. Similar mattress stitches are placed on the lateral corners of the graft. The posterior suture is then run around both sides of the graft as a continuous everting over-and-over stitch.

9

Proximal anastomosis—suturing anterior half

The anterior half of the aortic cuff is cut transversely to the lateral mattress stay-sutures. The posterior stitch is then continued around the stay-sutures to the anterior mid-point of the anastomosis and tied.

10

Testing of proximal anastomosis

Regardless of whether woven or preclotted knitted grafts are used, it is helpful to test the anastomosis and control bleeding through the graft interstices after completion of the proximal anastomosis. The limbs of the graft are occluded and the proximal clamps slowly released. Any significant bleeding between sutures is controlled with mattress stitches. The graft is then allowed to fill, the clamp occluded and the graft allowed to sit until there is no further bleeding through the interstices.

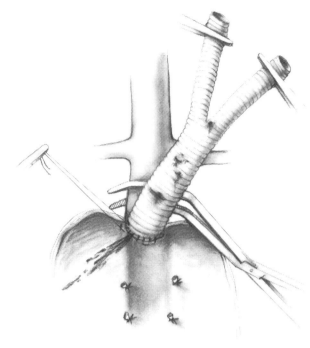

10

11

Distal anastomosis to the aorta or iliac artery

When possible a straight graft is used. The distal anastomosis being to the aorta just proximal to the bifurcation, this technique is possible in about 66 per cent of patients. When the proximal iliac arteries are severely diseased a bifurcation graft is used. One limb of the graft is then occluded with a non-crushing vascular clamp. The opposite limb is then cut to the length necessary to reach the site of the distal anastomosis. A suction catheter is then introduced into the limb and loose thrombi removed. It is preferable to make the anastomosis to the common iliac artery end-to-end if possible. If the common iliac is severely diseased and the external iliac artery soft-walled, the anastomosis should be made end-to-side to the external iliac artery. The common iliac is divided and the distal end oversewn which allows retrograde filling of the internal iliac artery.

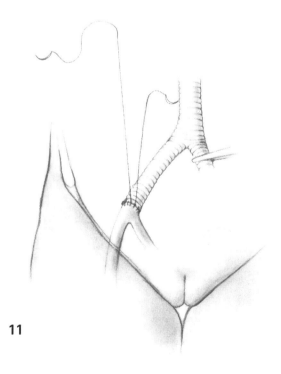

11

12

Distal anastomosis to common femoral artery—groin incision

After completing the anastomosis of one limb of the graft, the distal clamp is removed allowing retrograde filling of the graft. The clamp on the opposite limb is then removed and the limb with the completed anastomosis is occluded as the proximal clamp is removed to flush any debris from the graft. Flow is then gradually restored to the leg with the completed anastomosis while carefully monitoring the blood pressure. Sudden drops in blood pressure can be expected unless the clamps are slowly and intermittently removed over a 2—5-min period.

If it is necessary to carry the graft to the groin, a clamp is passed from the groin incision over the femoral artery and retroperitoneally to the sacral promontory. The limb of the graft is carefully oriented and passed to the groin.

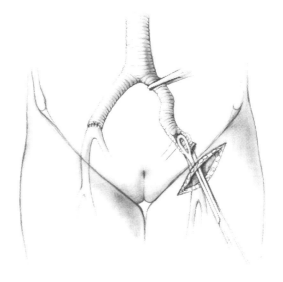

12

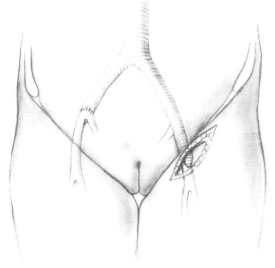

13

13

Distal anastomosis to common femoral artery

The common femoral artery is mobilized from the inguinal ligament to the profunda femoris artery. An end-to-side anastomosis is made to the occluded common femoral artery. Backflow from the femoral artery is checked prior to completion of the anastomosis. If the backflow is unsatisfactory, a Fogarty thrombectomy catheter is passed distally and thrombi removed if present (*see* Chapter on 'Arterial Embolectomy', pages 35—39). Flow is also gradually re-established to this limb. Protamine sulphate is then administered intravenously in doses of 1 mg for each 100 units of heparin sodium given when the vessels were clamped.

14

Closure of peritoneum

The sac of the aneurysm is then wrapped around the graft after removing any excess. The cut edge of the sac may bleed and require oversewing, cauterization, or multiple ligatures. A one or two-layer closure is made with a continuous stitch of 1/0 chromic catgut which includes both walls of the aneurysm sac and the posterior peritoneum. Care is taken to avoid injury to the mesenteric vein and duodenum. A special effort is made to separate the anastomoses and graft from direct contact with the duodenum and jejunum to avoid aorto-enteric fistulae.

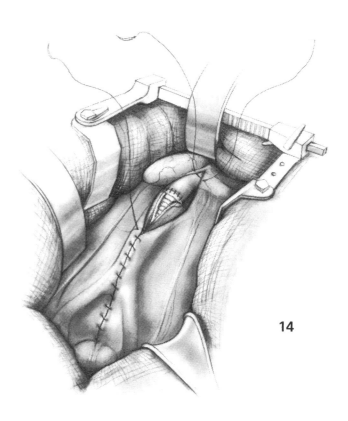

14

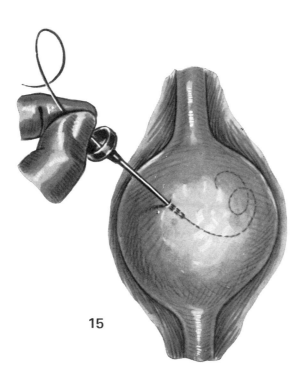

15

Wiring of aneurysms

15

Introduction of wire

This is recommended if the aneurysm cannot be resected, but the results are inferior to those obtained by the resection and reconstruction. When the aneurysm has reached the superficial tissues introduction may be performed directly through the skin. Otherwise it is wise to expose the aneurysm over a portion of its surface, but no attempt should be made to isolate or dissect the aneurysm from neighbouring structures. No. 82 or 86 stainless steel wire is used and this is introduced through a fairly wide bore (gauge 18) needle. If necessary a number of needle punctures can be made. The procedure takes a long time and a good length of wire (200–1000 ft; 61–305 m) should be introduced, depending on the size of the aneurysm. Linton of Boston has designed a simple apparatus for the introduction of the wire.

16

Function of wire

When fine wire, such as No. 86 stainless steel, is introduced into an aneurysm it bends and curls up as soon as it encounters the opposite wall of the sac or any other obstruction. This means that the whole aneurysm is gradually filled with a bundle of wire; around this the blood clots, leaving ideally a channel for the blood flow in the centre. It is important to use only fine wire; if wire of a greater size than No. 82 is used it may not remain in the sac of the aneurysm passing up and down the arterial tree.

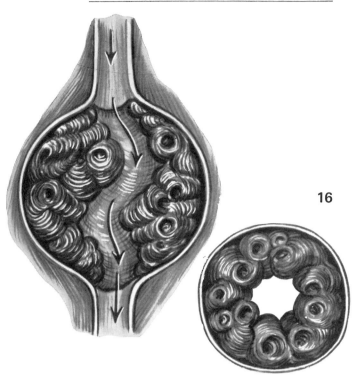

16

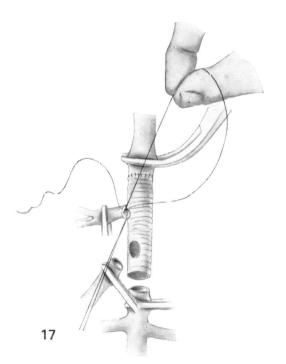

17

ANEURYSMS IN CERTAIN SPECIAL SITES

17

Upper abdominal aorta

This area is best approached through a left thoraco-abdominal incision along the bed of the ninth rib and extending to the mid-line of the anterior abdominal wall. It is wise to set up a bypass from the left atrium to the left femoral artery so as to ensure adequate perfusion of the distal arterial tree. The aneurysm is then mobilized together with the aorta proximal and distal, the coeliac, superior mesenteric and both renal arteries. After the aneurysm has been excised reconstitution is performed serially from above down, the clamps being moved distally after each branch has been anastomosed.

18

Splenic arteries

These may be single or multiple and appear to be more common in hypertensive than normotensive individuals. If the aneurysms are multiple or if they are situated in the hilum of the spleen, splenectomy is the best procedure. If they involve the main splenic artery then this vessel can be ligatured on each side of the aneurysm and the aneurysm removed, the spleen being left *in situ*. Under these circumstances the spleen receives sufficient blood from the short gastric arteries.

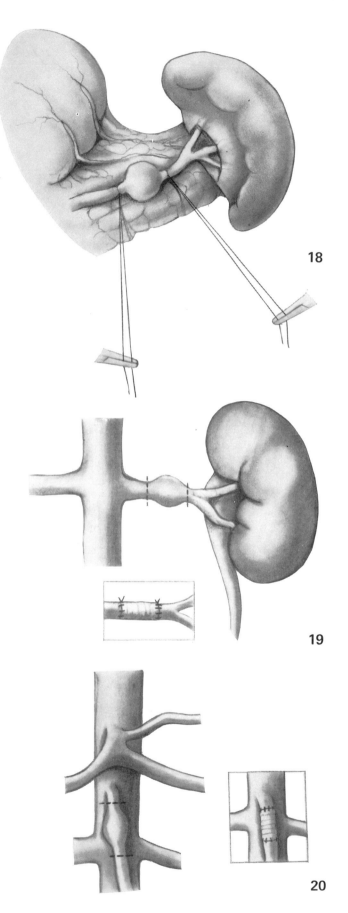

18

19

Renal arteries

These are often placed on the branches of the renal artery and fortunately are frequently saccular. If the main renal artery is involved, resection and graft replacement is the best treatment. If on a branch, resection and ligature of the involved vessel, combined if necessary with a partial nephrectomy, may be satisfactory. Saccular aneurysms of the main artery or of its branches can be treated by resection of the aneurysm and closure of the defect in the artery by an autogenous venous patch graft or occasionally by simple lateral suture.

19

20

Coeliac and mesenteric arteries

Aneurysms of some of the minor branches of these arteries can be resected and the artery tied. But aneurysms which involve the main stems of either of these arteries, or vital branches such as the hepatic artery, require both resection and arterial reconstruction. Reconstruction of these arteries may be performed in one of two ways. First by a standard end-to-end anastomosis with or without an intervening graft of Dacron or autogenous vein, and second, by a bypass from the aorta to the artery distal to the aneurysm, the vessel being ligated on each side of the aneurysm.

20

21

Carotid arteries

The surgery of aneurysms of the intracranial arteries will be described in the volume on *'Neurosurgery'*, to be published later on in this *Operative Surgery* series. Aneurysms of the cervical portions of the carotid arteries occur most frequently at the bifurcation of the common carotid artery, although a tortuous artery may mimic a true aneurysm, particularly on the right side of the neck. Resection of one proximal and two distal vessels is performed. The external carotid artery is tied and in many patients it is then possible to restore continuity by anastomosing the common carotid to the internal carotid artery. If this is not possible, the gap may be bridged by an autogenous vein graft or a plastic prosthesis.

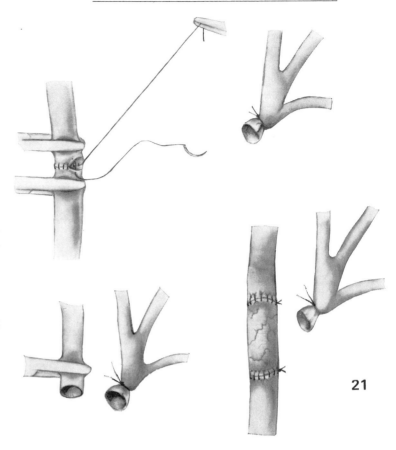

21

22

Vertebral arteries

These are uncommon. A special type occurs after direct puncture arteriography of the vertebral artery when either an arteriovenous fistula or aneurysm may develop. These aneurysms are usually located on the artery after it has entered the vertebral canal. An incision is made along the anterior border of the sternomastoid muscle, the carotid sheath is identified and retracted medially to expose the anterior surface of the transverse processes of the cervical vertebrae. The muscles are stripped from the bone with a periosteal elevator and the bone on the anterior wall of the vertebral canal removed with rongeurs to expose the vertebral artery and vein proximal and distal to the aneurysm. In many patients it is sufficient to ligature the artery at each of these two sites. If excision of the aneurysm and an arterial reconstruction procedure is to be performed, more bone is removed to expose the whole of the lesion, and the appropriate procedure carried out.

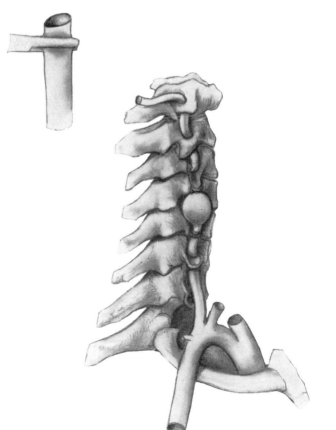

22

Main arteries of the limbs—femoral, popliteal, axillary

23

Resection and reconstruction

The approach to these vessels has already been described. The usual procedure is to resect the aneurysm dividing the main artery as close to the sac as possible so that the maximum number of collateral vessels are preserved. Continuity is then restored by inserting an autogenous vein graft or Dacron prosthesis anastomosed end-to-end to the host artery.

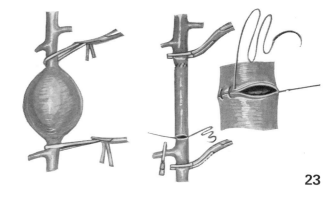

23

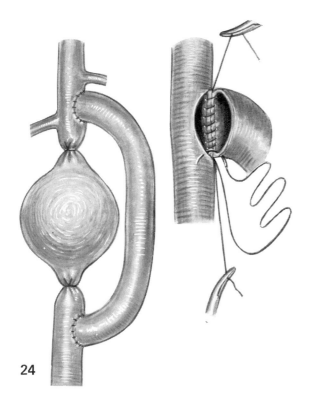

24

24

Bypassing the aneurysm

An alternative and perhaps a better method is to bypass the aneurysm with a Dacron prosthesis or vein graft. The main artery is first ligated immediately above and below the aneurysm. The bypass arterial transplant is then inserted with an end-to-end anastomosis above and below the points of ligature. No attempt is made to interfere with the sac of the aneurysm. The bypass procedure avoids dissection of the artery from the very adherent popliteal vein and also the incision causes less morbidity since less exposure is required.

SPECIAL POSTOPERATIVE CARE

The first essential is to maintain an adequate blood pressure to prevent clotting in the transplant or at another site such as the coronary arteries. This is achieved by continuing the blood transfusion if indicated and sometimes the intravenous infusion of noradrenaline at a rate sufficient to maintain the blood pressure at its pre-operative level. The blood pressure should be recorded at half-hourly intervals until it is stable.

Anticoagulants

In our view these are dangerous in the immediate postoperative period and should be avoided if possible during the first 72 hr. Even with meticulous control serious bleeding can occur. On the other hand, long-term oral anticoagulant therapy using Coumadin may be recommended in some patients after the first 72 hr.

Paralytic ileus

This follows nearly every transperitoneal operation upon the abdominal aorta and should be treated by gastric aspiration by means of an indwelling tube plus intravenous fluid and electrolyte replacement until intestinal mobility has been re-established.

Bedrest and care of wound

The patient is nursed flat until the blood pressure is stable. After this most patients can be allowed to sit in a chair by the second postoperative day. In the case of the abdominal aneurysms it is wise to leave the deep tension sutures in for 10 or more days. Patients, after temporary clamping of the aorta, are liable to develop sacral pressure sores; these are best prevented by careful cushioning with thick foam rubber pads during the operation and careful nursing afterwards.

Oliguria

Some patients develop oliguria after the abdominal aorta has been cross-clamped. A pre-operative water load plus adequate hydration during and after this procedure usually controls the problem. Some surgeons recommend mannitol.

References

Colt, C. H. (1927). *Q. Jl Med.* **20**, 331
DeBakey, M. E., Cooley, D. A. and Creech, O. (1955). *Symposium on Cardiovascular Surgery*, Henry Ford Hospital, p. 468. Philadelphia: Saunders
Erickson, J. E. (1844). *Observations on Aneurysms.* London. (For historical references)
Lexer, E. (1907). *Archs klin. Chir.* **83**, 459
May, A. G., DeWeese, J. A., Frank, I., Mahoney, E. B. and Rob, C. G. (1968). *Surgery* **63**, 711
Pringle, H. (1913). *Lancet* **1**, 1795
Rob, C. G. (1954). *Ann. R. Coll. Surg.* **14**, 35
Rob, C. G. (1963). *Surgery* **1**, 87
Rob, C. G., Eastcott, H. H. G. and Owen, K. (1956). *Br. J. Surg.* **43**, 449

[*The illustrations for this Chapter on Treatment of Arterial Aneurysms were drawn by Mr. R. Wabnitz and Miss D. Elliott.*]

Intrathoracic Aneurysms

James A. DeWeese, M.D., F.A.C.S.
Chairman of the Division of Cardiothoracic Surgery,
University of Rochester Medical Centre, and
Professor and Surgeon, Strong Memorial Hospital,
Rochester, New York

and

Charles Rob, *M.C.,* M.D., M.Chir., F.R.C.S.
Professor and Chairman of the Department of Surgery,
University of Rochester School of Medicine and
Dentistry, Rochester, New York

PRE-OPERATIVE

Indications

Fusiform or saccular aneurysms may occur in the ascending aorta, arch aorta and descending thoracic aorta, as well as its major branches. The usual causes are arteriosclerosis, lues and trauma. Dissecting aneurysms occurring in the presence of cystic medial necrosis present unusual problems in diagnosis and treatment and will be discussed elsewhere.

Surgical treatment should be considered whenever the diagnosis is made since, in general, the lesions are progressive to rupture and death. Surgical treatment becomes imperative in the presence of pain secondary to erosion of the spine or compression of nerves. Other indications include: (*1*) phrenic nerve or recurrent laryngeal nerve involvement; (*2*) compression or erosion of the trachea or oesophagus; and (*3*) rupture.

Contra-indications

Age alone is not a contra-indication to surgery. In fact, the lesions are most commonly found in patients over 60 years of age. Arteriosclerotic heart disease, chronic lung disease, or other significant medical illnesses may contra-indicate surgery in the asymptomatic patient.

Special preparations

Patients are admitted to hospital 2–7 days prior to surgery for a final medical evaluation. Attention should be directed towards improvements of the respiratory tract, particularly in those with chronic lung diseases. Smoking should be discontinued. Hyperventilation exercises should be prescribed. Bronchodilators, secretagogies, detergents, positive pressure breathing and even prophylactic antibiotics may be indicated.

Special techniques

When the thoracic aorta is clamped special equipment is needed to prevent left ventricular failure and to assure adequate circulation to the heart, brain, kidneys and viscera. The bypass procedures vary according to the site of clamping and will be discussed separately.

Special techniques for suturing the thoracic aorta are also necessary. The diseased thoracic aorta is more friable than the abdominal aorta or peripheral arteries. The simpler techniques of anastomosis used for the abdominal aorta, therefore, may be unsatisfactory in the thoracic aorta. Bleeding from suture lines or through needle holes is further accentuated by the fact that the patient must be heparinized for the bypass procedures and until the catheters used for the bypass procedures are removed. For these same reasons woven grafts and not knitted grafts are preferred.

THE OPERATION

ANEURYSMS OF ASCENDING THORACIC AORTA

1

Total cardiopulmonary bypass with coronary perfusion

Resection of an aneurysm of the ascending thoracic aorta requires clamping of the aorta proximal to the innominate artery. Total cardiopulmonary bypass is necessary. The superior and inferior vena cavae are cannulated through the right atrium. Venous blood is thereby returned to a pump oxygenator and heat exchanger. Arterialized and cooled blood is then returned to the femoral artery for retrograde perfusion of the visceral, renal and cranial arteries. A separate line from the pump oxygenator leads to the coronary arteries which are cannulated through a transverse incision in the base of the aorta.

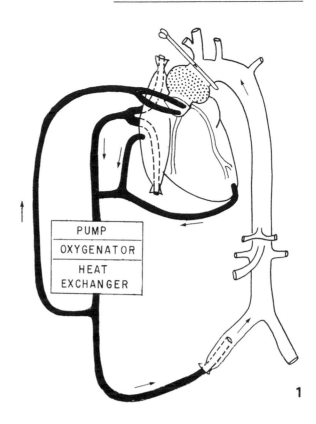

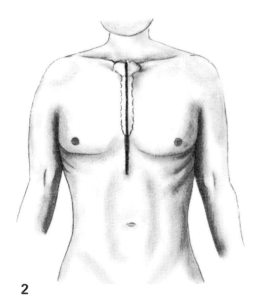

2

Median sternotomy incision

A short transverse incision is made just below the supraclavicular notch. A longitudinal incision is made along the entire length of the sternum beyond the xiphoid process. The sternum is then split longitudinally with an electric saw and Lebsche knife. To establish haemostasis, it is advisable to use cautery for cutting the periosteum of the manubrium and bone wax to control marrow bleeding.

3

Exposure of aorta and heart

The pericardium is incised longitudinally after dividing the thymus. It is advisable to peel the pleura laterally, with care, and avoid entering either pleural space. The innominate vein is carefully retracted superiorly. The aorta is mobilized under direct vision to avoid injuring the right pulmonary artery which passes directly behind it. Catheters are inserted into the superior and inferior vena cava and the right atrium through small right atriotomies for the return of venous blood to the pump oxygenator. A catheter has been placed in the femoral artery through an incision in the groin for the return of arterialized blood from the pump oxygenator.

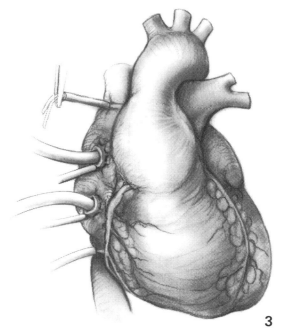

3

4

Preparation of artificial valve and graft

Aneurysms of the ascending aorta are usually associated with aortic valvular insufficiency. An artificial valve replacement as well as the insertion of a woven Dacron graft is therefore required. An appropriate-sized valve is sutured to the end of the Dacron tube using a continuous suture.

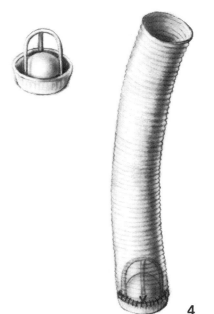

4

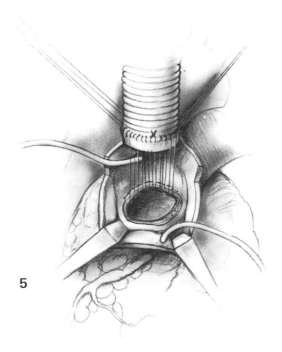

5

5

Cardiopulmonary bypass and excision of aortic valve

The patient is placed on cardiopulmonary bypass and the body temperature lowered to 20°C. A left ventricular sump is inserted. A longitudinal incision is made in the aneurysm without excision of any of the aortic wall. The aortic valve leaflets are excised at least 3 mm from the annulus. Small catheters are inserted into the orifices of the right and left coronary arteries for perfusion.

6

Seating of artificial valve

Mattress stitches of a No 0 braided plastic suture are placed through the annulus of the aorta and the base of the artificial valve which has been sutured to the graft. When all the sutures have been placed, the valve is glided down the sutures and seated in the aortic annulus.

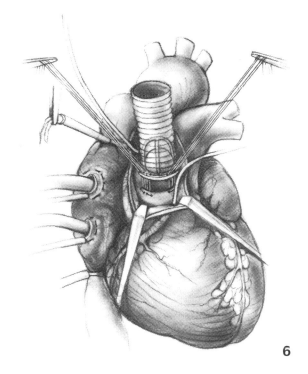

6

7

Distal anastomosis

Holes, 1 cm in diameter, are cut out of the Dacron tube at the estimated level of the coronary orifices. The coronary perfusion catheters are repositioned to pass through these holes and the distal end of the graft. The posterior edge of the distal end of the graft is then sutured to the posterior wall of the aorta from within. A mattress stitch is placed directly posteriorly taking generous bites of the aortic wall.

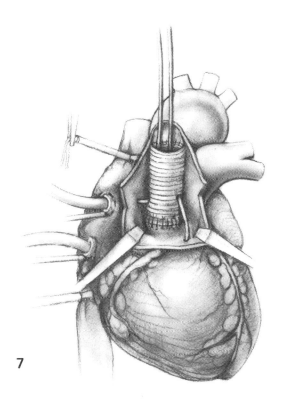

7

8

Completion of distal anastomosis

An over-and-over continuous stitch is then brought around both sides of the graft and the sutures are tied anteriorly. Both the proximal and distal anastomoses have been made from within the aorta.

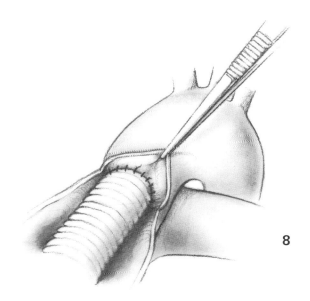

8

9

Suturing of new coronary orifices

The edges of the holes in the graft are now approximated to the aortic wall 2–3 mm from the coronary orifices. This is all accomplished from within aorta using a continuous stitch and taking generous bites of the aortic wall.

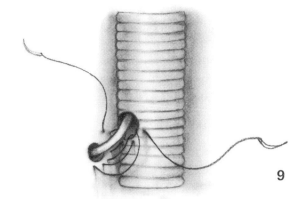

9

10

Closure of aorta

Strips of Teflon felt 1·5 cm are placed along the edges of the aortotomy. A horizontal mattress stitch of 0/0 silk suture is placed through the felt pad about 1 cm from the edge of the aortotomy. A second layer is made using a continuous stitch about 5 mm from the edge of the aortotomy. The patient is then slowly taken off cardiopulmonary bypass taking care to evacuate air from the aorta and heart before the heart contracts forcefully.

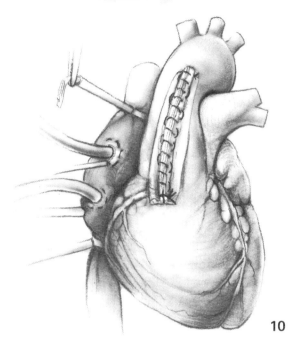

10

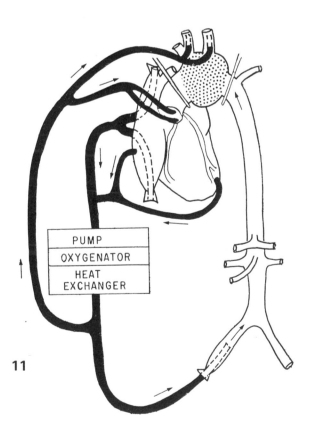

PUMP

OXYGENATOR

HEAT EXCHANGER

11

ANEURYSMS OF THE AORTIC ARCH

11

Cardiopulmonary bypass, coronary perfusion and cerebral perfusion

The resection of aneurysms of the aortic arch involving the origins of the innominate and left carotid artery require occlusion of the thoracic aorta both proximal and distal to these important cerebral vessels. In addition to perfusion of the coronary arteries, it is also necessary to perfuse the cerebral vessels. This perfusion is accomplished by the insertion of catheters from the oxygenator into the appropriate vessels.

12

Exposure and preparations for excision

The initial steps are the same as those used for treatment of aneurysms of the ascending aorta. A median sternotomy incision is made. If the aneurysm extends to or distal to the left subclavian artery it may be necessary to extend the incision into the left fourth or fifth interspace for additional exposure, and preparations for cardiopulmonary bypass are made. The proximal thoracic aorta is occluded and coronary perfusion established. The mobilized innominate and left carotid artery are then cannulated with catheters from the pump oxygenator and cerebral perfusion is begun. The aorta distal to the aneurysm is then occluded.

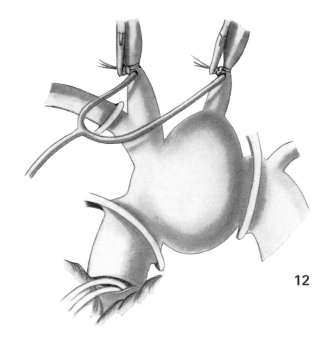

12

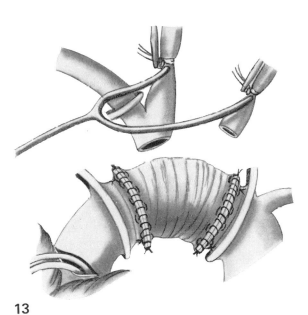

13

13

Excision and replacement

The aneurysm is excised, taking care to avoid injury to the innominate vein, phrenic nerve and vagus nerve. A woven prosthesis is used to re-establish continuity. The anastomoses are two-layered, with a first layer of continuous mattress stitch and a second layer of a continuous over-and-over stitch.

14

Re-anastomosis of arch vessels

The proximal left carotid artery in this case is involved in the aneurysmal degeneration. Therefore, a short small prosthetic graft is sutured end-to-side to the larger graft and end-to-end to the carotid artery. The innominate artery is not involved and is sutured end-to-side to the prosthesis. The carotid perfusion catheters are removed and the arteriotomies closed. The distal aortic clamp is removed allowing retrograde perfusion of the cerebral vessels. The coronary perfusion catheters are removed, aortotomy closed, cardiopulmonary bypass discontinued and incisions closed with drainage as previously described.

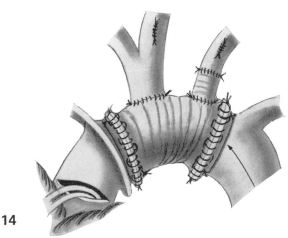

14

15

Aneurysms of the descending thoracic aorta

Occlusion of the descending thoracic aorta results in a proximal hypertension with left ventricular failure and possible cerebral haemorrhage and a distal hypotension with probable renal and hepatic failure. Left heart bypass provides a means for the controlled equalization of proximal and distal pressures. Inclusion of a heat exchanger in the circuit allows cooling of the body for further protection of the kidneys and spinal cord. The rate of flow required to equalize the pressures is usually between 1000 and 1500 ml/min but accurate monitoring of both the proximal and distal pressures is necessary to guarantee adequate distal perfusion. The proximal catheter can be inserted into the left subclavian artery or pulmonary veins but the left atrium is the most satisfactory site. The distal catheter is inserted retrogradely into the femoral artery.

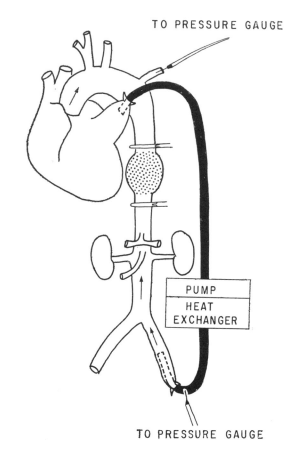

TO PRESSURE GAUGE

PUMP
HEAT
EXCHANGER

TO PRESSURE GAUGE

15

16

The incision

With the patient in a lateral position with the left side up, an incision is made along the course of the fifth rib beneath the nipple and tip of the scapula. The latissimus muscle and the posterior portion of the serratus anterior muscle are divided. The serratus anterior and pectoral muscles are then divided anteriorly to the nipple line. The chest is entered through the fourth or fifth intercostal space. Additional exposure can be obtained by division of the necks of the adjacent ribs posteriorly.

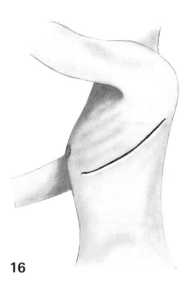

16

17

Exposure and preparations for left heart bypass

The lung is retracted anteriorly and downward. The phrenic nerve, vagus nerve, subclavian artery and thoracic aorta are visualized. The pericardium is incised longitudinally just anterior to the phrenic nerve to expose the left atrial appendage. A purse-string suture of heavy silk is placed around the appendage and the tip excised. A catheter is inserted through the appendage and connected by plastic tubing to the pump and heat exchanger which, in turn, is connected to a catheter inserted into the femoral artery through a groin incision.

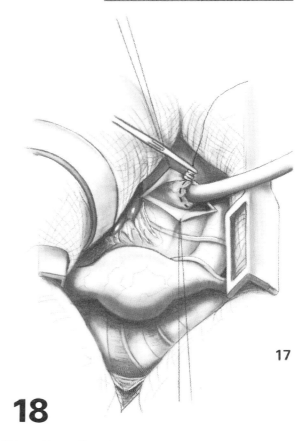

17

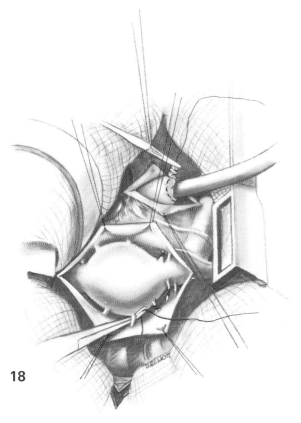

18

18

Dissection of aorta

The mediastinal pleura is incised over the aneurysm and to normal aorta proximally and distally. Under careful direct vision the proximal and distal aorta is encircled with tapes. Intercostal arteries just proximal and distal to the aneurysm are carefully dissected free and ligated in continuity and divided. It is important to sacrifice only those intercostal arteries which must be divided since the important spinal arteries arise from the intercostals.

19

Resection of aneurysm

After the patient is heparinized, the aorta is occluded proximally and distally at the same time that left bypass is begun. Following equalization of the proximal and distal pressures, the aneurysm is resected. It is not necessary to resect the aneurysm totally. A portion of the wall can be left where it is adherent to important structures such as the oesophagus or vagus nerves.

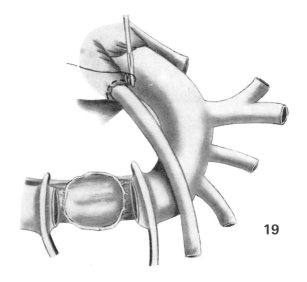

19

20

Replacement

A woven Dacron graft is sutured end-to-end to the ends of the divided aorta. A two-layered anastomosis is made. The first layer is a continuous everting horizontal mattress stitch and the second layer a continuous over-and-over stitch. The patient is given protamine to counteract the heparin after bypass is discontinued and the catheters in the atrium and femoral artery are removed. If possible the pleura is approximated over the graft. The wound is closed in layers after inserting a catheter through the seventh interspace for postoperative drainage of the pleural space.

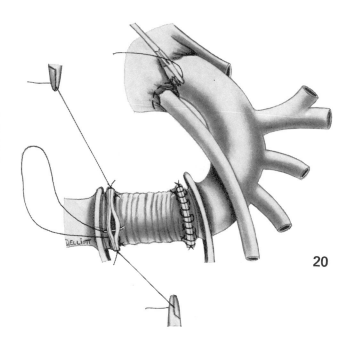

20

21

ANEURYSMS NOT REQUIRING BYPASS TECHNIQUES

21

Saccular aneurysm

Excision

A saccular aneurysm whose neck is relatively narrow can be excised without using bypass procedures. The neck of the sac is dissected free of surrounding tissues and a large clamp placed longitudinally across it. A continuous horizontal mattress suture is placed 1–2 mm outside of the clamp prior to excising the aneurysm.

22

Aortorrhaphy

Following excision of the aneurysm a second layer of a continuous suture is placed between stay sutures. The clamp is then removed.

22

23 & 24

Postcoarctation aneurysm

Localized aneurysms may develop distal to coarctations of the aorta. A left heart bypass is rarely needed. The well-developed collaterals present as a result of the coarctation provide sufficient blood flow to the distal aorta and prevent proximal dilatation from occurring. Tape control of the subclavian artery and proximal and distal thoracic aorta is obtained.

The portion of the aorta containing the aneurysm and the coarctated segment is excised. Only those intercostal arteries are excised which absolutely interfere with the anastomoses. A woven prosthetic graft is sutured end-to-end to the aorta. A continuous horizontal mattress stitch and a second over-and-over stitch is used.

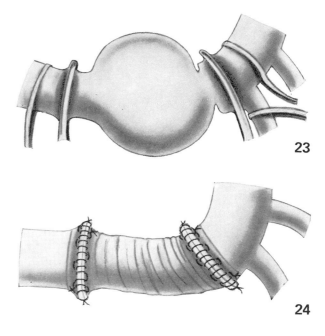

23

24

25

Aneurysms of subclavian artery

Distal control of the extrathoracic portion of the subclavian artery is difficult to obtain from within the chest and the following incision is recommended.

The incision is begun at the mid point of the clavicle extending to the suprasternal notch, carried down the middle of the sternum to the fourth interspace and then brought out through the fourth interspace. The sternocleidomastoid muscle is divided just above the clavicle and sternum. The scalenus anticus muscle is divided taking care to preserve the phrenic nerve. The sternothyroid and sternohyoid muscles are divided. The upper sternum is divided longitudinally with an electric saw and Lebsche knife. The pectoralis major muscle is divided along the fourth interspace and the serratus anterior muscles divided in the direction of their fibres. This flap of the upper thoracic cage can now be retracted laterally to expose the superior mediastinum and thoracic space.

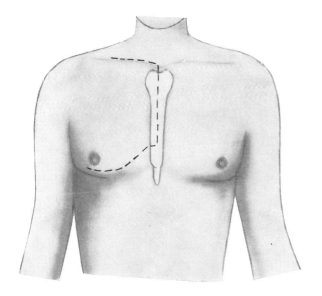

25

26

Dissection

Proximal tape control of the subclavian artery is obtained just distal to the innominate artery. Control of the subclavian artery is obtained distal to the aneurysm. The right innominate, jugular and subclavian veins are compressed by and adherent to the aneurysms and need not be dissected from the wall. Similarly, the phrenic and vagus nerves should be identified but need not be dissected from the aneurysm.

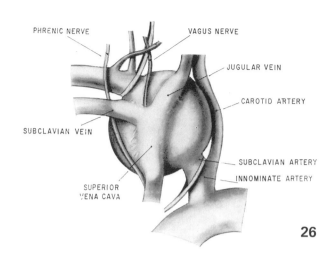

26

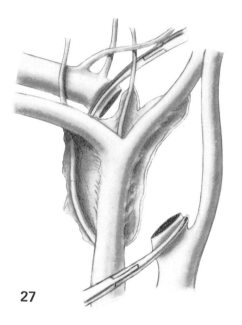

27

27

Partial excision

The artery is occluded proximally and distally. The aneurysm is then divided or opened. Any portion of the aneurysm which is easily dissected from the surrounding tissues can be excised. Any portion which is firmly adherent to important structures, such as major veins or nerves, can be left in place.

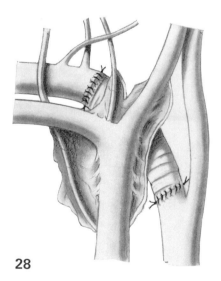

28

28

Graft replacement

A knitted plastic prosthesis is sutured end-to-end to the proximal and distal cut subclavian artery. A simple continuous suture is sufficient for these anastomoses.

POSTOPERATIVE CARE

These patients all require careful post-thoracotomy management. Catheters are inserted into the thoracic cavity and mediastinum and are brought through stab wounds, and connected to negative pressures of 10–20 cm of water to ensure drainage of blood and expansion of the lungs during the first 2–3 post-operative days. Oxygen by mask is recommended during the first 1–2 days. Atelectasis is prevented by hyperventilation and stimulation of coughing by means such as the intratracheal injection of saline, endotracheal suctioning, or breathing of bronchial irritants. The use of prophylactic antibiotics is recommended.

No anticoagulants are administered postoperatively. The patient receives heparin during the operation when on bypass or when major vessels are clamped, but protamine is administered to reverse this effect before the wound is closed.

References

DeBakey, M. E., Cooley, D. A., Crawford, E. S. and Morris, G. C., Jr. (1958). 'Aneurysms of the thoracic aorta: analysis of 179 patients treated by resection.' *J. thorac. Surg.* **36,** 393
Edwards, W. Sterling and Kerr, A. R. (1970). 'A safer technique for replacement of the entire ascending aorta and aortic valve.' *J. thorac. cardiovasc. Surg.* **59,** 837
Joyce, J. W., Fairbairn, J. F., Kincaird, O. W. and Juergens, J. L. (1964). 'Aneurysms of the thoracic aorta: a clinical study with special reference to prognosis.' *Circulation* **29,** 176
Moulder, D. G., Dilley, R. B. and Joseph, W. L. (1966). 'Surgical management of aneurysms of the thoracic aorta.' *Surgery* **60,** 142
Steenburg, R. W. and Ravitch, M. M. (1963). 'Cervico-thoracic approach for subclavian vessel injury from compound fracture of the clavicle: considerations of subclavian-axillary exposures.' *Ann. Surg.* **157,** 339

[The illustrations for this Chapter on Intrathoracic Aneurysms were drawn by Miss D. Elliott and Mr. R. Wabnitz.]

Dissecting Thoracic Aortic Aneurysms

James A. DeWeese, M.D., F.A.C.S.
Chairman of the Division of Cardiothoracic Surgery,
University of Rochester Medical Centre, and
Professor and Surgeon, Strong Memorial Hospital,
Rochester, New York

The pathologic process is best described as a dissecting haematoma within the media of the aorta rather than an aneurysm. It is only when the haematoma communicates with the aortic lumen and blood flows through this second channel that aneurysmal dilatation develops. This second channel also distorts the intima causing compression of the lumen and can occlude branches of the aorta. Smaller branches may be sheared off by the dissection.

Classically the patients present with severe chest and back pain. They may have central neurologic deficits secondary to occlusion of extracranial vessels, or be paraplegic from involvement of the anterior spinal arteries. They may be oliguric or anuric from renal artery occlusion. Ischaemia of an extremity secondary to peripheral arterial compression is commonly seen. The dissection may loosen the support of the cusps of the aortic valve allowing prolapse and aortic insufficiency. Rupture through the thin adventitia may occur into the pericardial, pleural, or abdominal cavities. The mortality rate in untreated patients is 50 per cent within 48 hr, 70 per cent within 1 week, and 90 per cent at 3 months.

Initial treatment

Almost 90 per cent of patients with dissecting haematomas are hypertensive. Except for patients who have suffered rupture the initial therapy should be aggressive drug control of the hypertension with the intravenous administration of trimethaphan or nitroprusside and propanol. The parenteral administration of reserpine or Aldomet should begin at the same time. Guanethidine and oral preparations of propranolol, reserpine and Aldomet may be useful later. The blood pressure must be significantly lowered, preferably below 120 mmHg. Close monitoring of the arterial pressure requires an intra-arterial line. Indwelling nasogastric tubes and urinary catheters are usually necessary. Endotracheal tubes or tracheostomies may be required for the control of tracheobronchial secretions in heavily sedated patients.

1

Diagnostic procedures

The diagnosis of dissection may be suspected or demonstrated with echocardiography, but angiography is usually required to prove the diagnosis. Only angiography can demonstrate a patent second channel and establish the sites of communication of the aortic lumen with this second channel. The extent of the dissection can also be demonstrated. It is of practical importance to know if it includes both ascending and descending aorta (Type I), ascending aorta only (Type II), or descending aorta only (Type III).

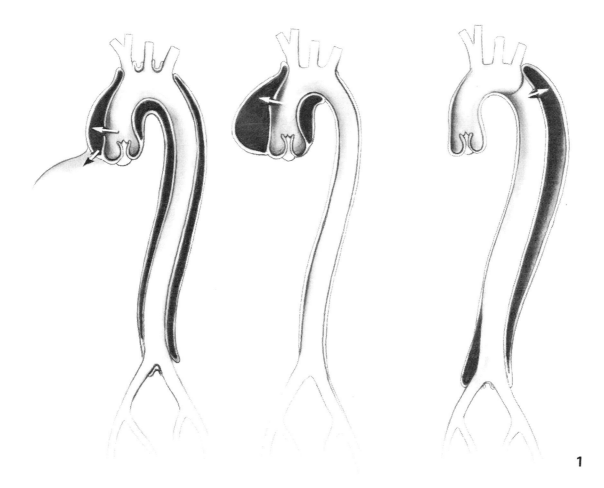

1

Indications

Patients with Type I, II and III dissections require immediate operations if rupture has occurred. Significant aortic insufficiency or the occlusion of major arteries is an indication for operations on Type I and II dissections. The operation is preferably delayed until the hypertension is under control and for at least 2 weeks if possible. Patients with Type III dissections require operation if major vessels are occluded and also if a patent second channel results in localized aneurysmal dilatation, which usually occurs just distal to the subclavian artery.

The entire extent of the disease cannot be resected. The operation is designed to obliterate the intimal tear which allows communication between the aortic lumen and second channel. At the same time, the second channel is circumferentially obliterated preventing progression of the dissection.

OPERATION FOR TYPES I AND II

2

Division of aorta

Operations on Type I and II dissections require total cardiopulmonary bypass (*see* Chapter on 'Intrathoracic Aneurysms', pages 84–95). In addition, the body is cooled to 20°C. The aorta is partially divided about 1 inch (2·5 cm) distal to the coronary arteries. The intimal tear is usually found at this level and the division of the aorta completed through the tear if possible. Catheters are then inserted into one or both coronary artery orifices for their perfusion with cooled blood from the pump oxygenator.

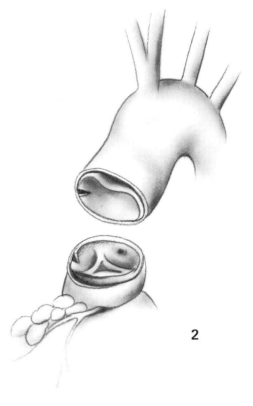

2

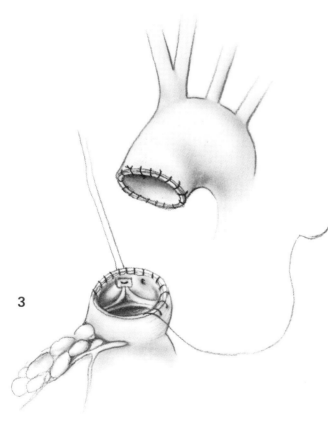

3

3

Obliteration of second channel

The dissection usually involves only a portion of the circumference of the vessel. The separated intima and adventitia are re-approximated and the remaining circumference of the vessel strengthened by a continuous over-and-over stitch of a fine 4/0 or 5/0 monofilament suture on a fine needle.

The aortic valve leaflets usually appear normal, but the intima and attached commissure and cusp are unsupported. The commissure is resuspended by placing a mattress stitch through a pledget, through the aortic wall, and then through a second pledget over which it is tied.

4

Aortic valve replacement

The aortic valve may be deformed as a result of co-existing disease or in the presence of a chronic dissection. The valve may then be excised and replaced with an artificial valve. Mattress sutures over pledgets are used to secure the valve in a subcoronary position.

In the presence of a chronic dissection and an aneurysmal aorta, the valve and an attached graft may be inserted within the aorta as described in the Chapter on 'Intrathoracic Aneurysms'.

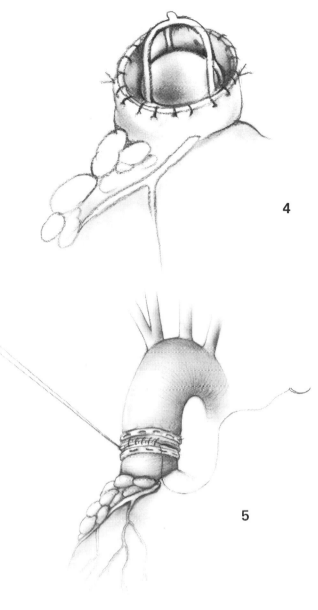

4

5

Re-approximation of aorta

If the aorta has an acceptably thick adventitia and is mobile so that the ends can be brought together without tension the aorta may be merely re-approximated. A 1–3 cm cuff of a synthetic plastic graft or plastic felt is placed about the ends of the aorta. A continuous mattress stitch of a 3/0 or a 4/0 mono-filament plastic suture is placed through all layers to evert the edges. Great care must be taken in placing these stitches to avoid leaving suture holes or needle tears in the thin intima. A second layer of fine sutures using an over-and-over continuous stitch is placed.

5

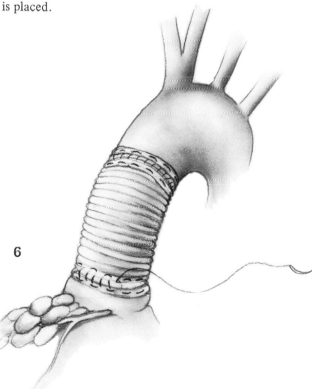

6

6

Insertion of graft

A graft is inserted if the dissection is sharply localized proximal to the innominate artery so that it can be totally excised, or if the edges of the divided aorta cannot be re-approximated without tension. A woven plastic tube graft is anastomosed end-to-end to the ends of the excised or divided aorta. An everting mattress stitch of 3/0 suture over a plastic cuff with a second over-and-over continuous stitch of 4/0 suture is used at each end. Any anastomotic leaks of suture holes must be controlled before the patient is taken off cardiopulmonary bypass. These leaks cannot be controlled when the aorta is distended by normal arterial pressures.

OPERATION FOR TYPE III

7

Exposure of descending aorta

Operations on Type III dissections require left heart bypass (*see* Chapter on 'Intrathoracic Aneurysms', pages 84–95). A left fourth interspace thoracotomy is performed. The mediastinal pleura is incised to expose the transverse aortic arch, the subclavian artery and the descending thoracic aorta. The first three pairs of intercostal arteries are carefully mobilized and taped. After left heart bypass has been initiated the aorta, and subclavian artery are clamped.

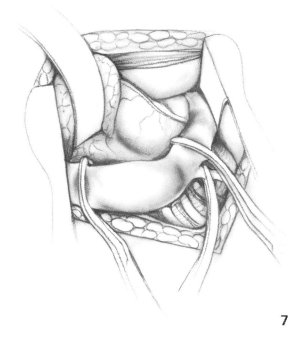

7

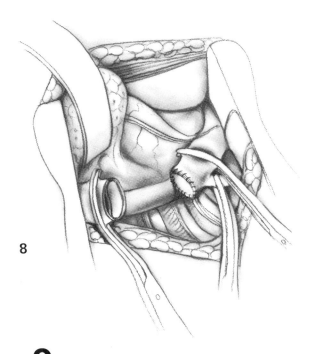

8

8

Division and oversewing of aorta

The aorta is divided at the level of the ligamentum arteriosum. The intimal tear allowing communication between the aortic lumen and second channel is usually found at this level. The ends of the aorta are then oversewn circumferentially to approximate the intima and media which obliterates the second channel.

9

Insertion of grafts

Unless the aorta is very mobile, a woven graft is interposed between the cut oversewn ends of the aorta. A 3-cm cuff of Dacron is placed around both ends. A continuous mattress stitch using a 3/0 monofilament suture with a fine needle is used to approximate the graft and aorta. The suture is passed through graft, aorta, and the short cuff of graft. An over-and-over continuous stitch of fine suture is then run as a second layer. When this first anastomosis is completed the clamp is removed allowing the graft to fill. The anastomosis, particularly its posterior half, is carefully inspected for leaks. The second anastomosis is completed and the graft and aorta carefully covered with pleura.

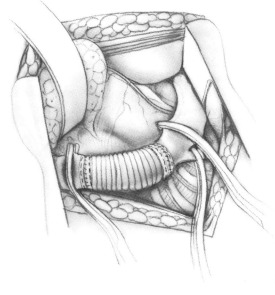

9

POSTOPERATIVE CARE

It is just as important to maintain the systemic arterial pressure in the normotensive range following operation as it was prior to operation to protect suture lines and to prevent progression of the dissection.

Endotracheal intubation with assisted ventilation is required for at least 18 hr following operation to allow for improvement in mechanics of respiration and gaseous diffusion.

The status of oxygenation, blood volume and ventricular function is followed closely by the monitoring of the blood gases, left atrial pressure, systemic arterial pressure, and cardiac output respectively.

Prophylactic antibiotics are indicated.

References

Austen, W.F. *et al.* (1967). 'Therapy of dissecting aneurysms.' *Archs Surg.* **95**, 835
DeBakey, M.E. *et al.* (1965). 'Surgical management of dissecting aneurysms of the aorta.' *J. thorac. cardiovasc. Surg.* **49**, 130
McFarland, J. *et al.* (1972). 'The medical treatment of dissecting aortic aneurysms.' *New Engl. J. Med.* **286**, 115
Wheat, M.W. (1973). 'Treatment of dissecting aneurysms of the aorta: current status.' *Prog. cardiovasc. Dis.* **16**, 87

[*The illustrations for this Chapter on Dissecting Thoracic Aortic Aneurysms were drawn by Mr. R. Wabnitz.*]

Aortocoronary Bypass Grafts

James A. DeWeese, M.D., F.A.C.S.
Chairman of the Division of Cardiothoracic Surgery,
University of Rochester Medical Centre, and
Professor and Surgeon, Strong Memorial Hospital,
Rochester, New York

Bypass grafts of occluded coronary arteries were first performed on a significant number of patients by Favoloro in 1968–1969. The bypass principle, so successful in operations for treatment of atherosclerotic lesions of other arteries, has become the most effective form of treatment for many patients with coronary artery disease.

Indications

Chronic angina which is preventing a patient from doing things he needs to do or wants to do despite an optimal medical programme of coronary vasodilators and propranolol is the most common indication for operation. Unstable angina as characterized by recent onset of angina or sudden exacerbation of chronic angina is an indication for urgent evaluation for operation. Complications of myocardial infarctions including mitral insufficiency, ventricular septal rupture, cardiogenic shock, or aneurysms not responding to optimal medical care are also indications for urgent operative intervention with correction of pathologic defects as well as the bypass of occlusive coronary artery lesions. Angina in patients with aortic valvular disease is also an indication for valve replacement as well as an aortocoronary bypass if coronary artery disease is present.

Patients require rather extensive evaluation including serial electrocardiograms, periodic measurement of the cardiac enzymes, coronary arteriography and ventriculography.

Contra-indications

Elective operations are not indicated on patients with advanced arteriosclerosis, particularly if it involves the smaller branches of the coronary arteries. Operation is not advised for patients with uncontrolled systemic disease or cancer. Poor ventricular function, as evidenced by ventriculographic evidence of significant myocardial akinesia, end diastolic ventricular pressure over 25 mmHg and ejection fractions less than 20 per cent are also contra-indications for elective operation.

The major contra-indication to operation in the more emergency situations, like cardiogenic shock, is the absence of bypassable lesions visible on coronary arteriograms. The lesions may not be bypassable because of the absence of occlusions of the major arteries, extensive visible calcification of all vessels, or extensive occlusive involvement of the smaller run-off vessels.

Preparation

The general preparations for these patients are those for any patient undergoing an operation on cardiopulmonary bypass and include discontinuance of smoking at least 1 week prior to admission, preoperative training in breathing and coughing exercises, provision for typed and cross-matched blood, and the administration of prophylactic antibiotics.

Propranolol should be discontinued at least 48 hr prior to operation.

THE OPERATION

1

Preparation

The patient is anaesthetized in the supine position with at least one arm at his side. The chest and both groins and legs are prepared and draped. A needle is inserted percutaneously into the radial artery for the monitoring of blood gases and systemic arterial pressures. A catheter is inserted into the bladder for the monitoring of urine flow.

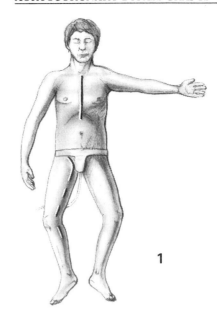

2

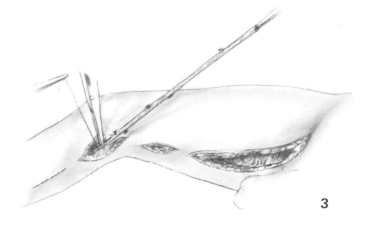

The groin incision

The greater saphenous vein is most commonly used as the bypass graft. A curved incision is made in the groin to expose the saphenous vein and the common femoral artery. The vein is divided at the sapheno-femoral junction. The course of the vein is identified with the index finger and additional incisions made. The branches of the vein are carefully ligated 1 mm from the vein, taking care not to catch adventitia of the vein in the tie which causes localized narrowing.

3

Removal of vein

The vein is removed through multiple incisions and, if necessary, it can be removed as far as the ankle. In fact, if the vein is more than 1 cm in diameter in the thigh it is preferable to obtain the vein from the lower leg where it is closer to the size of the coronary arteries.

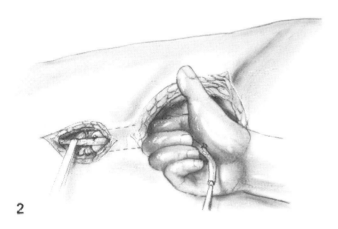

4

Preparation of vein

The vein is reversed and filled with heparinized saline or blood. Care is taken not to over-distend the vein which can cause tissue disruption. The vein is also handled very carefully to avoid intimal damage. Clamps or forceps are used to pick up the adventitia but not the whole thickness of the vein wall.

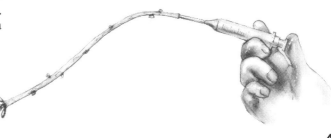

4

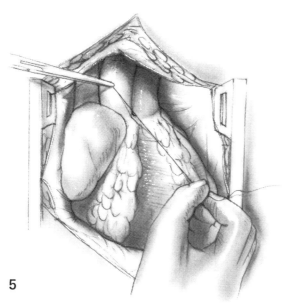

5

5

Exposure of heart and coronary arteries

A median sternotomy is performed and the pericardium incised in the mid-line and along the diaphragm to expose the entire anterior surface of the heart. The coronary arteries are carefully palpated and a soft area of artery identified which is distal to the area of stenosis or obstruction previously demonstrated on coronary arteriograms. While the heart is in its normal position, a string is cut the length of the proposed grafts.

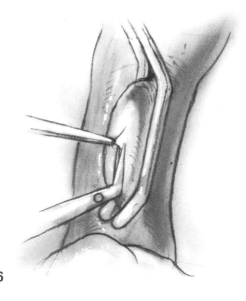

6

AORTIC ANASTOMOSIS

6

Partial occlusion of aorta

The patient is given 5000 units of heparin sodium intravenously. At least 1 min later a vascular clamp is applied to partially occlude the ascending aorta. The systemic arterial pressure is carefully observed during the application of the clamp. A generous portion of the aorta can be partially occluded before the blood pressure is affected. A small area of peri-adventitial tissue is removed.

7

Aortic preparation

A No. 18 needle is then inserted into the occluded aorta to remove any blood present and to assure that the clamp is applied tightly enough.

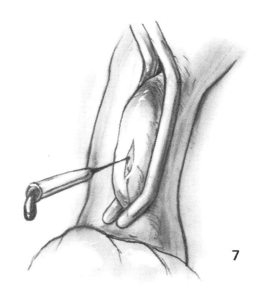

7

8

Aortotomy

The aorta is then pinched together with fingers while a narrow-tipped pituitary rongeur is used to grasp a 3—4-mm in diameter edge of the aortic wall.

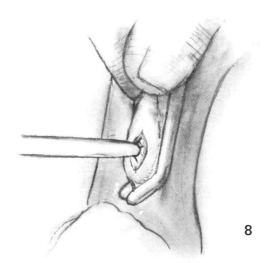

8

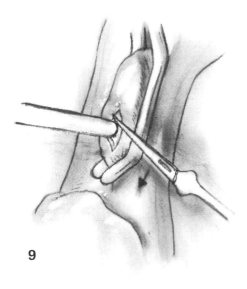

9

9

Circular opening

A straight-edged knife is then used to excise a 4-mm in diameter button of the aortic wall.

10

Preparation of vein

The distal end of a segment of the saphenous vein is then prepared for the proximal anastomosis. Excess adventitial tissue is removed. The end of the vein is enlarged with a short longitudinal incision.

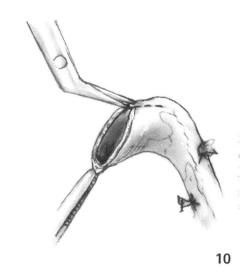

10

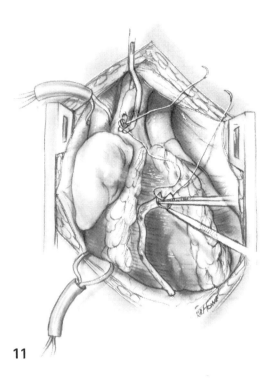

11

11

Initial stitches

The end-to-side anastomosis is begun by passing a fine 5/0 or 6/0 monofilament suture through the vein at the tip of the longitudinal incision and continuing the stitch from inside to outside the aorta near the distal end of the aortotomy.

12

Over-and-over stitch

The suture line is continued as an over-and-over inverting stitch for a short distance. The tip of the needle is kept in direct vision at all times to prevent the suture from catching the posterior or opposite wall of the vein or aorta.

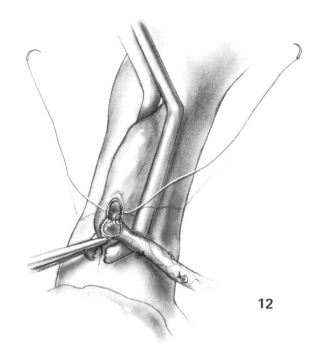

12

13

Completion of anastomosis

One end of the stitch is carried around the end of the aortotomy. The stitch is completed and tied in the mid-portion of the aortotomy.

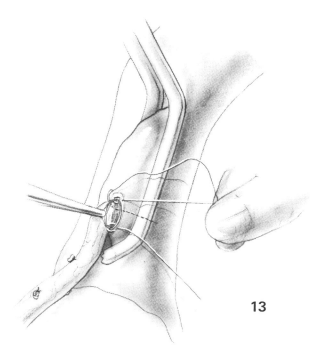

13

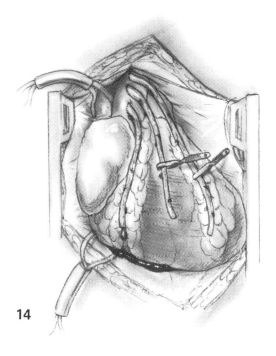

14

14

Checking for anastomotic bleeding

All of the proximal anastomoses are completed. The aortic clamp is removed and the flow through each graft is checked. The anastomoses are also inspected carefully for any leaks. If additional sutures are needed, very small mattress stitches using 6/0 or 7/0 sutures are used.

DISTAL ANASTOMOSIS TO RIGHT CORONARY ARTERY

15

Cardiopulmonary bypass and exposure of right coronary artery

The patient is placed on cardiopulmonary bypass and a sump catheter inserted into the left ventricle for decompression. The patient's body temperature is then cooled to 20°C. The diaphragmatic surface of the heart is exposed by placing stitches into the right ventricle, elevating the heart, and attaching the stitches to the drapes. The distal end of the right coronary artery is exposed by grasping the fat on either side of the artery and incising the overlying tissue.

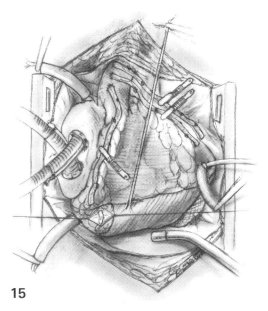

15

16

Arteriotomy

An incision is made in the right coronary artery with the tip of a pointed knife. The ascending aorta is then occluded preventing blood flow through the coronary arteries. The anastomosis can be performed in a relatively dry field.

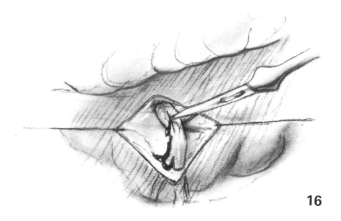

16

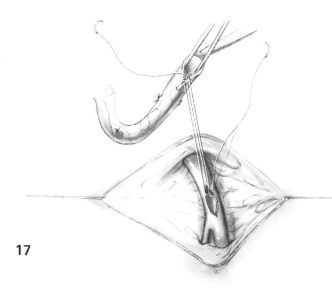

17

17

Initial stitch

The end of the vein is enlarged with a longitudinal incision. The anastomosis is begun by passing a 6/0 or 7/0 monofilament suture through the vein at the tip of the longitudinal incision and continuing the stitch from inside to outside the right coronary artery near the proximal end of the arteriotomy.

18

Over-and-over continuous stitch

The suture is continued for a short distance on either side as a continuous over-and-over everting stitch.

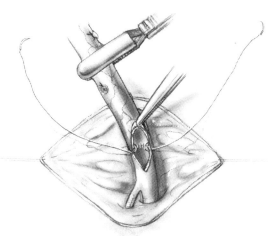

18

19

Distal stitch

An everting mattress stitch is then made at the distal end of the anastomosis. The stitch starts from outside the vein near its distal end and then comes from inside to outside the coronary artery near the distal end of the arteriotomy.

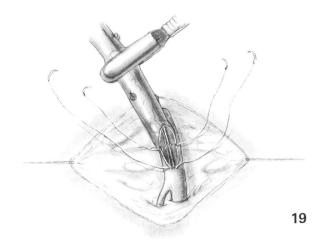

19

20

Exposure of tip of needle

The ends of the suture are then run as an over-and-over stitch to the middle of the arteriotomy where they are tied. A forceps grasps the adventitia of the vein holding the anastomosis open so that the tip of the needle can be visualized throughout the course of its passage. This prevents the suture from catching the posterior wall of the artery and narrowing the anastomosis.

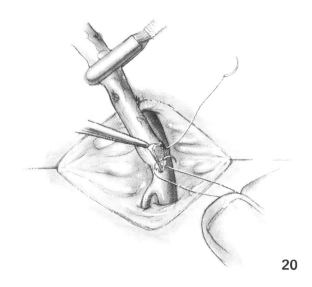

20

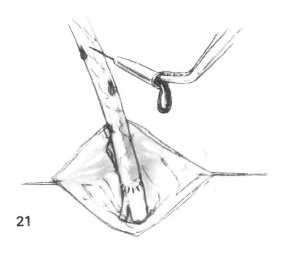

21

21

Evacuation of air from graft

The aortic clamp is removed allowing some retrograde flow into the vein graft. The clamp on the vein is also removed but only after placing a 25-gauge needle into the graft at its most superior position to remove any trapped air.

22

Exposure of circumflex artery

The circumflex artery and its three major branches can be visualized by retracting the heart upward and to the right. An opened moist loose-meshed gauze is placed on the heart and the fingers spread to expose the branch chosen for the anastomosis. The anterior descending artery is easily visualized by placing a pad in the pericardium under the apex of the heart.

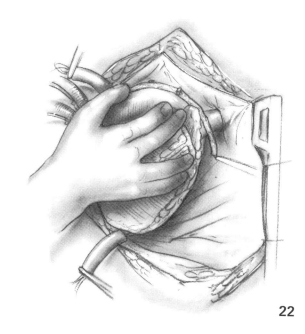

22

THROMBO-ENDARTERECTOMY OF RIGHT COR-ONARY ARTERY

23

Establishing plane

There are frequently atherosclerotic plaques of the distal right coronary artery, which cause a severe stenosis, or obstruction but which end abruptly within a few millimetres of the bifurcation. An incision is made over the plaque and a plane of dissection established which is usually just external to the diseased media.

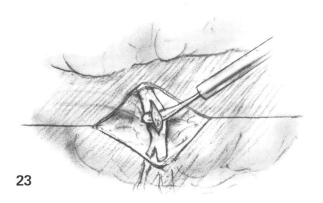

23

24

The endarterectomy

The endarterectomy is then performed with blunt dissection and eversion of the vessel to a point where the plaque has tapered to near normal intima. At that point the intima generally tears leaving adherent intima distally. If there is any question about the endarterectomy ending in that fashion, a small arteriotomy is made and more intima removed or tacked to the normal media. The distal end of a saphenous vein bypass graft is then anastomosed to the arteriotomy in the right coronary artery.

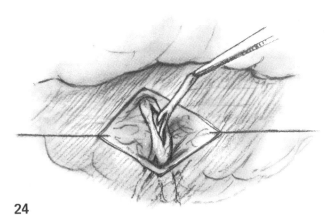

24

25

Measurement of blood flow in grafts

Following completion of each distal anastomosis the aortic clamp is removed for 5 min. Rewarming of the patient is begun when the aorta is occluded for the final anastomosis. When the oesophageal temperature reaches 37°C, the patient is taken off cardiopulmonary bypass.

The blood flow through each graft is measured with an electromagnetic flowmeter. If the flow is less than 25 ml/min the graft is carefully inspected for correctable technical errors, such as twisting, excessive tension or strictures secondary to the catching of adventitia by ties or sutures.

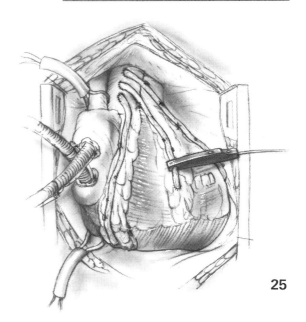

25

26

Internal mammary artery for bypass grafts

The internal mammary artery can also be used as a bypass graft either by leaving its proximal end *in situ* or as a free graft. The artery is mobilized from its origin to the fifth intercostal space and all of its branches divided. The artery must be handled with great care to avoid intimal damage. The distal end of the artery will usually reach the proximal right, left and circumflex arteries. For more distal anastomoses, the proximal end of the artery can be divided and transposed to the ascending aorta.

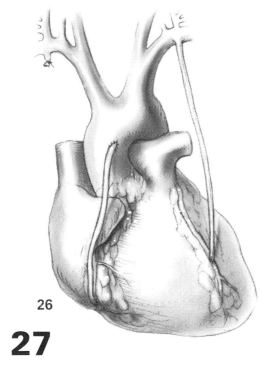

26

27

Aortocoronary bypass graft and resection of ventricular aneurysm

Ventricular aneurysms result from myocardial infarction as they are usually associated with significantly occlusive lesions of the coronary arteries. The aneurysms usually involve the apical anterior and anterolateral aspects of the left ventricle. The anterior descending artery is frequently completely occluded and involved in the aneurysm. The right and circumflex arteries may demonstrate proximal occlusive lesions. Indications for operation include angina, heart failure, ventricular arrhythmias, and emboli from mural thrombus.

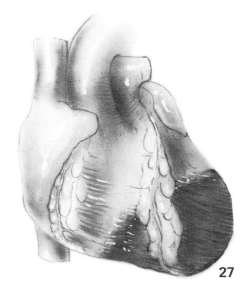

27

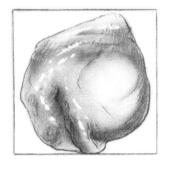

28

Resection of ventricular aneurysm

The limits of the aneurysm can be determined by observing the invagination of its fibrous wall when a left ventricular sump is inserted and suction applied. The aneurysm is excised leaving a 1-cm margin of the sac. Care is taken not to excise the papillary muscles of the mitral valve.

29

Closure of ventriculotomy

The ventricle is then closed in two layers. The first layer is a continuous horizontal mattress stitch of a heavy suture over a plastic felt pad. The second layer is a continuous over-and-over stitch of the same suture. Any occlusive lesions of the right or circumflex are bypassed with either autogenous vein or mammary artery.

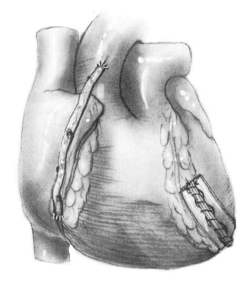

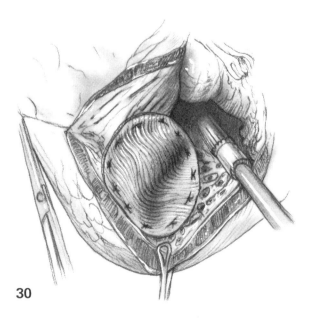

30

Closure of ruptured ventricular septum

Anteroseptal myocardial infarctions may result in rupture of the ventricular septum. Congestive heart failure may necessitate early resection of the infarct and patching of the defect. If the patient's condition permits, operation is delayed for at least 6 weeks and an aneurysmectomy and patching of the defect performed when the septum can be sutured with more confidence. A large plastic patch is placed over the defect and held with mattress sutures. A second patch can be placed on the right ventricular side of the defect if the entire septum feels friable.

31

Aortocoronary bypass graft and mitral valve replacement

Myocardial infarctions may cause severe mitral insufficiency due to rupture of papillary muscles or chorda tendineae. An operation is indicated in the presence of heart failure. In the presence of an infarct or aneurysm, the mitral valve should be replaced through the left ventricle. Following infarctectomy or aneurysmectomy, the mitral valve is excised and replaced with an artificial valve.

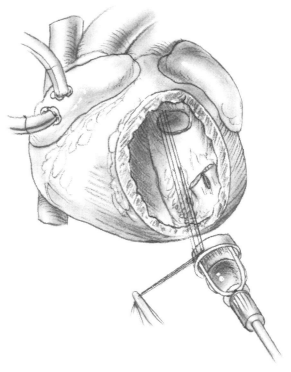

31

POSTOPERATIVE CARE

For the first 12–26 hr after operation intratracheal tubes connected to a respirator for assisted ventilation, are essential. Adequacy of ventilation is determined by frequent analysis of the blood gases (pH, pO_2, pCO_2 and total CO_2).

Cardiac function and the status of fluid replacement are monitored by the continuous measurement of left atrial pressure and systemic blood pressure and intermittent measurement of the urinary output and cardiac index. Accurate measurements of these four parameters provides the information necessary for the logical use of inotropic drugs, fluids, blood and diuretics during the critical first 36 hr after operation.

Vigorous respiratory therapy and ambulation is indicated following removal of the intratracheal tube to prevent pulmonary complications.

Antibiotic therapy is continued for the first 5 days for prophylaxis against significant pulmonary, urinary, blood stream, and wound infections.

The electrocardiogram is monitored continuously during the first 7 days after operation for the early detection of any arrhythmia. Temporary atrial and ventricular pacemaker wires are in place for 5 days for treatment of wandering atrial pacemakers, and heart-block. Atrial fibrillation is treated vigorously with digitalis and quinidine or DC conversion. Ventricular arrhythmias are treated promptly with lidocaine and external defibrillation is immediately available.

References

Barner, H. B. (1974). 'Double internal mammary-coronary artery bypass.' *Archs Surg.* **109**, 627
DeWeese, J. A., Moss, A. J. and Yu, P. N. (1972). 'Infarctectomy and closure of ventricular septal rupture following myocardial infarction.' *Circulation* **45, 46** 1–97
Favaloro, R. G., Effler, D. B., Groves, L. K., Sheldon, W. C. and Sones, F. M., Jr. (1970). 'Direct myocardial revascularization by saphenous vein graft: present operative technique and indications.' *Ann. thorac. Surg.* **10**, 97
Flemma, R. J., Johnson, W. D., Lepley, D., Auer, J. E., Tector, A. J. and Blitz, J. (1971). 'Simultaneous valve replacement and aorta-to-coronary saphenous vein bypass.' *Ann. thorac. Surg.* **12**, 163
Green, G. E., Spencer, F. C., Tice, D. A. and Stertzer, S. H. (1970). 'Arterial and venous microsurgical bypass grafts for coronary artery disease.' *J. thorac. cardiovasc. Surg.* **60**, 491
Groves, L. K., Loop, F. D. and Silver, G. M. (1972). 'Endarterectomy as a supplement to coronary artery-saphenous vein bypass surgery.' *J. thorac. cardiovasc. Surg.* **64**, 514

[The illustrations for this Chapter on Aortocoronary Bypass Grafts were drawn by Mr. R. Howe.]

Aorto-iliac Reconstruction Bypass Graft. Thrombo-endarterectomy

Charles Rob, *M.C.,* M.D., M.Chir., F.R.C.S.
Professor and Chairman of the Department of Surgery,
University of Rochester School of Medicine and
Dentistry, Rochester, New York

and

James A. DeWeese, M.D., F.A.C.S.
Chairman of the Division of Cardiothoracic Surgery,
University of Rochester Medical Centre, and
Professor and Surgeon, Strong Memorial Hospital,
Rochester, New York

PRE-OPERATIVE

Indications

These procedures are indicated in symptomatic stenosis or thrombosis of the abdominal aorta and iliac arteries when the general condition, particularly the cardiac condition, is satisfactory.

Principles of thrombo-endarterectomy

Although both operations had been performed previously, dos Santos (1947) is rightly credited with the development of the open operation and Cannon, Barker and Kattas (1958) with the development of the semi-closed procedure. The basic technique is to develop a plane of cleavage in the media. This results in the surgeon removing the intima, the plaques of atheroma, any thrombus, the internal elastic lamina and the inner layers of the media. The adventitia, the external elastic lamina and the outer layers of the media remain and form the wall of the reconstructed artery.

Thrombo-endarterectomy versus a bypass graft

The ideal situation for a thrombo-endarterectomy is a localized occlusion of the common iliac artery or a localized occlusion of the aorta. Here the severely diseased segment is short and the immediate distal artery usually has a nearly normal wall. When the disease involves the aorta and iliac arteries, a thrombo-endarterectomy gives excellent results and so does a bypass procedure; here the choice will depend upon the individual characteristics of the patient and the surgeon, but we have a strong preference for the bypass graft. The procedure is simpler and can be performed more rapidly. The dissection is minimal. In the male retrograde ejaculation is less common (May, DeWeese and Rob, 1969) and the long-term results have been good (Minken *et al.*, 1968). In some of these patients the bypass may be combined with a thrombo-endarterectomy of the proximal hypogastric artery.

Anticoagulant drugs

About 5 min before the arterial clamps are applied, the anaesthetist gives the patient 50–100 mg of heparin intravenously (depending upon the patient's body weight). Then at the time the proximal arterial clamp is removed, after the artery has been sutured, he gives 50–100 mg of protamine sulphate to neutralize the action of the heparin. Apart from this we do not use anticoagulant drugs in these patients.

THE OPERATIONS

The incision

The abdominal aorta and iliac arteries may be exposed through either an extraperitoneal (Rob, 1963) or a transperitoneal route. The extraperitoneal route has the advantage that it disturbs the patient less and the convalescence is shorter. It is preferred for occlusions of the common iliac arteries and localized occlusions of the abdominal aorta in whom it is planned to do a thrombo-endarterectomy. The transperitoneal is preferred if an aorto-iliac or aorto-femoral bypass is planned.

1a & b

The extraperitoneal route. Division of the muscles

The incision follows the lines of the creases on the abdominal wall and should pass between the segmental vessels and nerves. The incision is usually about 8 inches (20 cm) long and begins at the mid-line about 0·5 inches (1·3 cm) above or below the umbilicus extending laterally across the rectus abdominis muscle towards the flank. The rectus muscle is transected and at its outer margin the surgeon locates the segmental neurovascular bundle. The oblique and transversus muscles are then divided either above or below this bundle.

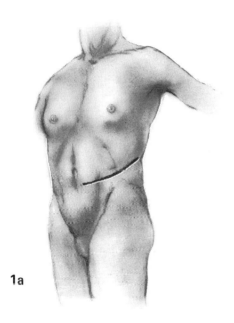

1a

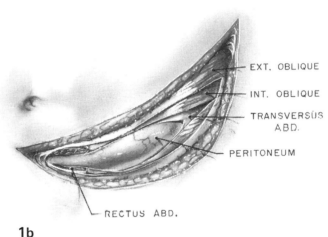

EXT. OBLIQUE

INT. OBLIQUE

TRANSVERSUS ABD.

PERITONEUM

RECTUS ABD.

1b

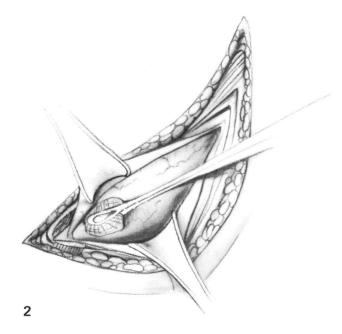

2

2

Stripping the peritoneum

After division of the muscles the surgeon incises the outer edge of the posterior sheath of the rectus abdominis muscle to expose the peritoneum. This incision is then extended with scissors medially and laterally throughout the length of the incision. Sometimes the rectus sheath medially is firmly attached to the peritoneum in these patients, this sheath is not incised over this section. If the surgeon makes a hole into the peritoneum, it is immediately closed with sutures. The peritoneum is now stripped from the abdominal wall for a distance of about 2 inches (5 cm) above and below the incision. It is then stripped laterally and posteriorly and retracted medially with the ureter to expose the abdominal aorta and iliac arteries.

3a & b

In many patients adequate exposure can be obtained without dividing the inferior mesenteric artery. But if greater exposure is required, this vessel is exposed extraperitoneally and divided between ligatures. This allows the peritoneum to be retracted further to the opposite side and greatly increases this exposure. If the patient has an intraperitoneal lesion which requires examination, the peritoneum can at this point be incised, the lesion explored, and perhaps treated and the peritoneum closed before the surgeon proceeds with the extraperitoneal part of the operation. In these two illustrations a small aortic aneurysm has been exposed extraperitoneally. The inferior mesenteric artery arises from this aneurysm.

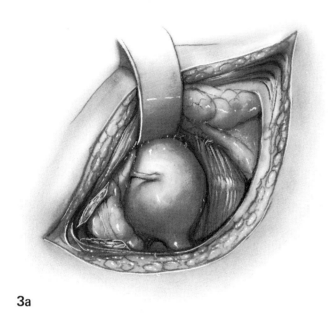

3a

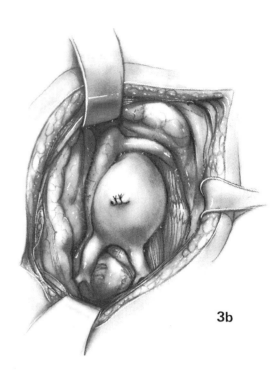

3b

THE INTRAPERITONEAL ROUTE

4

The incision

This may be mid-line, paramedian or transverse. We prefer the mid-line incision which should extend from below the umbilicus to the tip of the xiphoid. After exploration of the abdomen, the peritoneum over the aorta and iliac arteries is incised to the right of the inferior mesenteric artery. Proximally the surgeon should leave an adequate cuff close to the duodenum for later closure. He must then identify and avoid first the inferior mesenteric and higher the left renal veins. Distally he should identify and avoid the ureters as they cross the iliac arteries. If an aortofemoral bypass graft is to be inserted, separate incisions are made over the common femoral arteries. These vessels and the femoral canals are exposed.

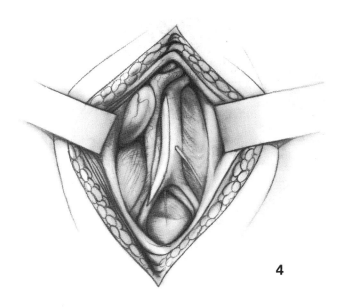
4

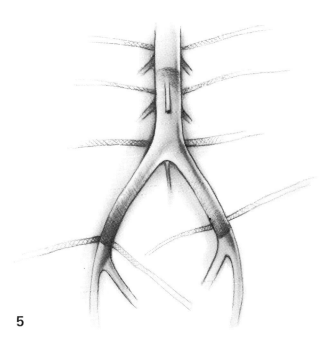
5

5

Mobilization of the aorta and iliac arteries

A major difference between an aortofemoral bypass and an open thrombo-endarterectomy is that complete mobilization of the artery and its branches is required for a thrombo-endarterectomy whilst only a short segment of the anterior and lateral surfaces need be freed for a bypass graft. For an open thrombo-end-arterectomy the artery throughout the involved segment and for about 2–3 cm proximal and distal must be fully mobilized and all branches identified and freed. In the aorto-iliac segment this will include the distal abdominal aorta, the distal lumbar arteries, the middle sacral artery, the common iliac and proximal external iliac and hypogastric arteries. In some patients the mobilization will extend proximally to include the inferior mesenteric artery, further pairs of lumbar arteries, and perhaps the renal arteries. A lesser dissection is required if the occlusion is localized to one common iliac artery.

THROMBO-ENDARTERECTOMY (OPEN METHOD)

Mobilization of the aorta and iliac arteries.

6

The arterial incision

With the open method an incision is made from one end of the proposed thrombo-endarterectomy zone to the other. The incision is carried through the arterial wall into the lumen if this is patent; otherwise it is carried at least to the intima. If the bifurcation of the abdominal aorta is being repaired in this way, two incisions are recommended: a long incision extending from the aorta down over one common iliac artery, and a short separate incision into the opposite common iliac artery. The pre-aortic plexus of autonomic nerves cannot be completely preserved, but as many of these nerves as possible should be left intact.

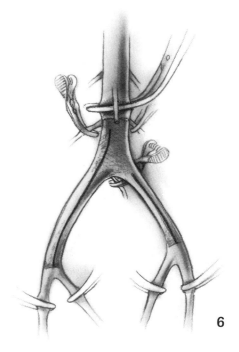

6

7

The plane of cleavage

This is the key to the operation. The surgeon must establish and carry out his dissection in the correct plane. Immediately superficial to the intima a plane can be established; this is not the correct layer. Slightly superficial to this the correct plane lies in the media. This is a definite layer and, once entered, blunt dissection easily removes the inner core. This consists of the intima, the internal elastic lamina, and the inner layers of the media, the atheromatous plaques and the thrombus if present. The residual arterial wall consists of the adventitia, the external lamina and the outer layers of the media.

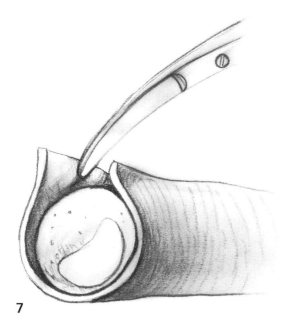

7

8

The thrombo-endarterectomy

The dissection in the plane of cleavage in the arterial wall is now continued circumferentially and longitudinally until the whole of the diseased segment has been freed. Proximally and distally the inner core is now divided with scissors and the diseased inner layers are removed. The area is flushed with saline and all loose fragments are removed. The clamps are loosened for a moment to confirm a good flow from each end of the vessel and then the whole area is flushed with saline for a second time.

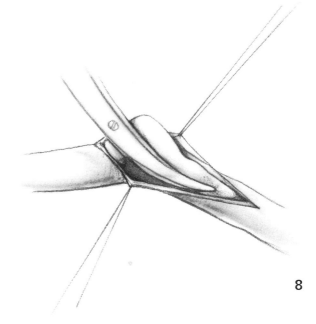

8

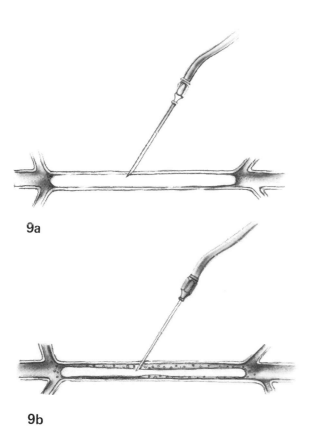

9a

9b

9a & b

Gas endarterectomy

This is of particular value in small vessels but also may be used in very large arteries such as the aorta or iliacs. A 26-gauge needle is introduced into the arterial wall and carbon dioxide gas is injected at pressures of up to 400 mmHg at gas flows of approximately 5–15 l/min. This gas naturally finds the plane of cleavage in the media so that inner core consisting of the thrombus, the intima, any plaques of atheroma, the internal elastic lamina and the inner layers of the media is fully mobilized. Small incisions are then made at each end of the diseased segment and the inner core is removed. The area is then flushed with saline, any loose tags or fragments are removed and the proximal and distal intima is inspected if possible.

10

The distal intima

It is important to cut the distal intima in such a way that no loose flaps remain. When possible the distal section should be close to a branch or bifurcation; a bridge of intima at this point serves to anchor the inner layers and then, combined with the attachment of the intima by the anterior suture line, prevents distal dissection when the blood flow is restored. The bifurcation of the common iliac artery is a good example of this, a bridge of intima passing from the inferior wall of the hypogastric artery to the posterior wall of the external iliac artery acts as such a bridge. In some instances it may be necessary to anchor the intima with mattress sutures placed circumferentially and tied outside of the vessel.

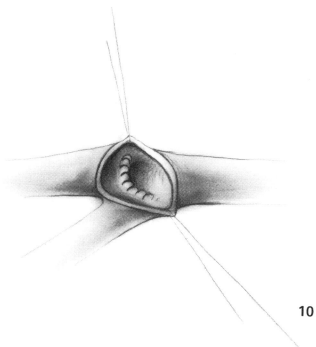

10

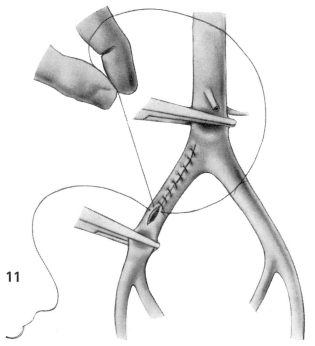

11

11

Closure of arterial incision

A continuous suture of 4/0 silk or Prolene with a simple over-and-over stitch is used for all except the smallest vessels. The suture should extend for a short distance beyond each end of the incision so that the intima is firmly anchored at this point. It is important not to pull the suture too tight because constriction of the lumen can be produced in this way. A suture inserted under slight tension tightens when the arterial flow is restored to the vessel. At this point the sutured vessel may be wrapped in surgical absorbable haemostatic gauze.

12

Removal of clamps; additional sutures

The distal clamps are removed first and the reconstructed segment allowed to fill with blood. At this time any large defects in the suture line are repaired with additional interrupted sutures. The proximal clamp is then removed and a gauze pack is held on the under suture line for 5 min. If necessary, further interrupted sutures are inserted after this but if only slight bleeding persists a further period of pressure is usually preferable to additional sutures.

13

Eversion technique

An alternative method is to transect the artery proximal or distal to the diseased area and to remove the inner core by everting and rolling the outer layers until the whole inner diseased core of the artery can be removed back from the proximal to the distal clamps. The divided ends of the artery are then anastomosed together with a continuous silk or Prolene suture. This technique is particularly useful for occlusions of the proximal hypogastric (internal iliac) arteries.

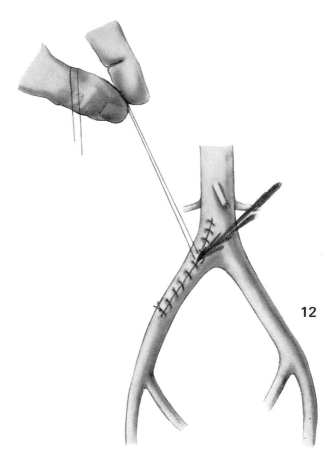

12

SEMI-CLOSED METHOD

Principles

The basis of this technique is to open the artery proximal and distal to the occluded area. At the distal end the correct plane of cleavage is established; a ring stripper is then introduced into this plane at the distal end and passed up the vessel to the proximal end. The inner core is then removed and, after flushing with saline and trimming of the divided intimal ends, the arterial incisions are closed. In the aorto-iliac segment this technique is particularly useful for occlusions of the external iliac arteries.

14

The incisions

The artery is exposed proximal and distal to the diseased area. At each end about 4 cm of the vessel is mobilized and all branches are carefully preserved. Clamps are then applied and the vessel at each level is incised transversely. Approximately two thirds of the circumference of the vessel is opened in this way.

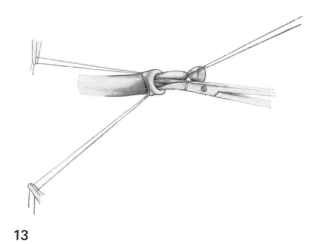

13

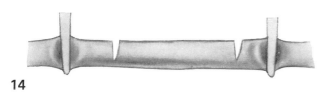

14

15

Introduction of stripper

At the distal incision the thrombo-endarterectomy is started. The inner core is dissected free and completely transected. Two sutures are then placed through the inner core and the ring of the stripper passed over these two sutures and the inner core.

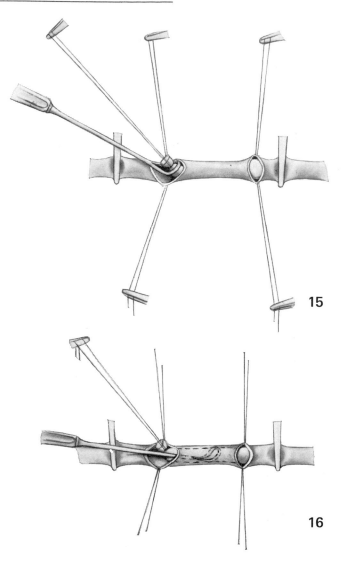

15

16

The actual stripping

Gentle traction is applied to the sutures attached to the inner core and the stripper is advanced in the plane of cleavage in the media in a proximal direction. The stripper is moved proximally by a combination of rotary and gentle pushing movements; it is found that it usually advances easily for the first few centimetres. For long occlusions, multiple incisions in the artery may be necessary. This technique may be combined with a gas endarterectomy.

16

17

17

Removal of the inner core

When the stripper reaches the proximal incision, the inner core is carefully divided so that a flap of loose intima does not remain in the vessel. Traction is then applied to both the inner core through the sutures previously placed in it and to the stripper. Both are then removed together through the distal incision.

18

Removal of loose fragments

A polyethylene tube attached to a syringe is then introduced into the vessel. The whole area is thoroughly irrigated with saline on several occasions and as much as possible of the lumen inspected to reduce to a minimum the number of loose fragments remaining in the lumen of the artery.

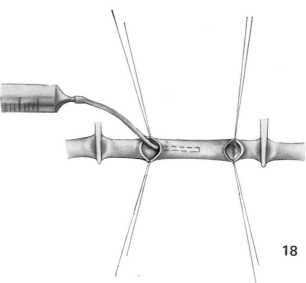

18

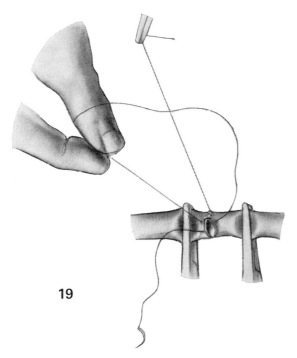

19

19

Closure of the arterial incisions

An over-and-over suture of 4/0 silk or Prolene produces a satisfactory closure and because the incisions are transverse the lumen is not narrowed. The clamps are then removed from the distal artery and from all branches. This allows the reconstructed segment to fill with blood. After it has filled, the proximal arterial clamp is removed and a pulsatile flow restored to the artery.

AORTO-ILIAC OR AORTOFEMORAL BYPASS GRAFT

20

Exposure of the aorta

The peritoneum is incised to the right of the inferior mesenteric vessels and the anterior and lateral surfaces of the abdominal aorta are exposed so that all but the posterior quarter of the circumference of the aortic wall is freed. This means that the origin of the inferior mesenteric artery is freed and this vessel carefully preserved. The lumbar arteries need not be exposed for an end-to-side anastomosis. It is usually best to attach the bypass graft to the anterior surface of the abdominal aorta between the renal vein above and the inferior mesenteric artery below. Sometimes there is not sufficient room for this and there the inferior mesenteric artery should be divided between ligatures.

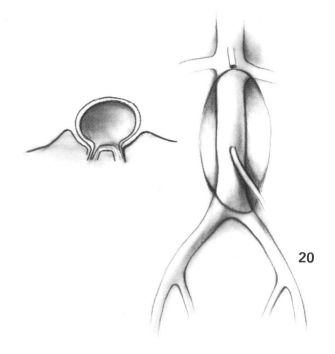

20

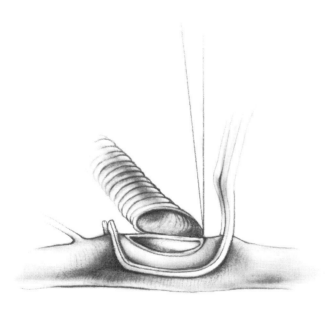

21

21

The proximal anastomosis end-to-side

A side clamp is applied to the abdominal aorta of sufficient size to permit an incision at least 2·5 cm long in the anterior aortic wall. If the aortic wall is diseased, it may be necessary to perform a thrombo-endarterectomy of that part included in the clamp. The main stem of the aortic prosthesis is cut obliquely to fit the size of the aortic opening and the prosthesis is then sutured to the aorta with a continuous suture of 4/0 Dacron. For the average-sized patient we use a woven Dacron bifurcated prosthesis with a mainstem 20 mm in diameter. In our hands the long-term results have been identical when either a knitted or woven Dacron prosthesis has been used in this situation; and the initial blood loss has been less when a woven prosthesis was used.

22

The proximal anastomosis end-to-end

We prefer the end-to-side technique but sometimes it is necessary to perform an end-to-end anastomosis between the abdominal aorta and the graft. For this the aorta must be fully mobilized and clamped between the renal arteries and the diseased segment. One or two pairs of lumbar arteries will be isolated and clamped. It may be necessary to divide one pair of these vessels between ligatures, but they should be preserved if possible if they are open. The aorta is then divided and the distal stump oversewn with large, interrupted sutures and sometimes an additional continuous over-and-over suture. The proximal aorta is then prepared by removing all debris and calcified plaques. It is then anastomosed to the Dacron prosthesis with a continuous 4/0 Dacron suture.

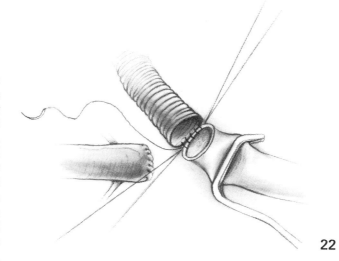

22

23

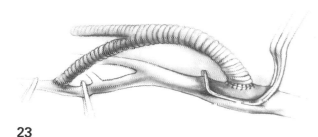

23

The distal anastomosis to the external iliac arteries

This should only be performed when the external iliac artery is nearly normal, an anastomosis at this site often fails if the artery is too diseased. The peritoneum over the artery is incised just above the inguinal ligament and the vessel mobilized for a distance of about 4 cm. A tunnel is then made behind the sigmoid colon and the ureter on the left. On the right side the ureter is retracted proximally and the graft placed in front of it. The limbs of the Dacron prosthesis are then placed in these tunnels and anastomosed end-to-side to the external iliac arteries with continuous sutures of 4/0 Dacron or Prolene.

24

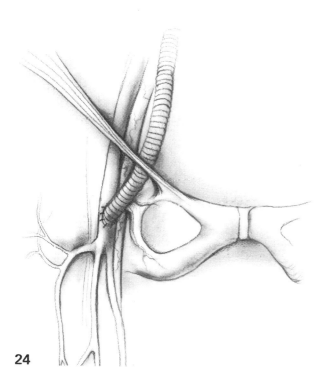

24

The distal anastomosis to the common femoral arteries

This is frequently the site because this artery often has a good lumen and flow can be restored at least into the profunda artery and often into all the arteries of the limb. A transverse incision is made below the inguinal ligament and about 4 cm of the common femoral artery is exposed and mobilized. All branches of the artery and the saphenous vein are carefully preserved. Tunnels are then made through the femoral canals and behind the peritoneum, the limbs of the Dacron prosthesis are placed in these tunnels. They are then anastomosed end-to-side to the common femoral arteries with continuous sutures of 4/0 Dacron or Prolene.

SPECIAL TECHNIQUE FOR A HIGH OCCLUSION OF THE ABDOMINAL AORTA

25

The exposure

An upper mid-line abdominal incision is made to expose the abdominal aorta just below the pancreas. The duodenum is retracted upwards and to the right and the inferior mesenteric vein to the left. The left renal vein is identified and mobilized. Tributaries such as the ovarian or testicular and the left adrenal veins are divided between ligatures. Both of the renal arteries and the abdominal aorta just above them are isolated. The aorta is occluded by the disease to the level of the renal arteries. It is now divided below the point where the left renal vein crosses it. Clamps are not required at this time because the aorta is thrombosed. The end of the distal segment is oversewn.

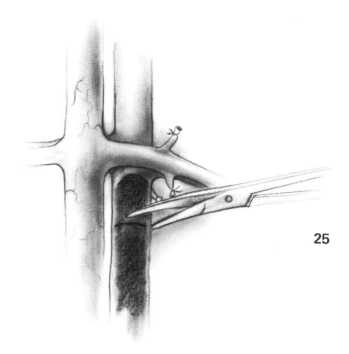

25

26a, b & c

Thrombo-endarterectomy of the proximal aorta

The stump of the occluded and divided aorta is now freed from behind the left renal vein and hooked up so that it lies in front of this vein. A clamp is now placed around the aorta above the renal arteries. but it is not closed. A thrombo-endarterectomy

of the occluded aortic stump is now begun. As soon as bleeding begins, this clamp above the renal arteries is closed and the thrombo-endarterectomy completed. The surgeon inspects the origins of the renal arteries from within the aorta to make certain that they are open and that no tags or debris remain to obstruct them. A second clamp is now placed across the aorta just distal to the renal arteries and the first clamp is removed to restore a flow to both renal arteries. If there are lumbar arteries distal to this clamp, they must be clamped separately with bulldog clamps.

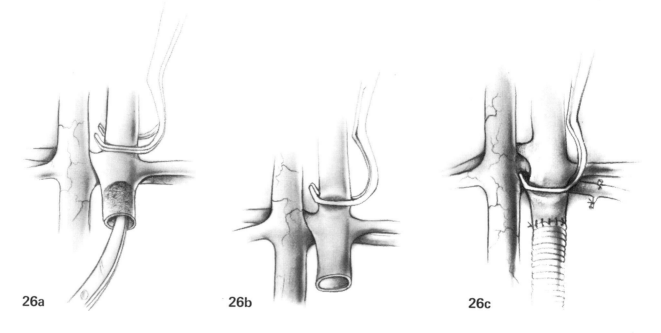

26a   **26b**   **26c**

27

The anastomosis

A bifurcated woven prosthesis is now anastomosed end-to-end to the stump of the divided and previously thrombo-endarterectomized aorta with a continuous suture of 4/0 Dacron or Prolene. When the anastomosis is complete it is wrapped in 'Surgicel' gauze and the whole prosthesis is now threaded back behind the left renal vein so that the aorta, the anastomosis and the prosthesis are returned to the correct anatomical position. If this is not done, the renal vein usually thromboses. The limbs of the prosthesis are now placed in retroperitoneal tunnels and are anastomosed to either the common femoral or external iliac arteries.

28

Unclamping

In some ways this phase of any arterial reconstruction operation requires the most experience. Extra sutures may be needed but unnecessary sutures can be harmful. In most instances when an aortofemoral or aorto-iliac bypass graft has been inserted, it is possible to restore the flow to first one lower limb and then the other. As soon as one distal anastomosis has been completed, it is wrapped in Surgicel gauze, the opposite limb is clamped close to the main stem with a Kelly or Fogarty clamp and the distal clamps are removed. Protamine sulphate is now given in the appropriate dose to counteract the heparin and after the prosthesis has filled with blood the proximal clamp is removed. If after 5 min of firm pressure, bleeding from either anastomosis persists, then further sutures may be required.

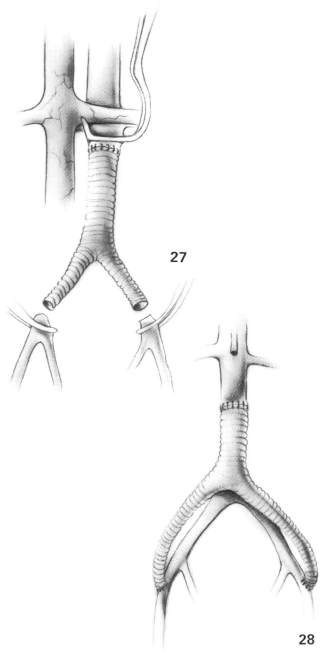

27

28

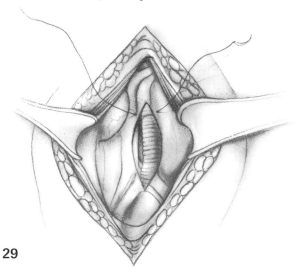

29

29

Closure of the posterior peritoneum

This is an important step particularly if a prosthesis has been used because the prosthesis must be isolated from the peritoneal cavity. The whole length of the posterior peritoneal incision is closed and great care is taken to avoid including either the inferior mesenteric vein or the inferior mesenteric artery in the suture line. It is also important to place as much tissue as possible between the duodenal flexure and the prosthesis.

30

The problem of mesenteric ischaemia

Whenever the inferior mesenteric artery is divided, it is important to avoid damage to the collateral circulation but sometimes this is not enough. If the coeliac and superior mesenteric artery are thrombosed or severely stenosed, ligature of the inferior mesenteric artery will cause alimentary tract ischaemia. The first step is to palpate the coeliac and superior mesenteric arteries to determine if they are diseased. The next step is to inspect the origin of the inferior mesenteric artery. If this vessel is large, more than 0·5 cm in diameter, it is an important vessel and must be preserved. This is best accomplished by resecting a ring of aortic wall around the origin of the inferior mesenteric artery and anastomosing this to the aortic prosthesis.

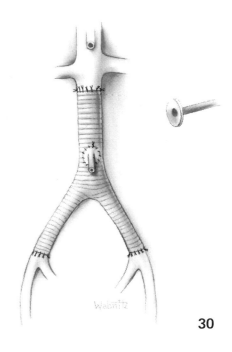

30

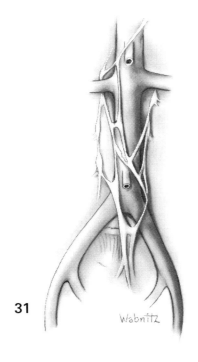

31

31

The problem of sexual function in the male

In the male patient division or excision of the pre-aortic plexus of nerves is frequently followed by retrograde ejaculation. Due to loss of control of the internal urethral sphincter which fails to contract during ejaculation with the result that the seminal fluid passes into the urinary bladder instead of through the urethra to the exterior. These nerves should, therefore, be preserved if possible.

32

An open thrombo-endarterectomy or an excision of the abdominal aorta (*see Illustration 32 A and C*) are the procedures most likely to destroy the pre-aortic autonomic nerve plexus. A bypass graft (*see Illustration 32 B*) is the least likely. For aneurysms of the abdominal aorta preservation of the aortic and iliac arterial walls to wrap around the graft at the conclusion of the procedure often preserves this nerve plexus whilst excision of the aneurysm results in their destruction.

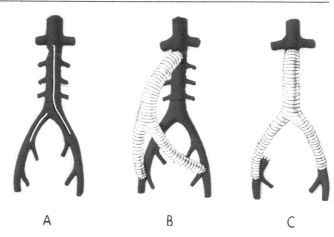

A   B   C

This illustration may also be seen in colour, facing page 130

32

SPECIAL POSTOPERATIVE CARE

Cardiac function

A definite complication of an aorto-iliac reconstruction operation is a myocardial infarction. This means that the cardiac function should be monitored during and after the operation and treatment commenced as soon as any change is observed.

Blood pressure

After an arterial reconstruction operation, it is important to maintain a satisfactory blood flow through the reconstructed segment. The maintenance of an adequate blood pressure and cardiac output is the best way of achieving this. Adequate but not excessive blood and fluid replacement with monitoring of the arterial and central venous is recommended.

Paralytic ileus

This occurs after every operation on the abdominal aorta. The treatment is continuous gastro-intestinal aspiration and fluid replacement until bowel sounds return and the patient begins to pass gas per rectum.

Antibiotics

These drugs are not required if the patient has an uncomplicated thrombo-endarterectomy, but should be given for 5 days beginning 12 hr before surgery in every patient who has a plastic prosthesis inserted.

Anticoagulant drugs

In our view these drugs should not be used after operations of this type. The complications largely due to haemorrhage outweigh every possible benefit.

Early thrombosis

This is very unusual in vessels of this size. If it occurs, immediate re-operation is usually required.

Urinary output

An important complication of aortic surgery is oliguria or anuria. Adequate fluid replacement with osmotic diuretics if necessary is the best method of preventing this complication.

References

dos Santos, J.C. (1947). 'Sur la desobstruction des thromboses arterielles anciennes.' *Mem. Acad. Chir.* **73,** 409
Cannon, J.A., Barker, W.F. and Kattas, A.A. (1958). 'Femoral popliteal endarterectomy in the treatment of obliterative atherosclerotic disease.' *Surgery* **43,** 76
May, A.G., DeWeese, J.A. and Rob, C.G. (1969). 'Changes in sexual function following operation on the abdominal aorta.' *Surgery* **65,** 41
Minken, S.L., DeWeese, J.A., Southgate, W.A., Mahoney, E.B. and Rob, C.G. (1968). 'Aorto-iliac reconstruction for atherosclerotic occlusive disease.' *Surgery Gynec. Obstet.* **126,** 1056
Rob, C.G. (1963). 'Extraperitoneal approach to the abdominal aorta.' *Surgery* **53,** 87
Sobel, S., Kaplitt, M.J., Reingold, M. and Sawyer, P.N. (1966). 'Gas endarterectomy.' *Surgery* **59,** 517
Sawyer, P.N., Kaplitt, M.J., Golding, M.R. and Dennis, C. (1968). 'Analysis of peripheral gas endarterectomy in 127 patients'. *Archs Surg.* **97,** 859

[*The illustrations for this Chapter on Aorto-iliac Reconstruction Bypass Graft. Thrombo-endarterectomy were drawn by Mr. R. Wabnitz.*]

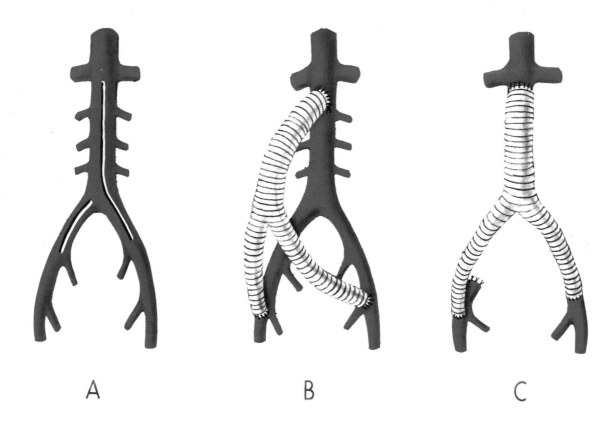

A   B   C

Illustration 32 from page 129

Arterial Reconstructions below the Inguinal Ligament

James A. DeWeese, M. D., F.A.C.S
Chairman of the Division of Cardiothoracic Surgery,
University of Rochester Medical Centre, and
Professor and Surgeon, Strong Memorial Hospital,
Rochester, New York

and

Charles Rob, *M.C.,* M.D., M.Chir., F.R.C.S.
Professor and Chairman of the Department of Surgery,
University of Rochester School of Medicine and
Dentistry, Rochester, New York

PRE-OPERATIVE

In the lower extremity severe atherosclerosis and thrombosis are usually centred in the femoral artery in the lower thigh where it passes beneath the rigid adductor magnus tendon to become the popliteal artery. The thrombosis may extend for some distance proximal and distal to that level, but the common femoral artery in the groin and the popliteal artery in the region of the knee usually remain patent.

The symptoms associated with chronic femoropopliteal thrombosis are intermittent claudication, rest pain, and gangrene or painful ulcerations. The symptoms are frequently progressive. At least 15 per cent of patients with claudication develop limb-threatening rest pain or gangrene within a few years of the onset of symptoms.

Pre-operative evaluation

When the superficial femoral artery is occluded the femoral pulses are present, but usually no pulses are felt at the popliteal or pedal level. There are some patients with femoral thrombosis who have weak pedal pulses but these pulses will disappear with exercise, proving the presence of arterial thrombosis.

Oscillometric examination and performance of an elevation-dependency test are helpful in determining the severity of the arterial insufficiency, but femoral arteriography is the most definitive and important of the studies. A general medical evaluation will frequently disclose diabetes or segmental atherosclerosis in other organ systems such as the extracranial cerebral vessels, and coronary or renal arteries.

Indications for surgery

All patients with limb-threatening rest pain and gangrene are advised to undergo arterial reconstruction if there are patent proximal femoral and distal popliteal or posterior tibial arteries visible on an arteriogram. The risk of the reconstruction operation is no greater than the risk of an amputation. All patients with significant claudication are also offered an arterial reconstruction operation if there are no serious medical contra-indications and if the distal anastomosis is proximal to the knee joint.

131

Choice of procedure (see Table 1)

The choice of operation is dependent upon the extent of the obstruction as determined by the arteriogram and the status of the greater saphenous veins. Every effort is made to use autologous tissue by performing a saphenous vein bypass (SVBP), thrombo-endarterectomy (TE) or a combination of these two procedures. Profundoplasties should be considered whenever there is stenosis or occlusion of the profunda femoris artery.

When the long saphenous vein is not available, too small or pathological then another method of reconstruction may be required if a thrombo-endarterectomy is also impossible. Table 2 gives a list of the alternatives to the long saphenous vein from the same limb in our order of preference.

Preparation for operation

A general anaesthetic or epidural anaesthetic is necessary. The opposite hip of the supine patient is elevated with a rolled sheet approximately 10°. The lower abdomen, groin and entire leg and foot is prepared and draped. The leg is externally rotated and the knee flexed and held in that position with padding beneath the knee joint.

Table 1

	Choice of operation	
Extent of thrombosis	First	Second
Less than 3 inches long	TE	SVBP
Length of superficial femoral	SVBP	TE
Femoral and proximal popliteal	SVBP	TE and SVBP
Femoral and entire popliteal	SVBP	TE and SVBP

Table 2

Saphenous vein not available or inadequate

Alternatives

1. Thrombo-endarterectomy
2. Saphenous vein from other leg
3. Cephalic vein
4. Composite graft
5. Dacron prosthesis if it does not cross the knee joint
6. Bovine heterograft
7. Sparks mandril
8. Homologous saphenous or umbilical vein
9. Homologous artery

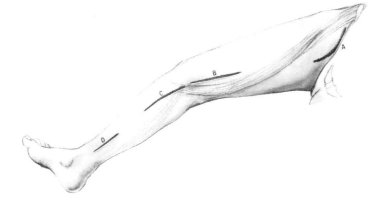

1

AUTOGENOUS VENOUS BYPASS PROCEDURES

1

Skin incisions

(A) For exposure of common femoral artery and proximal greater saphenous vein.

(B) For exposure of proximal popliteal artery and distal saphenous vein.

(C) For exposure of distal popliteal artery and distal saphenous vein.

(D) For exposure of posterior tibial artery.

OBTAINING AND PREPARING THE SAPHENOUS VEIN

2

Division of proximal saphenous vein

An incision is made in the inguinal crease from the mid-inguinal ligament to just below the pubic tubercle and extended distally if necessary. The branches of the vein are divided and ligated 1–2 mm from the saphenous vein. The saphenous vein is then doubly ligated at the saphenofemoral junction.

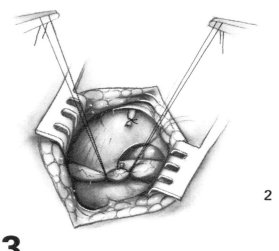

2

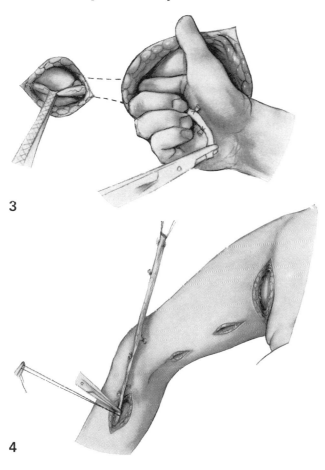

3

4

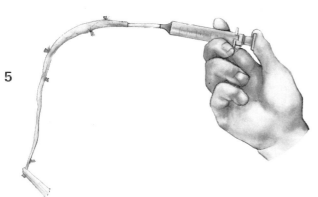

5

3

Dissection

The saphenous vein is then mobilized by sharp and blunt dissection, taking care to identify and ligate all branches. The course of the vein is identified with the finger and a short longitudinal incision made distally over the vein. The vein is dissected from the surrounding fat and a tape passed around it for traction. Branches are ligated and the freed proximal end of the vein is delivered into the incision. The proximal vein is divided close to the femoral vein.

4

Excision

Additional longitudinal incisions are made as necessary to obtain an adequate length of the vein. It is important that the incisions be made directly over the vein and undermining of the skin edges avoided or skin sloughs may occur.

5

Distension of vein

A cannula attached to a 50-ml syringe containing saline is inserted into the distal end of the resected vein. The proximal end of the vein is occluded with a clamp. The vein is then gently distended and untwisted by instilling saline. Unligated branches or tears are repaired with fine sutures, taking care not to narrow the vein by catching distant adventitia with the suture.

EXPOSURE OF THE ARTERIES

6

Exposure of common femoral artery in the groin

The incision made for ligation of the saphenous vein is deepened and the femoral artery mobilized. Tapes are passed around the common, deep and superficial femoral arteries. Any small branches are dissected free and carefully preserved.

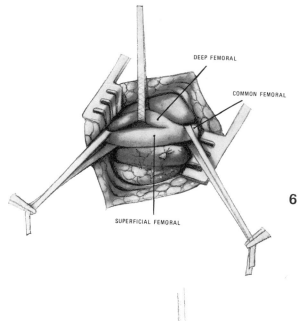

7

Exposure of popliteal artery proximal to the knee joint (for bypasses to proximal popliteal artery)

The skin incision is made 3 cm below the anterior border of the sartorius muscle beginning at the level of the knee joint and carried proximally for a distance of 15 cm. The popliteal artery is found in the fatty popliteal fossa just distal and posterior to the adductor magnus tendon and is mobilized to the level of the knee joint.

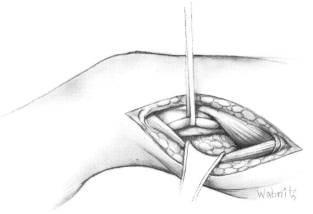

8

Exposure of popliteal artery distal to knee joint (for bypasses to distal popliteal artery)

The skin incision is made over the posterior border of the tibia from the level of the knee joint distally for 15 cm. The crural fascia and semitendinosis tendon is divided. The gastrocnemius muscle is retracted posteriorly to expose the fatty popliteal fossa and neurovascular bundle. The popliteal artery is mobilized and the thin-walled vena comitantes ligated at the proximal and distal extent of the dissection.

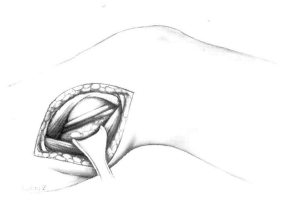

9

Exposure of entire popliteal artery (for bypasses to mid-popliteal artery)

The skin incision is made along the posterior border of the sartorius muscle. The sartorius, semimembranosus, semitendinosus, gracilis and gastrocnemius muscles are divided near their insertions and tagged. The adductor magnus tendon can be divided if needed for exposure of the distal femoral artery.

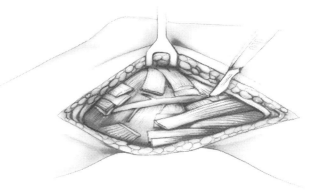

9

10

Exposure of distal vessels

The posterior tibial or peroneal artery is exposed through an 8-cm long incision just posterior to the tibia in the distal third of the lower leg. The soleus muscle is retracted posteriorly.

TUNNELLING OF THE VEIN

11

Passing of tunneller

The tunneller used is a 20-inch (50-cm) long slightly curved hollow tube and a long thick wire with one coned end and one flattened end containing two small holes. It is passed from the groin incision beneath the sartorius muscle to just above the knee joint where it is then passed along the course of the popliteal artery. The tunneller will reach from the groin to beyond the knee joint, if necessary.

Insertion of a twisted venous bypass graft usually results in early thrombosis of the graft. At this stage, therefore, it is important that the graft be distended with saline and its ends properly orientated.

12

Passage of vein through tunneller

The wire is passed through the tunneller and the orientated end of the vein sutured to the flattened tip and the vein is drawn through the metal tube to the groin. The tunneller is now withdrawn over the wire and vein. Both ends of the vein are now known to be properly orientated.

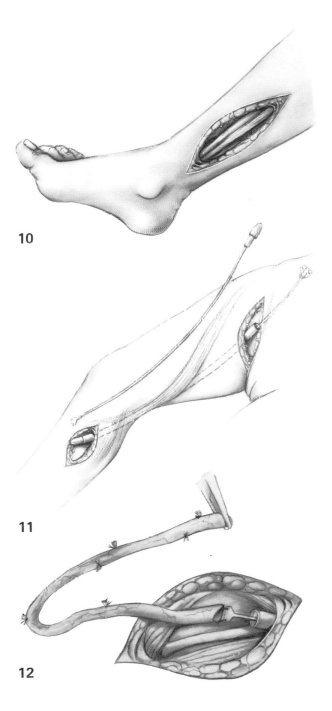

10

11

12

ANASTOMOSES

Prior to performing the proximal and distal anastomoses, 5000 units of heparin is given intravenously. The vessels are then occluded.

13

Enlarging the end of the vein

The proposed top of the vein is identified and the adventitia grasped with a fine forceps or clamp. A longitudinal cut is made in the opposite side of the vein with fine scissors. Using fine scissors, a longitudinal incision which is 1·5 times the diameter of the vein is made in the vein opposite the clamps.

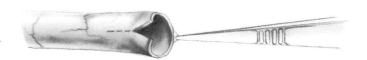

13

14

Arteriotomy and beginning the anastomosis

A longitudinal arteriotomy is made which is twice the diameter of the vein to be used. It is helpful to place traction sutures in the middle of each side of the arteriotomy.

A central horizontal mattress stitch is placed which passes from the outer side of the vein to its intimal surface and then from the intimal side of the artery to its outer side at the proximal end of the arteriotomy. A fine suture, preferably of the monofilament type, with double-ended needles is used. The stitch is continued as a simple over-and-over everting stitch.

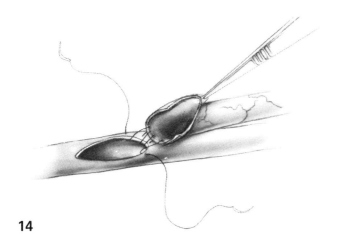

14

15

The distal stay suture

After the proximal suture has been carried a short distance, a stay suture is placed which approximates the tip of the vein to the distal end of the arteriotomy.

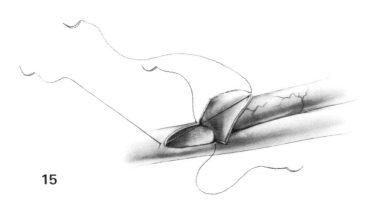

15

16

Completion of anastomosis

The sutures are then run to the distal end of the arteriotomy as a simple over-and-over stitch. A fine forceps grasps the adventitia to hold the vein edge away from the arterial edge so that the needle tip can be visualized as it passes through the intima of the artery. This assures approximation of intima to intima and also prevents catching the opposite wall of the artery with a needle and suture.

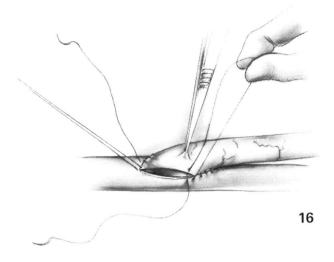

16

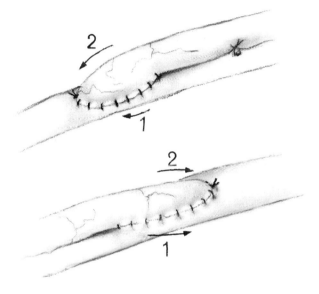

17

17

Completed anastomosis

The suturing of the anastomosis always begins at the end of the arteriotomy closest to the centre of the bypass graft. The distal anastomosis begins at the proximal end of the arteriotomy and the proximal anastomosis begins at the distal end of the arteriotomy. This allows for accurate placement of sutures in the critical corners of the anastomosis where the diameter of the entrance to and exit from the graft is determined.

All occluding clamps are removed and gentle pressure is applied directly over any bleeding points in the anastomosis for a period of 5 min. Heparin anticoagulation is reversed with 50 mg of protamine sulphate.

The wounds are closed in layers with interrupted silk sutures after obtaining meticulous haemostasis.

SYNTHETIC GRAFT BYPASS

If it is necessary to use a synthetic graft as a bypass, knitted Dacron tubes of at least 8 mm in diameter are preferred.

The incision for exposing the arteries and the technique of making the anastomoses are those described for use of an autogenous vein.

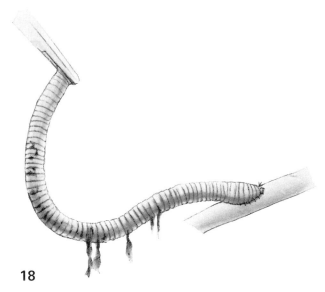

18

18

Synthetic tube bypass graft (preclotting)

Knitted and the higher porosity woven grafts require preclotting by immersion in 50 ml of blood which has been withdrawn from a nearby vessel. The graft is stretched and kneaded in the blood to promote clotting in the interstices of the graft. The proximal anastomosis is performed first. The proximal occluding clamp is briefly removed, the graft filled with blood which is again allowed to clot which may take 3–5 min and then the clot is expressed from the graft. The preclotting manoeuvre is important and prevents excessive blood loss through the interstices of the graft. The graft is then tunnelled to the distal incision and the anastomosis performed.

THE BOVINE HETEROGRAFT

The Bovine heterograft (Rosenberg *et al.*, 1970) is in our view less satisfactory as a femoral popliteal bypass than an autogenous vein, and gives results no better than those obtained with a Dacron prosthesis.

THE SPARKS MANDRIL TECHNIQUE

This is a two-stage procedure with an interval of 6 or more weeks between the stages. The long-term results are not known but the early results show promise. The mandril consists of a flexible silicone rubber rod covered with two layers of knitted Dacron. The Dacron fibres are a foundation upon which cellular deposition occurs and forms a tube of fibrous connective tissue upon the foundation of the Dacron fibres.

FEMOROPOPLITEAL THROMBO-ENDARTER-ECTOMY WITH PATCH GRAFT

19

Exposure of distal femoral and proximal popliteal arteries

The longitudinal skin incision is made along the anterior border of the sartorius muscle beginning at the knee joint and carried proximally for 2 cm. The adductor magnus tendon and its proximal membranous extension are divided near their insertions to expose the distal femoral and proximal popliteal artery. Care is taken to preserve the saphenous vein which accompanies the femoral artery in the adductor canal but pierces the adductor magnus aponeurosis to pass along behind the sartorius muscle. The popliteal artery is then mobilized until it is found to be circumferentially soft.

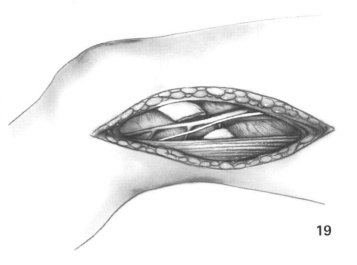

19

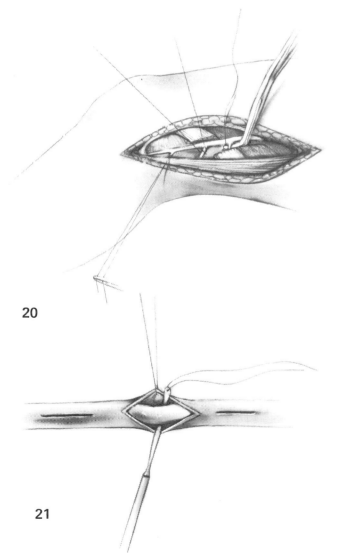

20

21

20

Control of branches

It is important to obtain control of all of the branches of the artery to at least 2 cm beyond the proposed length of the endarterectomy. Otherwise, unnecessary bleeding would occur when the arteriotomy is made or after the atherosclerotic core is removed. Small branches can be controlled by pulling a loop of suture material around the vessel and placing moderate tension on the suture. Atraumatic vascular clamps are used to occlude other vessels.

21

Arteriotomies and developing endarterectomy plane

A superficial longitudinal incision is initially made at the site of the severest disease which is usually at the level of the adductor tendon. The incision is deepened until the yellow atherosclerotic core is identified. This is usually within the media of the artery and the proper place is reached when the core can be easily bluntly dissected away from the outer wall of the artery. A blunt dissector is used to develop the plane proximally, distally, and around the core. The core is divided between two sutures which are gently tied to compress but not cut through the core.

22

Distal dissection

The plane of dissection is carried distally to a point where the core becomes adherent to the outer wall of the artery and is carefully incised. The endarterectomy should end distally within clear view of the arteriotomy even if it needs to be extended. This allows careful termination of the dissection and incision of the core at a point where it is adherent to the outer wall of the artery.

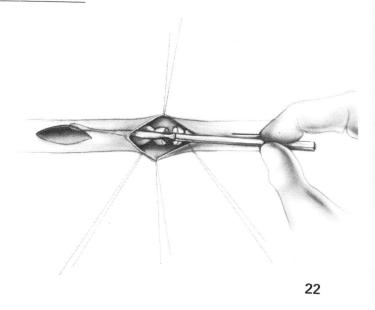

22

23

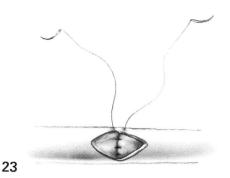

23

Tacking of intima distally

It is extremely important that the intima be tightly adherent to the media at the distal end of the endarterectomy to prevent the raising of a flap of tissue which could obstruct the vessel. If there is any question about the adherence, three or four sutures with double-ended needles are used to tack the intima to the arterial wall.

24

Proximal dissection

A ring stripper is then passed around the core and advanced in the plane of cleavage in the media in a proximal direction. It is moved proximally by a combination of rotary and gently pushing movements. Gentle traction can also be applied to the suture attached to the inner core which had been passed through the ring with the endarterectomized specimen. A straight haemostat is used to crush the vessel at the proximal extent of the endarterectomy. The crushing will separate the intima from the atherosclerotic core and the specimen can be easily removed. It is not necessary to tack the intima to the arterial wall proximally.

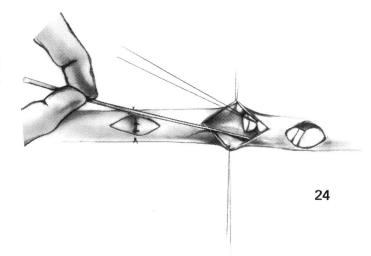

24

25

Patch grafting distal arteriotomy

A patch graft is used to cover the distal arteriotomy to ensure a widely patent outflow from the end-arterectomized vessel. A small rectangular piece of vein is obtained. The width of the vein should be no greater than one half of the diameter of the artery. Stay sutures are placed in the four tips of the patch anchoring it to the edges of the arteriotomy a few millimetres from the end.

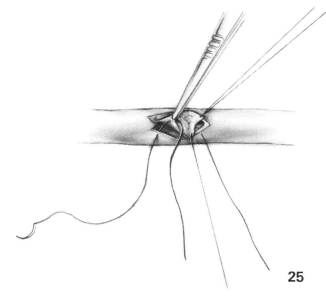

25

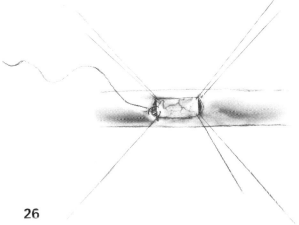

26

26

The suturing

A continuous everting stitch is run between the stay sutures. A monofilament synthetic suture material is preferred which avoids gathering of the adventitia of the vein.

27

Completed closures

The middle and proximal arteriotomies are closed with a simple over-and-over stitch between proximal and distal stay sutures. The completed patch on the distal arteriotomy has caused localized enlargement of the arterial lumen and prevented a stenosis at the critical distal end of the endarterectomy.

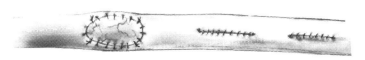

27

PROFUNDOPLASTY

28

Incision and exposure

A generous hockey-stick incision is made in the groin to expose the common femoral and superficial femoral arteries. The superficial femoral artery is retracted medially and the fascia overlying the profunda femoris artery divided to beyond its palpable atherosclerotic plaques.

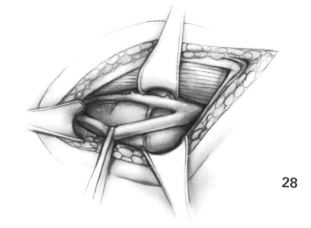

28

29

Arteriotomy for localized lesions

The circumferential or posterior atherosclerotic plaques frequently are localized to the distal common femoral artery and the profunda femoris artery proximal to its medial and lateral circumflex femoral branches. The longitudinal arteriotomy incision is made along the anterior wall of the common femoral artery and carried down the profunda femoris artery to at least 1 cm beyond the palpable plaque.

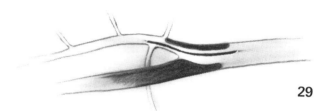

29

30

Endarterectomy of localized lesion

A plane of dissection is established within the media of the vessel and the atherosclerotic core removed under direct vision. Proximally the lesion is separated by the prior application of a straight haemostat which disrupts the lesion from the normal artery. Distally the endarterectomy is ended by sharply incising the intima at a point where it is adherent to the media.

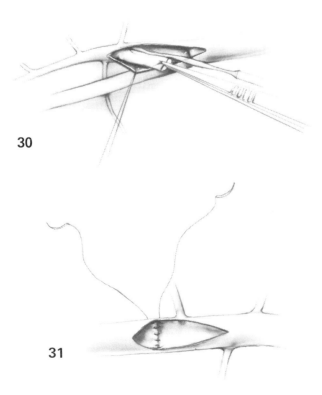

30

31

31

Tacking of intima distally

It is very important that intima at the distal end of the endarterectomy is tightly opposed to the media or a flap can be raised that obstructs the vessel or serves as a nidus for a thrombus. If there is any question about the adherence of the intima and media, double-ended sutures can be passed through the intima and media from within the vessel and tied on the outside of the vessel.

32

Arteriotomy for extensive lesions

The atherosclerotic lesions may extend beyond the circumflex femoral arteries and the first or even second branches of the profunda femoris artery. One short longitudinal incision is made in the common femoral artery and a second incision is made in the profunda femoris artery making sure to carry it at least 1 cm beyond the palpable plaque.

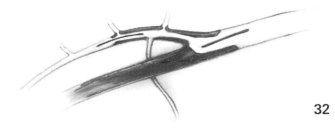

32

33

Endarterectomy of extensive lesion

A plane of dissection is established through the distal arteriotomy in the profunda femoris artery and the endarterectomy ended distally by sharply incising the intima where it becomes adherent. A ring stripper is then used to remove the core to the level of the proximal arteriotomy.

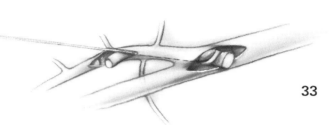

33

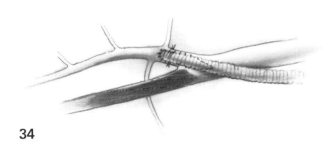

34

Closure of the common femoral arteriotomy incision

The incision in the common femoral artery can be used for the anastomosis of the distal end of an aortofemoral bypass graft. It could also be used for the proximal anastomosis of a femoropopliteal bypass graft.

34

35

Closure of profunda femoris vessel

A patch graft, preferably of autogenous vein, should always be used to cover the incision in the profunda femoris artery to ensure its wide patency (*see Illustration 25*). A patch graft may also be used for covering the incision in the common femoral artery but a simple over-and-over stitch between two stay sutures is usually sufficient.

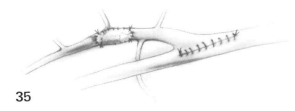

35

POSTOPERATIVE CARE

Following any arterial procedure on the lower extremity, particularly if the knee joint is crossed, it is important that for a period of 2 weeks the patient should not sit for longer than a few minutes at a time. Patients are allowed to be up walking or lying down. Elevation of the leg and use of elastic support is prescribed for those patients who develop oedema. No anticoagulants are used, but 500 ml of dextran twice daily for the first 48 hr may increase the blood flow through the bypass.

References

Bernhard, V. M., Militello, H. M. and Geringer, A. M. (1974). 'Repair of the profunda femoris artery.' *Am. J. Surg.* **127**, 676
Breslau, R. C. and DeWeese, J. A. (1965). 'Successful endophlebectomy of autogenous venous bypass graft.' *Ann. Surg.* **162**, 251
Gryska, P. F., Darling, R. C. and Linton, R. (1964). 'Exposure of the entire popliteal artery through a medial approach.' *Surgery* **118**, 845
Dale, W. A. and Lewis, M. R. (1965). 'Lateral vascular patch grafts.' *Surgery* **57**, 36
DeWeese, J. A., Barner, H. B., Mahoney, E. B. and Rob, C. G. (1966). 'Autogenous venous bypass grafts and thromboendarterectomies for atherosclerotic lesions of the femoropopliteal arteries.' *Ann. Surg.* **163**, 205
DeWeese, J. A. and Rob, C. G. (1971). 'Autogenous venous bypass grafts five years later.' *Ann. Surg.* **174**, 346
Martin, P. R. and Stephenson, C. (1968). 'On the surgery of the profunda femoris artery.' *Br. J. Surg.* **55**, 539
Morris, G. C., Edwards, W., Cooley, D. A., Crawford, E. S. and DeBakey, M. E. (1961). 'Surgical importance of the profunda femoris artery.' *Archs Surg. Chicago* **82**, 32
Rosenburg, D. M. L., Glass, B. A., Rosenburg, N., Lewis, M. R. and Dale, W. A. (1970). 'Experiences with modified Bovine carotid arteries in arterial surgery.' *Surgery* **68**, 1064
Sparks, C. G. (1971). 'Silicone mandril method of femoropopliteal artery bypass.' *Am. J. Surg.* **124**, 244

[*The illustrations for this Chapter on Arterial Reconstructions below the Inguinal Ligament were drawn by Mr. R. Wabnitz.*]

Axillofemoral and Cross-leg Bypass Grafts

Allyn G. May, M.D.
Associate Professor of Surgery,
University of Rochester and
Strong Memorial Hospital,
Rochester, New York

Some patients, who have severe ischaemia due to aortic or iliac obstruction, cannot safely undergo deep abdominal surgery. In these patients the axillofemoral or cross-leg bypass graft offers a technique for successful treatment.

AXILLOFEMORAL BYPASS GRAFTS

The particular indications for the axillofemoral bypass graft are: (*1*) an urgent need to bypass aorto-iliac obstruction in the presence of generalized peritonitis or of retroperitoneal infection; (*2*) as part of the treatment for infection of an aortic prosthesis; and (*3*) the urgent need to bypass aorto-iliac obstruction in the poor risk patient who cannot tolerate deep abdominal surgery or general anaesthesia.

Frequently a unilateral axillofemoral bypass will suffice even for bilateral severe lower extremity ischaemia. Thus, it is wise to drape the patient so that both feet can be observed for colour change and for venous filling (i.e. in sterile transparent plastic bags), and to revascularize the contralateral side only if necessary. If significant contralateral ischaemia persists after axillofemoral bypass grafting, the procedure may be extended by adding a femorofemoral bypass graft (*see* below). There is some evidence that the long-term patency is better after a femorofemoral graft is added to an axillofemoral graft. The flow appears to be greater through an axillofemoral graft if it supplies both lower limbs.

Technique

1

The axillofemoral bypass is constructed with the patient in the supine position and the arm abducted, and under general or local anaesthesia. A wide area of skin is prepared over the shoulder, base of the neck, anterior and lateral side of the chest, groin, and thigh. The femoral artery is exposed first. The skin incision begins at the level of the inguinal ligament about 4 cm lateral to the pubic tubercle and passes medially and inferiorly in a gentle curve. The greater saphenous vein may be seen and should be preserved. The incision is deepened lateral to the saphenous vein and widened by retraction. The pulseless femoral artery can be felt as it is approached and it will be found to lie immediately lateral to the femoral vein and to the termination of the greater saphenous vein. In mobilizing the femoral artery the posterior origin of the deep femoral artery should be remembered, for it is liable to injury in its un-obtrusive position. All branches of the femoral arteries should be preserved. Eventually tapes are passed about the common, superficial, and deep femoral arteries. These arteries are palpated for evidence of patency and to detect areas, relatively free of atheroma, which can satisfactorily take the graft.

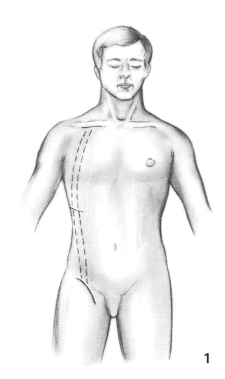

1

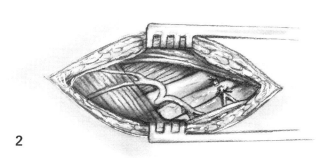

2

2

The incision to expose the axillary artery is then made. It is 8 cm long, parallel to and one finger's breadth below the clavicle with its centre at the junction of the medial and middle portions of the clavicle. The two portions of the pectoralis major muscle are re-tracted and the coracoclavicular fascia is incised. The axillary vessels are uncovered in the space beneath this membrane. Venous branches and the supreme thoracic artery should be tied and divided to allow adequate mobilization of the axillary artery. The axillofemoral tunnel is constructed between the pectoralis major and minor muscles, along the mid-axillary line in the deep subcutaneous space, passing towards the femoral triangle immediately above the inguinal ligament. It is made with an arterial tunneller or with an external vein stripper, using a small in-cision midway along the course of the tunnel.

3

The upper anastomosis is done first. A knitted Dacron prosthesis at least 10 mm in diameter is recommended. The artery is controlled with vascular clamps and a longitudinal incision is made on the inferior aspect of the vessel. An end-to-side anastomosis is made using 5/0 prosthetic arterial suture. After completion of the anastomosis, the vascular clamp is removed briefly at intervals to preclot the graft. Excess clot is sucked or milked out of the graft, and the vascular clamp is repositioned on the proximal graft to restore blood flow to the upper limb.

The prosthesis is placed in the tunnel without twisting and trimmed to reach the site prepared for femoral anastomosis. The femoral clamp is applied, an anterior arteriotomy made, and the end-to-side anastomosis made with the same suture material. On completion of the anastomosis, the proximal clamp is removed and the blood allowed to fill the prosthesis in order to exhaust air through the distal suture line. As soon as air-bubbles cease to appear, the femoral artery is declamped. Not until all bleeding has been controlled and excess clot expressed from the tunnel are the incisions closed. The patient is advised not to lie on the side of the graft or to wear constrictive clothing about the waist.

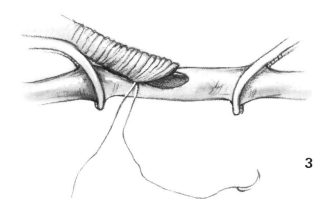

3

CROSS-LEG BYPASS GRAFTS

The cross-leg bypass is useful in the poor risk patient when there is: (*1*) unilateral iliac arterial obstruction significantly the cause of ischaemia; (*2*) good arterial blood flow to the contralateral lower extremity; and (*3*) a need to avoid deep abdominal surgery. It is possible and sometimes desirable to combine this procedure with the axillofemoral bypass graft.

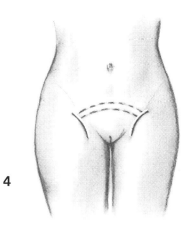

4

Technique

4

Many aspects of this procedure are the same as those for the axillofemoral bypass graft. The patient is supine and the anaesthesia may be general or local. The lower abdomen, groin, and upper thighs are prepared and draped to provide for bilateral femoral and suprapubic exposure. The femoral arteries of the ischaemic side are first exposed to permit evaluation of patency. Operative angiography may be helpful at this time, if prior aortography failed to show patency of the femoral arteries. Frequently, revascularization of a patent deep femoral artery, alone, will suffice to heal a serious lesion of the foot. The patent segment is mobilized so that vascular clamps can be applied.

The contralateral femoral artery is exposed and prepared for clamping. A subcutaneous tunnel is developed with the fingers cephalad from one femoral incision passing superior to the mons pubis and descending symmetrically to the contralateral femoral incision.

5

The upstream anastomosis is completed first. The arteriotomy should be longitudinal and on the anteromedial aspect •of the femoral artery. When the anastomosis is finished, the position of the vascular clamp is transferred to the prosthesis at the suture line and the prosthesis, if knitted Dacron, is preclotted by intermittent declamping. Excess clot is removed from the graft, and then it is passed through the tunnel without twisting in a gentle curve from one femoral artery to the other. Next the downstream anastomosis is completed. The upstream clamp is removed and the graft freed of entrapped air before downstream declamping is done.

When haemostasis is secured, the wounds are closed in layers and provided with simple dry dressings.

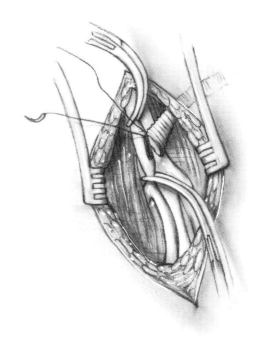

5

References

Blaisdell, F.W. and Hall, A.D. (1963). 'Axillary-femoral artery bypass for lower extremity ischaemia.' *Surgery* **54**, 563

McCaughan, J.J. and Kahn, S.F. (1960). 'Cross-over graft for unilateral occlusive disease of the ileofemoral arteries.' *Ann. Surg.* **151**, 26

Mannick, J. A. and Nabseth, D. C. (1968). 'Axillofemoral bypass graft.' *New Engl. J. Med.* **278**, 461

[*The illustrations for this Chapter on Axillofemoral and Cross-leg Bypass Grafts were drawn by Mr. R. Wabnitz.*]

Operations for Stenosis, Thrombosis and Embolism of the Mesenteric and Coeliac Arteries (Acute and Chronic Arterial Occlusion)

Charles Rob, *M.C.,* M.D., M.Chir., F.R.C.S.
Professor and Chairman of the Department of Surgery,
University of Rochester School of Medicine and
Dentistry, Rochester, New York

Occlusion of the mesenteric and coeliac arteries may be partial or complete and may present as an acute problem or with chronic symptoms. Acute symptoms may be due to an embolus or thrombosis. Chronic symptoms are usually due to arterial stenosis secondary to atherosclerosis or in the case of the coeliac artery external compression. Other causes of chronic symptoms include recovery from an acute episode, trauma, arteritis including Buerger's disease, involvement by an aneurysm and retroperitoneal fibrosis.

ACUTE OCCLUSION OF THE SUPERIOR MESENTERIC ARTERY

The patient presents as an acute abdominal emergency and in the case of an embolism has a cause for this event such as auricular fibrillation or a recent myocardial infarction. The pre-operative preparation must therefore consist of the resuscitation of the patient for the intestinal problem and special cardiac care and evaluation. Many patients with an arterial embolus have recently developed a change in their cardiac status often with increased decompensation. It is important that this is evaluated and if possible treated before surgery. Nonetheless, acute occlusion of the superior mesenteric artery is a surgical emergency requiring operation as soon as the condition of the patient permits.

THE OPERATION

1

The incision and exploration

An upper mid-line abdominal incision extending from below the umbilicus to below the xiphoid process gives satisfactory exposure. A full abdominal exploration is performed and the surgeon carefully inspects the region supplied by the superior mesenteric artery. This is the jejunum, ileum, appendix and colon to the splenic flexure. The pulse is palpated in the superior mesenteric artery. If this is absent, then the diagnosis is obvious. If the superior mesenteric arterial pulse is still present, then the whole length of the superior mesenteric arterial tree must be examined to determine the exact location of the arterial occlusion. It is also important to examine the origins of the coeliac and inferior mesenteric arteries to check the presence of pulsatile flow and the presence or absence of a thrill.

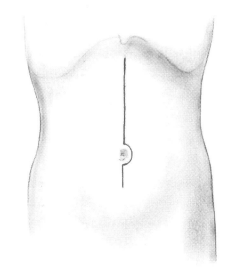

1

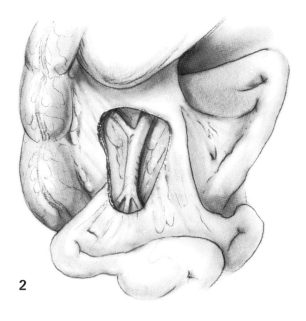

2

2

Exposure of the superior mesenteric artery

The aim is to isolate the superior mesenteric artery distal to the point where it emerges from behind the pancreas. The surgeon's assistant elevates the transverse colon. The superior mesenteric artery can then be identified at the base of the transverse mesocolon. The peritoneum is then incised over the superior mesenteric vessels. The superior mesenteric artery is carefully separated from the superior mesenteric vein and the dissection carried proximally until the superior mesenteric artery has passed behind the pancreas. The middle colic artery and the first two or three jejunal arteries are then freed. It is now possible to palpate the artery and locate the exact site of the embolus. This is usually just proximal to the middle colic artery.

3

Removal of the embolus

The artery is not actually clamped but a tape is passed around the artery and a curved vessel clamp of the DeBakey type is made available for immediate use if necessary. The anaesthetist gives the patient 50–100 mg of heparin intravenously. The artery is now incised transversely just proximal to the middle colic artery. This incision should pass a little more than half way round the circumference of the artery. The embolus and any associated thrombus is then allowed to extrude from the vessel and this process is assisted with gentle traction on the embolus. If a good flow from the proximal stump is now achieved, the arterial clamp is applied. If such a flow is not obtained, a Fogarty balloon catheter is passed proximally into the aorta and any thrombus or embolus removed. After a good flow has been obtained, the vessel is again clamped.

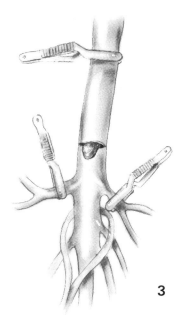

3

4

The establishment of distal arterial patency

The middle colic artery and other branches should be assessed for retrograde arterial flow. If necessary a small Fogarty balloon catheter is passed up each branch and any thrombus extracted. Unfortunately, if the embolus has been present for a long time, 36 hr or more, it may not be possible to remove all the thrombi from these arteries.

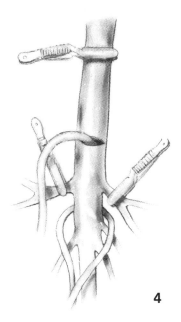

4

5

Closure of the arteriotomy; the 'second-look' procedure

The transverse arteriotomy incision is now closed with a continuous suture of 5/0 Prolene or silk. The distal clamps are then removed and the suture line wrapped in Surgicel gauze. The proximal clamp is removed and the return of pulsation to the branches of the superior mesenteric artery are carefully observed. At the same time the bowel is inspected and the rate and extent of revascularization noted.

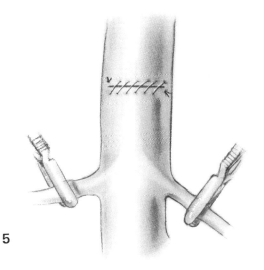

5

A 'SECOND-LOOK' OPERATION

Reconstruction of an acutely occluded superior mesenteric artery is a major indication for a 'second-look' operation. If the intestine is perforated, it must be immediately resected or exteriorized. But in many other patients, even those with apparently irreversible changes in the bowel, a second-look should be employed. The bowel is returned to the peritoneal cavity and the abdomen closed temporarily. Experience is required to decide if and when to take the 'second-look'. If the bowel was apparently successfully revascularized and appears to have recovered completely, then the 'second-look' should be deferred for 48–72 hr, but is often indicated. The reason is that small areas may still become necrotic and require resection. If on the other hand the bowel still looked ischaemic at the conclusion of the operation, the 'second-look' should be performed after 12–24 hr. It is surprising how an apparently gangrenous loop of intestine can recover and the length requiring resection be dramatically reduced.

6

Abdominal closure before the 'second-look'

If the surgeon proposes to re-explore the abdomen within 24 hr, all that is required is closure of the peritoneum with a continuous catgut suture and closure of the abdominal wall with a series of 'all-layer' or 'through-and-through' sutures of Dacron. These are tied in the usual manner over sponges. The fascia and skin are not closed in a formal manner. The wound is then dressed and arrangements made for the 'second-look' procedure, at which time the 'all-layer' sutures are removed together with the catgut. The intestine is inspected and any grossly ischaemic areas are resected. After the 'second-look', the abdomen is formally closed in layers. A frequent question asked by residents is, 'when is a third-look required?' The answer is only if the patient's condition demands it.

CHRONIC OCCLUSION OF THE COELIAC AND MESENTERIC ARTERIES

These patients have frequently been fully investigated for abdominal pain of obscure aetiology (Rob, 1966, 1967), but the definitive diagnosis depends upon arteriography. It is of interest that it is possible to have a complete thrombosis of both the coeliac and superior mesenteric arteries without any symptoms referable to the gastro-intestinal tract. But most patients are not so fortunate and stenosis or thrombosis of these arteries may cause crippling problems. In general stenosis or thrombosis of two of the three arteries supplying the alimentary tract is required before symptoms develop, but symptoms may develop from involvement of only one artery if the collateral circulation is inadequate.

In the past the following procedures have been employed in the management of these patients, but these have been abandoned because the results have been less effective than the procedures described in this chapter. These include a splenic artery-to-aorta bypass for thrombosis of the coeliac artery, thrombo-endarterectomy of the first part of the superior mesenteric artery and re-implantation of the superior mesenteric artery into the aorta.

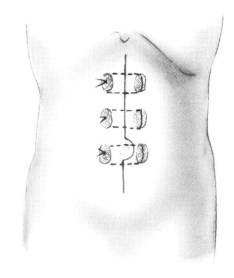

6

AORTA-TO-SUPERIOR MESENTERIC BYPASS GRAFT

This is the most widely used operation. If the patient also has disease of the coeliac and inferior mesenteric artery, it is usually sufficient to restore a flow to the superior mesenteric system only.

7

Preparation of the superior mesenteric artery

After a full abdominal exploration and careful palpation of the coeliac and both mesenteric arteries, the peritoneum over the root of the mesentery is incised to expose the superior mesenteric artery from the point where it emerges from behind the pancreas to beyond the origin of the middle colic artery. This section of the superior mesenteric artery is mobilized and inspected. In most patients the atherosclerotic plaques lie proximal to this point. The strength of the pulse in the superior mesenteric artery will depend upon the state of the stenosis at the origin of this vessel which may have progressed to total occlusion. The collateral circulation particularly the marginal artery of the colon must be inspected, but not damaged in any way. A site for the anastomosis is then selected usually just proximal to the middle colic artery.

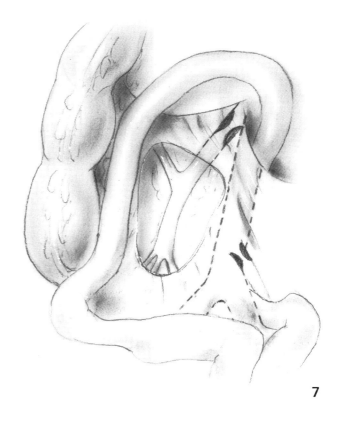

7

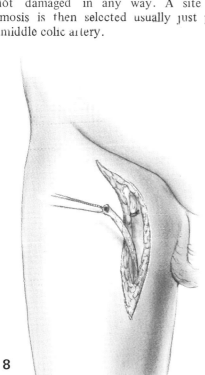

8

8

Preparation of the vein graft

In the past Dacron and other plastic prostheses have been used, but the results with autogenous vein graft have been better. The saphenous vein is exposed at the groin and 6–8 cm of the main trunk removed. This is then washed in saline, all branches are tied and the vein marked so that it will be reversed when placed in the patient. The distal end of the vein is then anastomosed to the side of the abdominal aorta and the proximal end to the side of the superior mesenteric artery.

9

The proximal or aortic anastomosis

This preferably is placed on the anterior wall of the abdominal aorta just below the renal arteries, but it may be placed on one common iliac artery. The anterior 75 per cent of the circumference of the abdominal aorta is exposed and isolated for a distance of about 5 cm. It is not necessary to mobilize the whole aorta or to identify and isolate the lumbar arteries. The anaesthetist injects 50–100 mg of heparin intravenously. A side clamp is placed on the aorta so that sufficient of the aortic wall is included in the clamp to perform a satisfactory anastomosis to the vein graft. The vein is then cut obliquely and the aortic wall incised so that the sides of the venous and arterial openings will be equal. The vein graft is then anastomosed to the side of the aorta using a 5/0 suture of silk or Prolene.

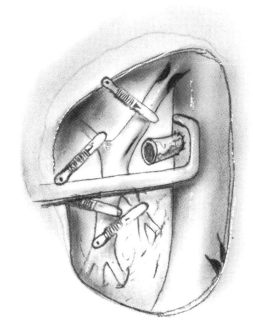

9

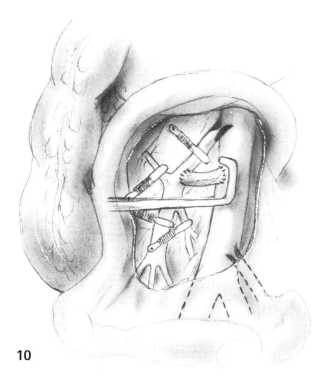

10

10

The distal or mesenteric anastomosis

The vein is best anastomosed to the superior mesenteric artery proximal to the middle colic branch, but it may be placed just opposite the origin of this vessel. The artery is clamped and incised on the surface facing the abdominal aorta. The surgeon then establishes that the distal vessels are open by observing the retrograde flow. The vein graft is then cut obliquely.

The length of the vein graft is important. If it is too long, it may kink and occlude. The correct length is such that it will lie straight between the aorta and superior mesenteric artery, a distance of about 4 cm in most patients. It is now anastomosed to the side of the superior mesenteric artery. A 5/0 suture is used, after which the clamps are removed and firm pressure applied for a few minutes to complete haemostasis.

RELEASE OF EXTERNAL COMPRESSION OF THE COELIAC ARTERY

The coeliac artery may be compressed by the median arcuate ligament of the diaphragm and the coeliac ganglion. These patients have a bruit in the upper abdomen and many have no symptoms or problems referable to the stenosis of the coeliac artery. For them neither investigation nor treatment is required. But others complain of postprandial pain. This pain is often intermittent and usually follows a large meal. The diagnosis is often made after studies of the gastro-intestinal tract, gall-bladder and pancreas have shown no abnormality. Arteriography confirms the presence of stenosis of the coeliac artery.

11a, b & c

The anatomical abnormality

The vertebral portion of the diaphragm arises from three aponeurotic arches, the lateral, medial and median arcuate ligaments. *Illustration 11a* shows their relationship to each other and to the aorta, vena cava and oesophagus. There is only one median arcuate ligament. It is this ligament which may compress the coeliac artery close to its origin from the abdominal aorta.

Illustration 11b is a lateral view showing how the median arcuate ligament crosses the front of the aorta just above the coeliac artery. If the artery arises at an abnormal height on the aorta or if the median arcuate ligament of the diaphragm is placed unusually low, then the upper surface of the coeliac artery is compressed and the artery stenosed. The coeliac ganglion surrounds the coeliac artery at this point (*see Illustration 11c*). It may be impossible to decide if the compressing agent is the coeliac ganglion or the median arcuate ligament of the diaphragm.

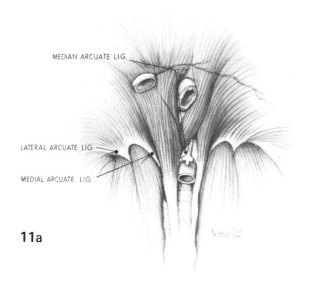

MEDIAN ARCUATE LIG.

LATERAL ARCUATE LIG.

MEDIAL ARCUATE LIG.

11a

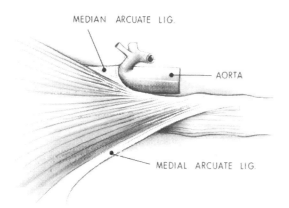

MEDIAN ARCUATE LIG.

AORTA

MEDIAL ARCUATE LIG.

11b

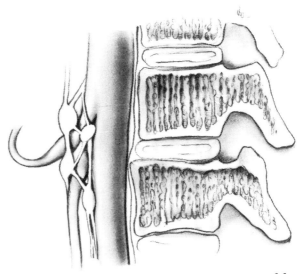

11c

EXPOSURE OF THE ORIGIN OF THE COELIAC ARTERY

12

This may be through a mid-line upper abdominal incision or a left, thoraco-abdominal incision. The thoraco-abdominal incision provides better exposure, but when possible we use a mid-line incision because this produces less postoperative problems. For the release of external compression a mid-line incision is preferred.

The gastrohepatic omentum is opened and the stomach displaced to the left. The left gastric artery is located and followed towards the coeliac artery. The coeliac artery is now exposed together with the adjacent abdominal aorta. The compressing agent is isolated around the circumference of the coeliac artery and either excised or divided to release the compression. We have found that excision is better. The coeliac ganglion and part of the median arcuate ligament are removed by dissecting carefully around the artery. The main compression is on the superior surface of the artery and here the surgeon must be careful to avoid injury to the vessel wall. Should it occur, repair is by simple suture or a patch-graft angioplasty.

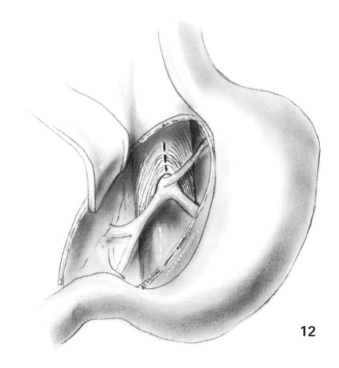

12

AORTA-TO-COELIAC ARTERY BYPASS

13

The best incision for this operation is a left, thoraco-abdominal incision through the ninth intercostal space to expose the coeliac artery and the adjacent aorta. The abdominal viscera including the spleen and pancreas are displaced forwards and to the patient's right side.

This is a good procedure if the patient has a complete thrombosis of the coeliac artery, but is unsatisfactory for a stenosis of the coeliac artery. The reason is that when the artery is stenosed, the flow through the narrowed segment may persist and result in thrombosis of the bypass. In the past the splenic artery was divided close to the spleen and used for this bypass, but in our patients this artery has usually been diseased and as a result has been unsuitable.

A segment of autogenous saphenous vein is the preferred vessel for the bypass. It is removed from the groin, reversed and anastomosed to the side of the abdominal aorta. An aortic side clamp of the

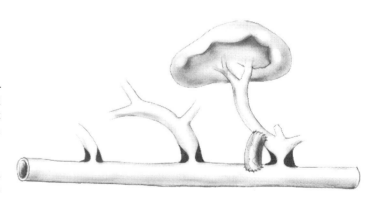

13

Derra type is used, so that the flow to the distal vessels is not completely interrupted.

The distal anastomosis is best placed on a branch of the coeliac artery rather than the main trunk. A good site is the side of the splenic artery close to the origin of this vessel from the coeliac artery. This will permit perfusion of the whole coeliac arterial system and it is simpler to place the anastomosis there than on the coeliac trunk.

THE INFERIOR MESENTERIC ARTERY

This vessel may require reconstruction under three main circumstances. Embolic occlusion, when the procedure is similar to that described for acute occlusion of the superior mesenteric artery. Stenosis associated with occlusion of the superior mesenteric and coeliac arteries, and as part of a procedure which requires division of the origin of the inferior mesenteric artery.

14

Thrombo-endarterectomy of the inferior mesenteric artery

Occasionally a patient presents with a thrombosis of the coeliac or superior mesenteric artery and a severe stenosis of the origin of the inferior mesenteric artery. After revascularization of the occluded coeliac or superior mesenteric artery, the surgeon can perform a thrombo-endarterectomy of the stenosed inferior mesenteric artery. A side clamp is applied to the aorta around the origin of the inferior mesenteric artery. A thrombo-endarterectomy is then performed of the proximal inferior mesenteric artery and of the adjacent abdominal aorta. The arterial incision is then closed with a patch graft of autogenous saphenous vein.

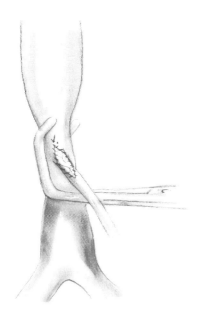

14

RE-IMPLANTATION OF THE INFERIOR MESENTERIC ARTERY

Occasionally a patient with severe occlusive disease of the coeliac and superior mesenteric arteries requires ligature of the inferior mesenteric artery, either as part of an operation upon the abdominal aorta or as part of a colectomy. This is usually without adverse effects, but if the inferior mesenteric artery is noted to be unduly large, then it is probably an important collateral vessel and should be preserved if possible. In these patients the surgeon should examine the coeliac and superior mesenteric arteries before he divides the inferior mesenteric artery. If they are diseased and the inferior mesenteric artery has to be divided, then two alternative procedures may be considered. These are an aorta-to-superior mesenteric arterial bypass graft (*Illustrations 8–11*) and re-implantation of the inferior mesenteric artery.

15

Re-implantation of the inferior mesenteric artery

The important step is to recognize that the inferior mesenteric artery is large and an important part of the blood supply of the intestinal tract before it is divided. The surgeon is then able to preserve a ring of aortic wall around the origin of this artery if he is operating for an aneurysm of the abdominal aorta. This ring should be about 1·5–2 cm in diameter. The aorta is clamped. The ring is excised and then the ring, including the inferior mesenteric artery is re-implanted into the aortic prosthesis in the manner illustrated. The actual sutures are placed just outside the orifice of the inferior mesenteric artery.

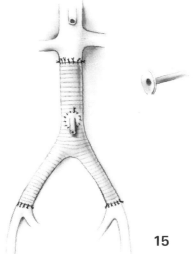

15

POSTOPERATIVE CARE AND COMPLICATIONS

The place of the 'second-look' abdominal exploration has been discussed. This is very important in the management of ischaemia of the intestine which is likely to become gangrenous and perforate. Another major problem is the massive water, electrolyte and even blood loss that can occur and persist for many days if there is widespread necrosis of the intestinal mucosa. These fluid, electrolyte and blood losses must be replaced so that the patient will maintain an adequate circulating blood volume, blood pressure, cardiac output and urine excretion.

Anticoagulants should not be used in the postoperative period because these will increase the risk of blood loss from the intestinal wall as well as from the surgical wounds.

Antibiotics are important and should be used during the postoperative period.

The surgeon must also follow the patient very carefully and if signs of local peritoneal irritation develop, it is likely that gangrenous bowel is present. The white blood count, serum enzymes and abdominal x-ray examinations are useful in following the patient during the postoperative period.

References

Bergan, J.J., Dean, R.H., Conn, J. and Yao, J.S.T. (1975). 'Revascularization in treatment of mesenteric infarction.' *Ann. Surg.* **182**, 430

Dunbar, J.D., Molnar, W., Beman, F.F. and Marble, S. (1965). 'Compression of the celiac trunk and abdominal angina.' *Am. J. Roentg.* **95**, 731

Lord, R.S.A., Stoney, R.J. and Wylie, E.J. (1968). 'Celiac-axis compression.' *Lancet* **2**, 795

Morris, G.C., Jr. and DeBakey, M.E. (1961). 'Abdominal angina—diagnosis and surgical treatment.' *J. Am. med. Ass.* **176**, 89

Rob, C.G. (1965). 'Disease of the abdominal aorta.' *Manitoba med. Rev.* **45**, 552

Rob, C.G. (1966). 'Surgical disease of the celiac and mesenteric arteries.' *Archs Surg.* **93**, 21

Rob, C.G. (1967). 'Stenosis and thrombosis of the celiac and mesenteric arteries.' *Am. J. Surg.* **114**, 363

Scott, J. Boley, Schwartz, S.S. and Williams, L.F. (1971). *Vascular Disorders of the Intestine.* New York: Appleton-Century-Crofts

[*The illustrations for this Chapter on Operations for Stenosis, Thrombosis and Embolism of the Mesenteric and Coeliac Arteries (Acute and Chronic Arterial Occlusion) were drawn by Mr. R. Wabnitz.*]

Stenosis of the Renal Arteries

Kenneth Owen, M.S., F.R.C.S.
Consultant Urologist, St. Mary's Hospital,
St. Peter's Hospital and King Edward VII
Hospital for Officers, London

and

Charles Rob, *M.C.,* M.D., M.Chir., F.R.C.S.
Professor and Chairman of the Department of Surgery,
University of Rochester School of Medicine and
Dentistry, Rochester, New York

PRE-OPERATIVE

Renal artery stenosis is now a well established if one of the less common causes of renal hypertension. It may be due to a number of causes but the most common are atheroma and fibromuscular hyperplasia. While external bands may cause obstruction, these may be associated with intrinsic arterial disease so that, should a band appear to be the cause of obstruction, the flow rate should be checked after division as a supplementary reconstruction may be needed.

The disease may be unilateral or bilateral but when it is bilateral it is rarely symmetrical so that there are usually functional differences between the two kidneys.

Evidence of the disease may rarely be given by an episode of pain in the loin (due to a small embolus) and suspicion of renal artery stenosis in a hypertensive patient may be aroused by the finding of a murmur on auscultation just above and to one side of the umbilicus or posteriorly over the renal artery. The majority of cases are, however, discovered from the hypertensive population after screening tests, the most important being the intravenous pyelogram and renogram. The pyelogram may show reduced size of the affected kidney, delayed excretion and increased contrast density in the later films. There may also be some evidence of collateral vessels shown by notching of the pelvis and ureter. The ^{131}I

Hippuran renogram shows a delayed peak and an impaired second phase and usually an impaired third phase.

Definitive diagnosis

Renal arteriography

Selective catheterization and injection of the renal arteries gives the exact anatomical definition of the disease but the apparent radiological obstruction may be disproportionate to the functional ischaemia. A plaque of atheroma on the anterior or posterior wall will be much less evident than a concentric narrowing or a plaque on the superior or posterior wall. The florid lesions of fibromuscular hyperplasias are easily seen but the finer intimal proliferations of this disease may only be detected after critical examination, particularly in the distal vessels.

Renin level

While peripheral vein renins may be useful in excluding hyperaldosteronism they are not particularly helpful in the diagnosis of renal artery stenosis. The ratio between the renal vein renin on both sides may however be helpful, a ratio of 1:5 or more being strongly suggestive of renal artery obstruction.

Divided function tests

The most widely used technique is that of Stamey (1961, 1966). This gives quantative confirmation of the functional changes seen on the pyelogram, with reduced urine flow, sodium concentration and creatinine, PAH and inulin clearances but increased concentrations of creatinine, PAH and inulin on the affected side. Stamey has also suggested that the test has prognostic importance in that a PAH clearance of less than 250 ml/min on the contralateral side indicates a poor outlook.

TREATMENT

Atheromatous lesions, although apparently solitary, are usually evidence of widespread disease and of a significant reduction in life expectancy from other lesions such as coronary and cerebral artery disease. It is usually better to treat these patients medically in the first instance and to reserve surgery for the more severe cases which fail to respond to medical treatment. Fibroplasia tends on the other hand to have a good prognosis. It is most common in young females and surgical treatment may be contemplated at an early stage providing the lesion is anatomically suitable. Arterial reconstruction is preferable to nephrectomy but the latter procedure may be indicated in poor risk patients or those with widespread disease of the peripheral arteries. Some type of bypass procedure is the usual reconstruction but thrombo-endarterectomy may sometimes be of value in atheromatous lesions.

THE OPERATION

1

The incision

An anterior incision is far preferable to a posterior renal exposure as it gives so much better exposure and control of the vessels. The incision may be either paramedian or a transverse upper abdominal incision and this latter incision is favoured in most instances as it gives an extremely good exposure and good healing with a very low incidence of hernia. The incision is about 1–1·5 inches (2·5–3·8 cm) above the umbilicus, the exact height depending upon the build of the patient and the subcostal angle. It is extended to the costal margin on the affected side and can be further extended into a thoraco-abdominal incision should greater exposure be required. In many patients of a favourable build the incision need only go a little beyond the mid-line but in more difficult cases or in bilateral lesions it should extend from one costal margin to the other. Both rectus abdominus muscles with their sheaths and linea alba are divided, as are the internal and external oblique muscles together with the transversus abdominis. The peritoneum is opened throughout the length of the incision and the ligamentum teres divided just above the umbilicus.

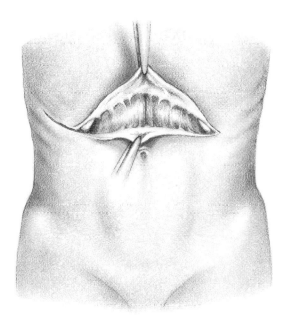

1

Exposure of kidneys, renal arteries and aorta

2

Right renal artery

After a full abdominal exploration the right renal artery is exposed by incising the posterior peritoneum lateral to the second part of the duodenum so that the head of the pancreas and duodenum can be retracted to the left and the liver upwards and hepatic flexure of the colon downwards. It is usually necessary to pass a tape around the vena cava and also the right renal vein before exposing the artery deep to the renal vein.

The stenosis, even if fibromuscular may lie deep to the vena cava and an atheromatous stenosis will lie very medially behind the vena cava. Palpation of the artery may give obvious evidence of the stenosis but on some occasions, particularly in fibromuscular hyperplasia lesions, there may be very little macroscopic evidence of a very florid radiological obstruction. Auscultation of the artery through a sterile stethoscope and/or pressure and flow measurements may occasionally be of help.

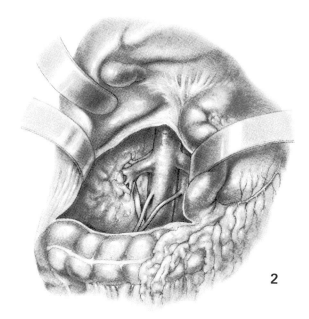

2

3

Left renal artery and aorta

The left renal artery is exposed by dividing the peritoneum along the lateral side of the descending colon and also lateral to the splenic flexure so that the splenic flexure and descending colon can be retracted medially. The tail of the pancreas is seen in the upper part of the incision and if use of the splenic artery is contemplated it may be useful to expose it at this stage. Small pancreatic branches of this artery may be found running into the pancreas and it is important to isolate and ligate these as, should they be divided accidentally, they may produce profuse bleeding. The left renal artery may be more easily exposed back to the aorta after taping the left renal vein.

The aorta is mobilized with care. It is usually necessary to divide at least one pair of lumbar arteries and often two pairs of these otherwise they run a risk of being torn during aortic clamping. The lower border of the superior mesenteric artery is identified and if a bypass graft is to be taken from the lower part of the aorta the inferior mesenteric artery may also need identification.

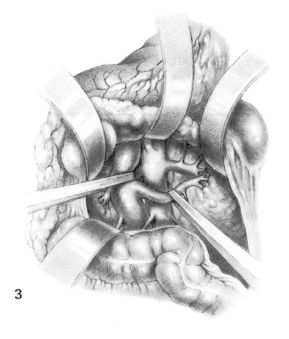

3

AORTA-TO-RENAL ARTERY BYPASS

A bypass graft is usually the method of choice on the right side and may also be needed on the left if the splenic artery is unsuitable for use. A saphenous vein graft has the advantage of using autogenous tissue and its long-term results are excellent. Although the ovarian or testicular vein may appear suitable the tensile strength of these vessels is not as great as the saphenous vein and their use should be avoided as it carries the risk of rupture.

4

Isolation of the saphenous vein

A longitudinal incision is made in the leg starting at the upper end of the saphenous vein about 1·5 inches (3·8 cm) below and lateral to the pubic tubercle. The vein is exposed and its branches ligated carefully with fine silk ligatures before being divided. It is advisable to remove a length about 1·5 times longer than is thought necessary so that there is adequate length to select a suitable place for a tension-free anastomosis. Care is taken to mark the distal end (B) which must be anastomosed to the aorta so that the direction of blood flow conforms with the arrangement of the valves.

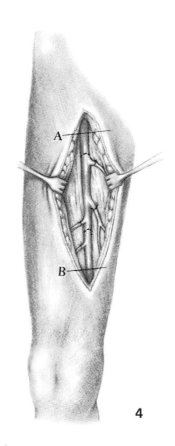

4

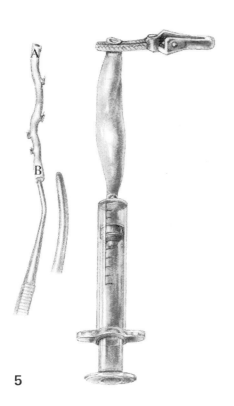

5

5

The vein contracts markedly on removal and it is essential to dilate it before making the anastomosis. This can be done initially with a small probe or Hegar's dilator. It is then possible to dilate it hydrostatically with saline using a syringe with one end of the vein clamped.

Anastomosis of vein to aorta

6a

The aorta is clamped transversely above and below the area selected for anastomosis. This should be a relatively disease-free part of the aorta and there seems to be no disadvantage in running the graft obliquely upwards from the lower aorta or, even in some instances where the aorta is grossly diseased using the common iliac artery. An oval window is cut in the aorta to match the obliquely-cut distal end of the vein graft so as to give as long a suture line as possible, A continuous suture of 6/0 plastic suture material is used. On completion of this suture line the renal end of the vein graft is clamped and blood allowed to distend the graft so that the optimum length for anastomosis to the distal renal can be chosen with the vein under arterial pressure.

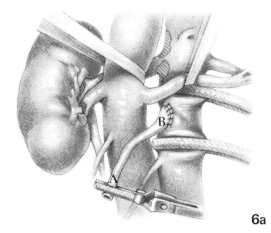

6a

6b

When the length is decided the bulldog clamp is moved from the end (A) (*see Illustration 6a*) of the vein graft to the other end so that the vein is clamped flush with the aorta. The renal artery is then divided, its proximal end being ligated securely and the distal end is turned up for anastomosis. There is often a considerable back-flow from capsular collaterals so that the distal artery of its terminal branches may need to be clamped.

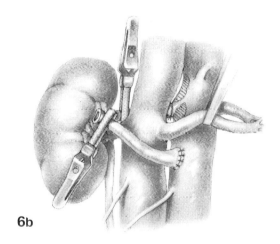

6b

6c

In cases of fibromuscular hyperplasia if there is any narrowing of the distal arteries these may be dilated at this stage using a metal dilator.

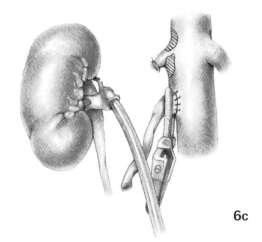

6c

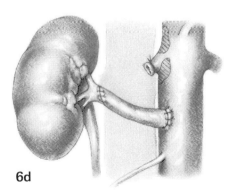

6d

6d

An end-to-end anastomosis is then made with 7/0 plastic suture material making an oblique suture line. On removing the clamps the vein takes up a natural curve in front of the vena cava.

7

A plastic prosthesis may be used instead of a vein graft but this is thought in most centres to have a greater risk of long-term failure. If a plastic prosthesis is used it is advisable to do the distal anastomosis first as there is no great problem in selecting the correct length and the greater rigidity of the plastic material may lead to tearing of the thin distal arterial wall if there is any degree of post-stenotic dilation should this suture line be done when the aortic end is fixed in position.

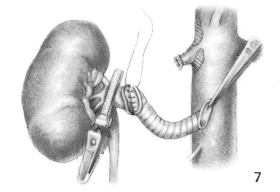

7

8

Splenorenal anastomosis

On the left side if the splenic artery is healthy it may be used in a similar way for anastomosis to the distal renal artery.

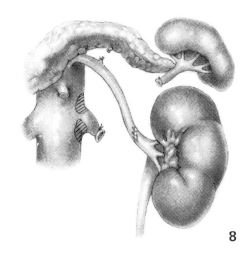

8

THROMBO-ENDARTERECTOMY

This operation is suitable for some cases of atheromatous obstruction where the disease is localized. It should be noted that, although the obstruction may appear radiologically to be within the renal artery it starts as a plaque in the aorta and should be approached from the aorta.

9a

The facility of this operation often depends upon the exact relationship of the left renal vein crossing the aorta and the position of the two renal arteries. The aorta is exposed and cross-clamped below the renal arteries. In some cases it may be possible to put the upper clamp obliquely so as to allow blood to continue flowing through the contralateral kidney. The aorta is then incised, usually through an oblique incision and the atheromatous plaque around the renal artery ostium is dissected away. It is usually possible to pull any obstructing plaque from the renal artery but if there is any doubt as to whether the distal part of the removal is clear then the renal artery may need to be opened.

9b

The incision is then closed with 6/0 plastic suture material. If the disease is bilateral or if there is any residual aortic plaque which may later obstruct the opposite side then the direction of the upper clamp can be reversed and a similar procedure carried out on the opposite side.

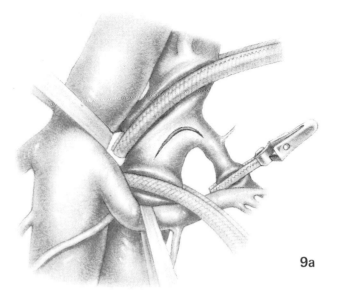

9a

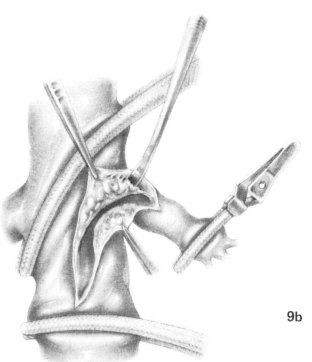

9b

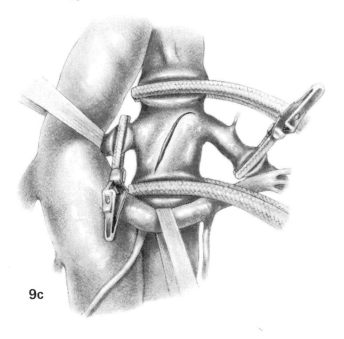

9c

9c

An alternative procedure is to cross-clamp the aorta above both renals but care must be taken if this is done to complete the procedure within 30 min to avoid ischaemic renal damage and it is wise to give an intravenous infusion of mannitol before removing the clamps to lessen this risk.

10

Alternative procedures

In young children any renal artery reconstruction must allow for growth. On the left side this is relatively easy using the splenic artery and interrupted sutures but can present a problem on the right side. In such young children with a healthy lower-limb vasculature the common iliac artery has been divided proximal to its division and swung up to anastomose to the distal renal artery using a long oblique suture line with interrupted sutures. A good collateral circulation very rapidly develops to the leg and this procedure produces no disability although its use must clearly be restricted to young children with a healthy circulation. Should there be any doubt about the circulation to the lower limb then a vein graft or prosthesis could be used to bridge the gap between aorta and distal common iliac artery.

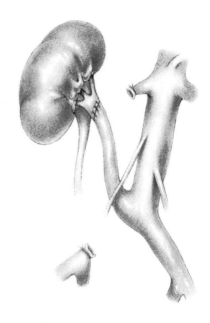

10

11

Internal iliac artery graft

In some instances of fibromuscular hyperplasia the disease may extend into the proximal part of the renal arteries, and dilation may not be possible, so that a branched replacement is necessary. A free internal iliac artery segment may be used for this replacement. Its main divisions are anastomosed to two renal artery branches and any further branch can be anastomosed to the side of the graft. The main trunk is anastomosed to the aorta. As with a plastic prosthesis it may be easier to do the distal anastomosis before doing the aortic end. Such a reconstruction can usually be done satisfactorily within a safe ischaemia time, particularly as there is some protection against ischaemic damage by the collateral capsular circulation. However, an alternative which allows of very prolonged ischaemia while a difficult technical reconstruction is done is to remove the kidney to perfuse and cool it and then to replace it as an autograft, anastomosed to the iliac vessel (*see* Chapter on 'Renal Hypothermia' in the volume on *Genito-urinary Surgery* to appear later on in the *Operative Surgery* series).

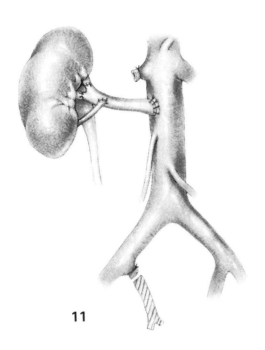

11

12

Re-implantation of the renal artery to the aorta

This procedure may often seem tempting on consideration of the radiological appearance but in practice it is very rarely possible to obtain an adequate length of renal artery to anastomose to the most suitable healthy portion of the aorta without undue tension of angulation so that this procedure is only very rarely practicable.

NEPHRECTOMY OR PARTIAL NEPHRECTOMY

This is the simplest operation and may be the procedure of choice in patients whose general condition is poor; it is also indicated when a conservative arterial reconstruction operation has failed. In most patients an arterial reconstruction operation is the best treatment because the kidney on the affected side may be the better kidney after a normal blood flow has been restored, having been protected by the arterial stenosis from secondary hypertensive changes.

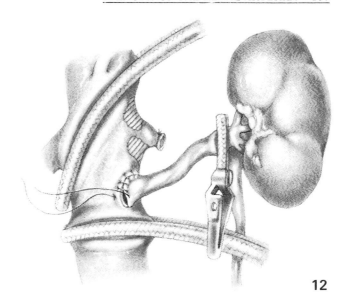

12

POSTOPERATIVE CARE

Prophylactic measures

Ischaemic renal damage

The risk of ischaemic damage is slight as these procedures can usually be done well within the safe ischaemia time limit and the tolerance of the kidney beyond a renal artery stenosis is probably significantly greater than normal in view of the considerable collateral circulation through capsular and other vessels as evidenced by the brisk back-flow from the distal end of the artery. However, if prolongation of the ischaemia period beyond, say, 30 min is necessary then it is wise to give an infusion of mannitol intravenously before releasing the clamps.

Paralytic ileus

Because of the extensive retroperitoneal dissection performed in operations for stenosis of the renal arteries it is essential to take prophylactic measures against paralytic ileus. Gastric suction and intravenous fluid replacement should be used until the patient has good bowel sounds and is passing flatus.

Anticoagulant drugs

Anticoagulant drugs are not used in the immediate postoperative period because of the danger of haemorrhage.

Blood pressure

The fall in blood pressure in successful cases usually occurs slowly after operation and it often takes a period of months before the blood pressure returns completely to normal and secondary hypertensive changes regress. Severe hypertensive retinopathy is seen to revert to almost normal within a period of 3 months after an operation for reconstruction of the renal artery. Occasionally there may be a more precipitate fall of blood pressure and, should this occur, a careful search should be made for the usual causes such as haemorrhage, lung infection, acute gastric dilation or gram-negative bacteraemia before assuming that such a fall is due to an overswing following correction of the renin-angiotensin stimulus.

References

Stamey, T. A. (1961). *Postgrad. Med.* **29**, 496
Stamey, R. A. (1966). *Anti-hypertensive Therapy*, Ed. by F. Gross, p. 555. Ciba Symposium, 1965. Berlin: Springer Verlag

[The illustrations for this Chapter on Stenosis of the Renal Arteries were drawn by Miss F. Wadsworth.]

Vascular Injuries

Charles Rob, *M.C.,* M.D., M.Chir., F.R.C.S.
Professor and Chairman of the Department of Surgery,
University of Rochester School of Medicine and
Dentistry, Rochester, New York

INTRODUCTION

Blood vessels may be injured by penetrating, blunt and deceleration forces. When the vessel wall is completely disrupted, haemorrhage occurs. This may be external or internal. If it is internal into a body cavity, the patient frequently develops shock and may present a difficult diagnostic problem. Alternatively the haemorrhage may be into the tissues of the body producing a haematoma. If the disruption of the arterial wall is partial, a false aneurysm forms as in the deceleration injury of the thoracic aorta or the artery thromboses which occurs for example after a fracture–dislocation or dislocation of the knee joint. Arteries and veins are close together and so an injury, particularly a penetrating wound with a small object may produce an arteriovenous fistula.

In many patients with a penetrating wound the diagnosis is obvious, but in others it may be difficult. Arteriography is then indicated and is of special value if a chest x-ray shows a widened mediastinum in a patient who has suffered a deceleration injury, or the presence of pulsation in the peripheral arteries is in doubt after a dislocation or fracture–dislocation of the knee, elbow or shoulder joints.

The first step is to control haemorrhage by a pressure dressing if possible. The patient is then resuscitated and urgent operation is required in most patients. The surgeon obtains proximal and distal control of the injured vessel. This may be a matter of extreme urgency if the bleeding has not been controlled. In patients with an associated fracture of a long bone, stabilization of the fracture should precede vascular repair because subsequent manipulations may disrupt an otherwise satisfactory vascular suture line.

For convenience the problems facing a surgeon in the management of vascular injuries will be covered by describing the management of: a stab wound of the inferior vena cava; a deceleration injury of the thoracic aorta; thrombosis of the popliteal artery after a fracture–dislocation of the knee joint; a gunshot wound of the femoral artery and a stab wound which has injured the internal mammary vessels.

It is stressed that heparin must be used with great caution in patients who are injured because bleeding may be increased from an injury at another site such as the brain, liver or spleen. Nevertheless, it is usually wise to give the patient 50–75 mg of heparin systemically just before the injured vessel is clamped provided it is reversed with an equivalent dose of protamine sulphate as soon as the vascular repair has been completed.

STAB WOUND OF THE INFERIOR VENA CAVA

1

Preparation for massive blood loss

The entry wound is frequently in the back or right flank. Other organs likely to be involved include the right kidney, duodenum, right colon, abdominal aorta, liver and small intestine. The haemorrhage from a stab wound of the inferior vena cava may be surprisingly moderate until the surgeon exposes the area when it can be catastrophic. In all patients suspected of having such a wound, preparation should be made before operation to deal with major venous bleeding during the procedure. Such preparation should include: confirmation with the operating room nurse that appropriate instruments are available including vascular clamps and sutures; confirmation with the anaesthetist that adequate amounts of blood are available for immediate transfusion and confirmation that an apparatus for autotransfusion is available in the operating room. We prefer our modification of the autotransfusion system.

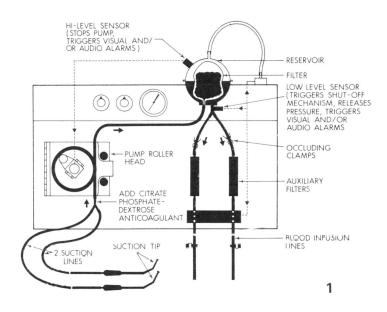

1

2a & b

Exposure of the inferior vena cava

This must be through an abdominal or thoraco-abdominal incision depending upon the location of the injury. It is a mistake to expose the injured inferior vena cava by enlarging the stab wound in the flank. After exploration of the abdominal organs, the surgeon examines the haematoma in the flank. If possible, he isolates and clamps the inferior vena cava below and above before he approaches the injured segment. He then opens the haematoma and using suction attached to the autotransfusion apparatus, he inspects the injured area. At this time lumbar, renal or gonadal veins opening into this segment are also clamped. Once haemostasis has been achieved, the surgeon repairs the defect or ligatures the inferior vena cava.

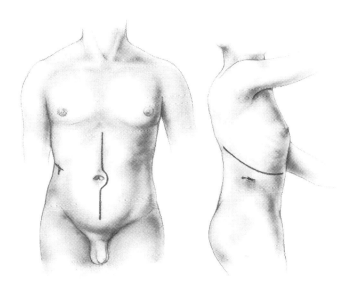

2a   2b

3a & b

Repair of ligature of the inferior vena cava

When the injury is below the renal veins, is extensive and when full control of the bleeding is difficult or impossible, simple ligature proximal and distal to the injury combined with suture ligature of any bleeding lumbar veins is the best treatment. But, in most patients the stab wound can be closed by simple suture using 4/0 silk or Prolene. Sometimes the knife will have crossed the vena cava and perforated both sides. Under these circumstances the posterior injury is closed from within the lumen of the inferior vena cava and the anterior injury by a simple over-and-over stitch. If a satisfactory closure of the posterior wound is to be achieved, the surgeon may have to enlarge the anterior wound. If the renal vein is also injured, it may be repaired, but simple ligature of a renal vein does not appear to change the function of that kidney.

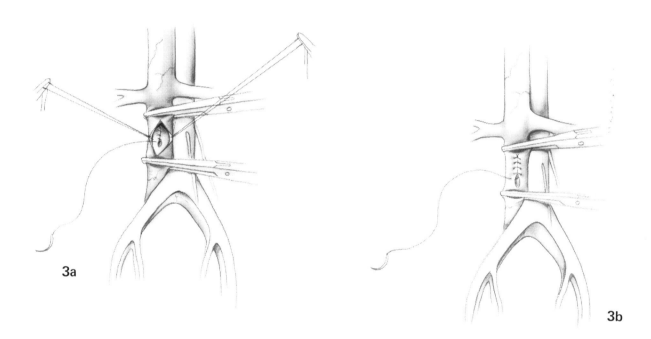

3a

3b

4a & b

Injury of the inferior vena cava and the hepatic veins

A right thoraco-abdominal incision is required to expose the part of the inferior vena cava which lies between the renal veins and the diaphragm. An injury to this part of the vena cava is one of the most difficult situations a surgeon ever has to face. If possible, a vascular side-clamp is applied and the defect closed by suture or with a venous patch graft angioplasty. At this level an indwelling shunt is required to maintain the return of sufficient blood to the heart to ensure a satisfactory cardiac output. The inferior vena cava at this level should not be cross-clamped except for a very short time.

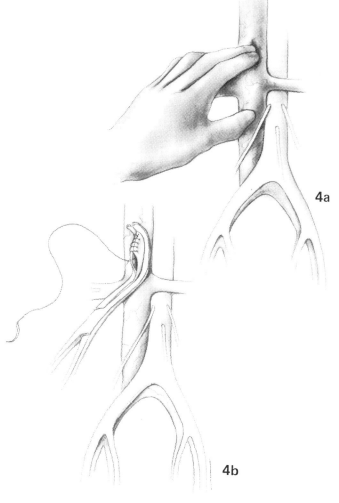

4a

4b

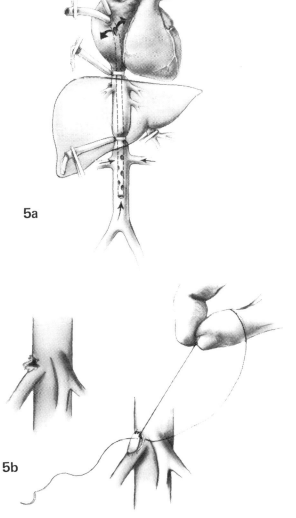

5a

5b

5a & b

An indwelling shunt in the suprarenal inferior vena cava

Through a purse-string suture in the right atrium a large, polyvinyl catheter bonded with tridodecyl-metrylammonium-heparin is passed into the inferior vena cava to a point close to the junction of the common iliac veins. As shown in *Illustrations 5 a* and *b* this catheter has holes in it which should be opposite the renal veins. Similar side holes are made in the portion which lies within the right atrium. Tapes are placed around the vena cava and catheter close to the right atrium and again just above the renal veins. The inflow to the liver may be temporarily controlled by a vascular clamp across the porta hepatis. The injury to the inferior vena cava which may also involve the hepatic veins is then repaired by suture or a patch graft angioplasty.

DECELERATION INJURY OF THE THORACIC AORTA

This injury is often fatal, the patient dying of haemorrhage before reaching hospital. But in many others the outer layers of the aorta hold and a false aneurysm results. Essentially the descending thoracic aorta is fixed whilst the heart, aortic arch and the great vessels have some mobility. Thus, deceleration may cause a tear of the point where those two zones meet. This is just distal to the origin of the left subclavian artery at the point where the ligamentum arteriosum is attached to the thoracic aorta.

A deceleration injury of the thoracic aorta is suspected in such a patient if an x-ray shows widening of the mediastinum. An arteriogram will confirm the diagnosis. These patients frequently have associated head, abdominal or bony injuries. Rupture of the liver or spleen is of special importance because these may also require surgical correction, and heparin used during the aortic repair may increase the bleeding from these other injuries.

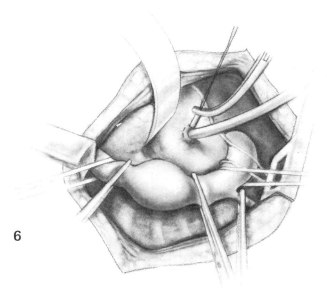

6

6

Obtaining proximal and distal control

It is important to isolate and control the aorta proximal and distal to the rupture before entering the haematoma or false aneurysm. It is usually best to obtain proximal control by isolating the aorta between the left common carotid and left subclavian arteries. During this part of the operation, the surgeon should identify and preserve the left recurrent laryngeal and vagus nerves. The aorta at this point and the left subclavian artery are then prepared for clamping. Often the first and second intercostal arteries are seen at this time. Their position is noted for future clamping. The descending thoracic aorta is then isolated distal to the lesion and prepared for clamping.

7a & b

Bypass during the period of aortic occlusion

Some surgeons proceed directly to repair the aortic injury by suture or a graft. In expert hands when the operation is performed rapidly, the results are excellent and complications such as paraplegia are rare. But most surgeons prefer to use a bypass during the period of aortic occlusion. The advantages include the prevention of proximal hypertension and of ischaemia of the distal spinal cord, kidneys and abdominal viscera. The disadvantages include the complications which may follow the insertion of a catheter into the left auricle if an auricular-to-femoral bypass is used and the increased risk of abdominal haemorrhage if heparin is given to a patient with an associated rupture of an abdominal organ such as the liver or spleen. An alternative is to place a bypass from the aortic arch to the common femoral artery. The tube is of polyvinyl bonded with tridodecyl-methylammonium-heparin. It is secured in the aortic arch with two purse-string sutures and placed into the common femoral artery through a transverse arteriotomy. At the conclusion of the procedure the aortic arch opening is repaired after a side-clamp has been applied and the femoral incision closed in the usual manner. The heparin effect if heparin has been given is reversed with protamine sulphate.

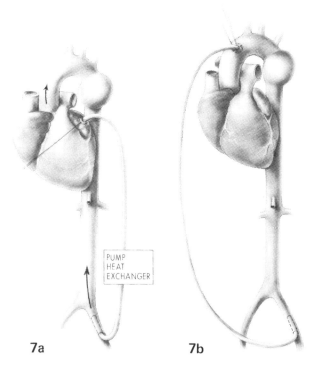

PUMP
HEAT
EXCHANGER

7a   **7b**

8

Suture repair of the aortic defect

A deceleration injury of the thoracic aorta produces a transverse rupture of the intima and inner layers of the media. For the patient to reach hospital alive, the adventitia and usually the outer layers of the media must hold. The result is a haematoma within the wall of the aorta. Untreated this may rupture or a false aneurysm may form. In some patients the aortic rupture may be repaired by simple suture taking large bites through all layers of the aortic wall. In others a graft is required to replace a few centimetres of the aorta; for this we recommend woven Dacron. The first step is to clamp the aorta above and below plus any other vessels which have been identified and which enter this segment such as the left subclavian or intercostal arteries are also occluded with clamps. The haematoma is now incised and the defect in the intima is identified. Frequently other intercostal arteries enter this segment of the aorta, they will be bleeding. They are either controlled with bulldog clamps or the orifices are oversewn with 4/0 vascular sutures. The aortic rupture is now repaired with a continuous 4/0 suture passing through the whole aortic wall. If there is any doubt about the effectiveness of this repair or if the injury is more than a few days old, so that a false aneurysm has formed, a graft of woven Dacron should be inserted.

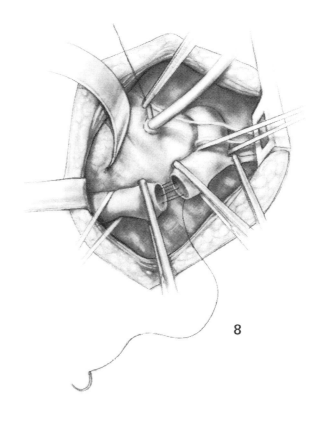

8

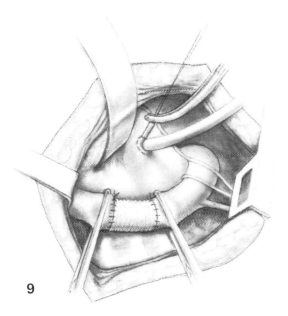

9

9

Repair with an aortic graft

The edges of the ruptured aorta are trimmed back so that a sound suture line is possible. This often requires the ligature and division of one or sometimes two pairs of intercostal arteries. A straight tube graft of woven Dacron usually about 20 mm in diameter is now sutured into position with a continuous 4/0 suture of Dacron or Prolene. We recommend placing the proximal suture line first. After completing both suture lines, any gaps are reinforced with additional sutures and the suture lines are wrapped in Surgicel gauze. The distal clamp is then removed followed by the proximal clamps and firm pressure is applied by the surgeon to the suture lines for 3–5 min. The heparin effect is next reversed with protamine sulphate. The shunt is then removed and the chest wound closed with drainage.

THROMBOSIS OF THE POPLITEAL ARTERY AFTER FRACTURE–DISLOCATION OR DISLOCATION OF THE KNEE JOINT

It is very important to check the dorsalis pedis and posterior tibial pulses in every patient who has suffered an injury of this type. In children particularly, the dislocation may have reduced spontaneously and the diagnosis then becomes difficult. It is surprising how often a hospital record shows that several observers have noted satisfactory pulsation in these arteries. The limb, however, becomes ischaemic or gangrenous. These observers were clearly wrong because a later arteriogram shows thrombosis of the popliteal artery. Whenever there is any doubt, an arteriogram should be performed immediately, and the popliteal artery repaired if it is occluded.

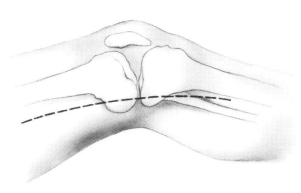

10

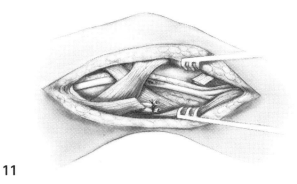

11

10

Exposure of the popliteal artery

The first step is to reduce the bone deformity. The popliteal artery will have thrombosed at the level of the knee joint. The artery at this point may be exposed by a posterior or medial incision. If the patient's condition permits, he or she is placed in the prone or face down position and the posterior approach is used. This provides excellent exposure without disturbing the muscular attachments. Often the injuries are multiple and the prone position is contra-indicated. The medial approach is then required. The incision for this approach is made just distal to the knee joint behind the tibia, the long saphenous vein is identified and preserved. It will probably be required for a graft. The fascia behind the tibia is incised and the popliteal space is entered. The surgeon dissects out the popliteal artery just proximal to its trifurcation. It will not be pulsating. He then dissects proximally until a pulsating artery is reached. This may require proximal extension of the incision with division of the semitendinous, semimembranous and gracilis muscles close to their tibial attachments.

11

Examination of the thrombosed artery

The injury consists of an intimal rupture with subsequent thrombosis. From the outside the artery may appear surprisingly normal, but the area of intimal damage may be quite large. All damaged intima must be excised and a good flow obtained from each end of the artery before it is repaired. This will require the resection of 2 or 3 cm of the vessel. It is always wise to pass a Fogarty catheter down both the anterior and posterior tibial arteries to the ankle. Even the presence of a brisk retrograde flow does not guarantee that there are not clots distally in these vessels. A Fogarty catheter is therefore used in every patient.

12

Repair of the arterial defect

End-to-end suture is rarely possible because of the length of the arterial injury and of the segment requiring resection. A vein graft is therefore used. The long saphenous vein has already been seen if the medial approach has been used. If at this level it is of sufficient size, a length slightly longer than the arterial defect is removed, washed with saline and reversed. It is then anastomosed end-to-end to the popliteal artery proximally and distally. Before the second anastomosis any excess vein is removed. If the saphenous vein at this level is too small or is duplicated, then a segment of the saphenous vein is taken from the groin. If the saphenous vein has previously been removed by stripping, a segment of cephalic vein is taken from the shoulder.

In some patients the popliteal vein will also have thrombosed. Providing the injury is less than 24 hr old, we recommend a thrombectomy through a transverse venotomy and sometimes repair with a vein graft.

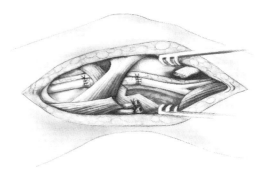

12

A GUNSHOT WOUND OF THE SUPERFICIAL FEMORAL ARTERY

This injury may occur in military or civilian practice. The management is similar in many ways, but differs in others. In this chapter civilian injuries will be discussed. The weapon may be a shotgun, large or small calibre hand gun, rifle or high velocity rifle. The femur is often fractured. The femoral and sciatic nerves may be severed or contused, and the muscle damage may be extensive if the weapon has been a high velocity rifle or a close-range shotgun blast. The first step is to control the bleeding after which the wound is excised and the fractured femur splinted. The stage is now set for the arterial repair.

13a & b

Exposure and control of the superficial femoral artery

This may have been achieved during the wound excision when the cut ends of the superficial femoral artery will have been controlled with vascular clamps. Some surgeons routinely obtain proximal and distal control through separate incisions. We sometimes do this if there is a large, pulsating haematoma but more often obtain control as described through the wound. The injury to the artery may be partial or a complete transection. In either case all of the damaged artery should be excised. We recommend the passage of a Fogarty catheter down the distal artery to the ankle in every patient, even if the retrograde flow is satisfactory. The adjacent femoral vein may also be injured, and sometimes the defect may be sutured, but more frequently a simple ligature is required. We do not recommend repair of the femoral vein with a venous graft in injuries of this type.

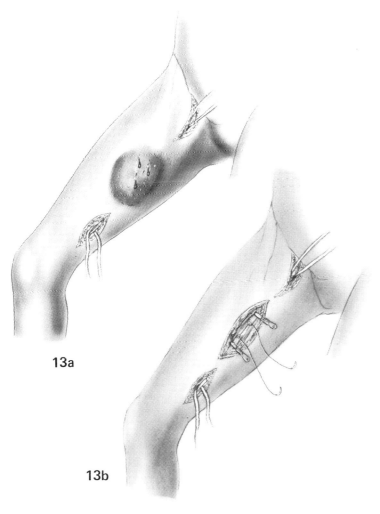

13a

13b

14

Repair of the superficial femoral artery

Simple suture is rarely possible in a gunshot wound of an artery. A venous graft is usually required. It is important not to place such a graft in an infected wound. If the injury is old and obviously infected, ligature is preferred with delayed graft if necessary after the wound has healed. But in most patients treatment is prompt and infection can be prevented by wound excision and antibiotics. The nature of this wound means that the saphenous vein should be preserved because the femoral vein has been ligatured. The best alternative is the saphenous vein from the other leg. If this is not available, a length of cephalic vein may be taken from either shoulder.

The segment of vein is then reversed and anastomosed end-to-end to the femoral artery proximally and distally. The second anastomosis being performed under slight tension to prevent redundancy.

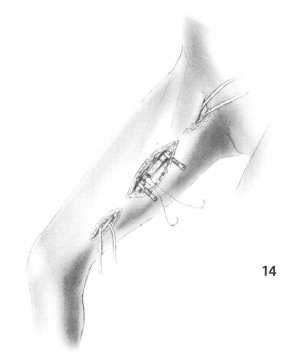

14

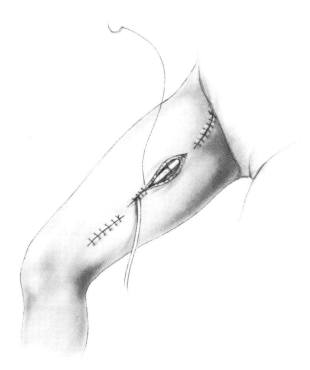

15

15

Closure of the wound

After the arterial repair has been completed and haemostasis achieved, we recommend irrigation of the wound with a solution containing a cephalosporin and kanamycin. Systemic antibiotics in the form of a cephalosporin, 2 g every 6 hr, and kanamycin 500 mg every 12 hr, are also commenced before the operation and given for 5 days after. The fascia and muscles are now sutured to cover the vein graft. The skin is closed very loosely and the wound drained. We recommend splinting the limb even if there has been no fracture. The more complete rest provided by splinting aids the healing of extensive gunshot wounds.

STAB WOUND OF THE INTERNAL MAMMARY VESSELS

A stab wound of the chest near either side of the sternum may injure the internal mammary vessels. Sometimes this is the only visceral injury; the heart, great vessels and lung being spared. The patient then develops a haemothorax which may become large, haemorrhagic shock develops and the mediastinum shifts to the opposite side as the haemothorax increases in size. The treatment is resuscitation combined with emergency ligature of the internal mammary vessels with drainage of the haemothorax.

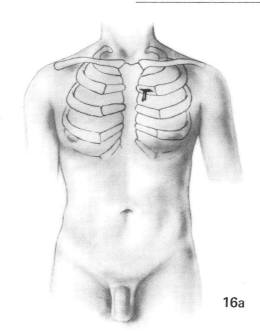

16a

16a & b

Ligature of the internal mammary vessels

As this is a stab wound the location of the wound gives an indication of which segment of the internal mammary vessels has been divided. Therefore, a wide excision of the wound with considerable enlargement transversely across the anterior thorax permits exposure of the divided vessels and their ligature. It may be necessary to excise part of the adjacent sternum and costal cartilages. Once the bleeding vessels have been ligatured, the haemothorax is aspirated completely by suction and a chest tube placed for drainage at the base of the pleural cavity.

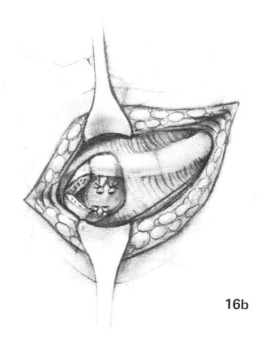

16b

References

Bergan, F. (1963). 'Traumatic intimal rupture of the popliteal artery with acute ischaemia of the limb in cases with supracondylar fractures of the femur.' *J. cardiovasc. Surg.* **4**, 300

Collins, J. A (1974). 'Problems associated with massive transfusion of stored blood.' *Surgery* **75**, 274

Connors, J. P., Ferguson, T. B., Weldon, C. S. and Roper, C. L. (1975). 'The use of the TDMAC-heparin shunt in the replacement of the descending thoracic aorta.' *Ann. Surg.* **181**, 735

Eastcott, H. H. G. (1963). 'A report on the management of various arterial injuries.' *J. Bone Jt Surg.* **47**, 394

Jordan, G. L. and Beall, A. C., Jr. (1971). 'Diagnosis and management of abdominal trauma.' *Curr. Probl. Surg.* 44—47, November

Morton, J. H., Southgate, W. A. and DeWeese, J. A. (1966). 'Arterial injuries of the extremities.' *Surgery Gynec. Obstet.* **123**, 611

Patman, R. P., Poulos, E. and Shires, G. T. (1964). 'The management of civilian arterial injuries.' *Surgery Gynec. Obstet.* **118**, 725

Spencer, F. C. and Tomplins, R. V. (1960). 'Management of acute arterial injuries.' *Postgrad. Med.* **28**, 476

Stoney, R. J., Roe, B. B. and Redington, J. V. (1964). 'Rupture of thoracic aorta due to closed chest trauma.' *Archs Surg.* **89**, 840

Szilagyi, D. E., Whitcomb, J. C. and Smith, R. F. (1959). 'Anteromedial approach to the popliteal artery.' *Archs Surg.* **78**, 647

[The illustrations for this Chapter on Vascular Injuries were drawn by Mr. R. Wabnitz.]

Iatrogenic Vascular Injuries

Charles Rob, *M.C.*, M.D., M.Chir., F.R.C.S.
Professor and Chairman of the Department of Surgery,
University of Rochester School of Medicine and
Dentistry, Rochester, New York

INTRODUCTION

Any artery or vein may be injured by a therapeutic procedure. Simple ligature is the treatment if the injured vessel is not essential. In all other cases repair should be considered. A vascular injury may cause haemorrhage, thrombosis or delayed effects such as the formation of an aneurysm, a dissecting aneurysm or an arteriovenous fistula.

Since the first descriptions of arteriovenous fistulas were made by Hunter in 1757 and 1762, iatrogenic vascuiar injuries have been too frequent. The arteriovenous fistulas described by Hunter were between the brachial artery and vein and were caused by barbers performing therapeutic phlebotomy. Today major causes of iatrogenic vascular injuries are surgery, angiography and injections of all types including needle biopsies. As these injuries occur in hospital or in a doctor's office, early diagnosis is both possible and important. This is aided by awareness of the problem and of its frequency. It is possible that arteriography is today the most common cause of traumatic arterial thrombosis.

The problems a surgeon faces when treating an iatrogenic vascular injury are numerous and will be illustrated by describing the management of brachial artery thrombosis due to coronary angiography; accidental injury to the femoral artery during a long saphenous ligature and stripping operation; injury to the inferior vena cava during the resection of an abdominal aortic aneurysm; and the correction of an arteriovenous fistula between the abdominal aorta and left common iliac vein caused by a lumbar disc operation. These examples illustrate therapeutic procedures which can be applied to all iatrogenic vascular injuries.

THROMBOSIS OF THE BRACHIAL ARTERY AFTER CORONARY ANGIOGRAPHY

This problem develops after approximately 2 per cent of coronary angiograms performed via the brachial route. In most patients the collateral circulation is adequate and few problems arise. But ischaemia may be severe and loss of the limb can occur. In our view thrombectomy followed by arterial repair with a venous patch graft angioplasty should be performed at once if there is evidence of peripheral ischaemia.

1

Exposure of the occluded artery

The thrombus begins at the point where the Seldinger catheter enters the artery and at first is localized. An incision is made over the artery to expose about 6 cm of the vessel. The patient is given 50–100 mg of heparin. A clamp is applied proximal to the thrombus but not distally. The artery is opened with a longitudinal incision which includes the site of needle puncture. A longitudinal incision is used because this arteriotomy will be closed with a venous patch.

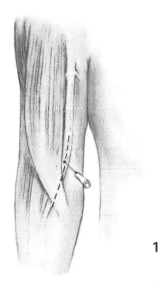

1

2

Removal of the thrombus and any damaged intima

The thrombus will extrude from the incision and is removed with suction and irrigation. If a retrograde flow develops from the distal vessel, it is clamped temporarily. The intima is now inspected; frequently there is a loose flap caused by the introduction of the Seldinger catheter. This is carefully removed until the interior of the artery consists either of intact intima or an arterial wall which has undergone a thrombo-endarterectomy.

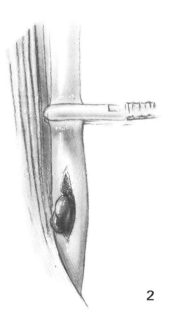

2

3

The establishment of distal arterial patency

The presence of a retrograde flow is not a guarantee of complete distal arterial patency. In our opinion after a traumatic arterial thrombosis, a Fogarty catheter should always be passed down the distal artery to remove, if possible, any residual thrombus or debris. In this situation it should, if possible, be passed down both the radial and ulnar arteries.

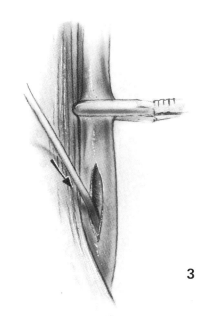

3

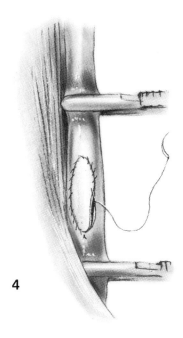

4

4

Closure with a venous patch graft angioplasty

The margin of the artery at the point of insertion of the Seldinger catheter may require excision. The amount of arterial wall removed should be as small as possible. A length of the basilic vein should now be mobilized and laid open. This piece of vein is then sutured to the margins of the arteriotomy incision with 5/0 silk or Prolene. It is important to use a venous patch graft because stenosis and recurrent thrombosis is likely to follow a simple closure of this arteriotomy. The clamps are now removed and the heparin neutralized with protamine sulphate. If pulses return to the wrist and the hand becomes pink and warm, all is well. If this does not occur, an intra-operative arteriogram is required to demonstrate the state of the arterial tree.

ACCIDENTAL INJURY TO COMMON FEMORAL ARTERY DURING LIGATURE OF THE SAPHENOUS VEIN

This unfortunate injury must be recognized at once. It is usually obvious because of the arterial bleeding. Then it is important not to increase the arterial damage by clamping with haemostats. The correct procedure is to control the bleeding with pressure and then deliberately clamp the injured artery with vascular clamps.

Sometimes a far worse and almost unbelievable situation develops. The surgeon mistakes the super-ficial femoral artery for the long saphenous vein, carefully dissects the superficial femoral artery and clamps it. A stripper is then introduced into the superficial femoral artery and is passed distally to the ankle. The whole length of the main arterial system of the lower limb is then removed by stripping. The inevitable result is massive gangrene. This error can be avoided by introducing the stripper into the long saphenous vein at ankle and passing it proximally and by the obvious step of performing an accurate dissection of the saphenofemoral junction in the groin.

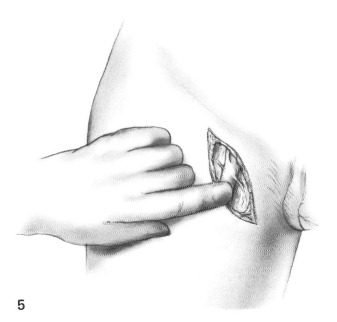

5

5

Control of the arterial haemorrhage

The first step is to apply firm pressure which is gradually reduced in size so that eventually only the actual bleeding point is compressed. The surgeon and his assistant then isolate the artery proximal to the injury. This artery is now clamped and the patient is given 50–75 mg of heparin by the anaesthetist. Pressure is still applied to the arterial wound and the distal vessel isolated and clamped. The area is then inspected and if bleeding persists, any unclamped branches are isolated and occluded with bulldog clamps. During this phase of the procedure great care is taken not to injure the femoral vein or femoral nerve.

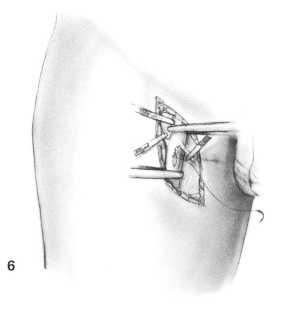

6

6

Repair of the arterial wound

If this is a clean, surgical knife wound, it can be sutured. But if haemostats have been used, the damaged arterial wall must be excised, the defect in the artery can then be repaired with an autogenous venous patch graft. The saphenous vein is available for this and can be used unless the segment is very large and dilated, when a small and thick-walled segment of vein, often from the ankle region, may be preferred. The heparin effect is now reversed with protamine sulphate and the arterial clamps are removed.

INJURY TO THE INFERIOR VENA CAVA OR COMMON ILIAC VEINS DURING AN OPERATION UPON THE ABDOMINAL AORTA

In the past, aneurysms of the abdominal aorta were excised. Today the aneurysm is not removed. For an aortofemoral bypass graft the aorta was cross-clamped. Today a side clamp is applied. Modifications of this type have greatly reduced the incidence of damage to the inferior vena cava or common iliac veins during operations upon the abdominal aorta. But this complication may still occur and its management will now be discussed.

7

Temporary control of the haemorrhage

The injury to the inferior vena cava or common iliac vein is usually small, but it may be made larger by inefficient attempts to control the bleeding. As a first step pressure is applied to stop the bleeding. The surgeon then inspects the area and reduces, if he can, the pressure point to a small area. Should he succeed in this, the next step is to apply a side clamp.

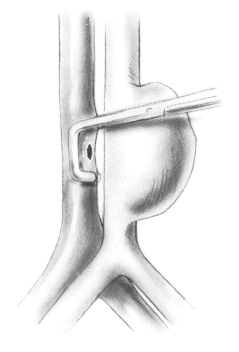

7

8

The management of a major defect which cannot be controlled with a side clamp

If the procedure described in *Illustration 7* is impossible or fails, the surgeon is presented with a very difficult and possibly disastrous situation. The first step is again to control the bleeding with firm pressure. The surgeon then proceeds in a step-by-step manner. He confirms with the anaesthetist that adequate blood is available for immediate transfusion. He confirms with the operating room nurse that all the instruments he will need are ready and available including instruments for clamping the vena cava, sutures for repairing the vena cava and ligatures for ligaturing the vena cava if his attempts at repair fail. He also has prepared and brought to the operating room a machine for autotransfusion. We prefer our modification of the autotransfusion system 100. The surgeon must be prepared for massive blood loss and its management.

Whilst continuing to control the haemorrhage with firm pressure, the surgeon carefully dissects out the vena cava for a distance of about 2 cm above and below the point of injury. The vena cava is then clamped with vascular clamps above and below the injured segment. If the bleeding persists, any lumbar veins entering the damaged segment of the vena cava must be controlled with bulldog clamps or suture ligatures. During the whole of this phase of the operation, the field is kept clear by pressure on the bleeding point and a suction device connected to the autotransfusion system so that the requirement for donor blood is kept to a minimum.

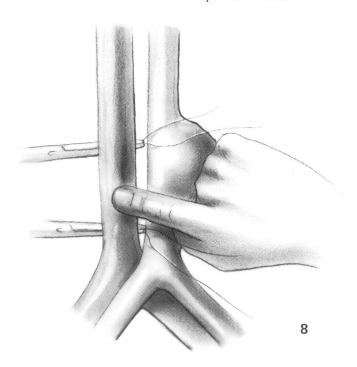

8

9

Ligature or repair of the inferior vena cava

The surgeon now inspects the injured vena cava. If he can repair the defect, he should do so. But the disability from ligature of the inferior vena cava in a patient without previous thrombophlebitis may be surprisingly slight. Therefore, if a doubt exists as to the effectiveness of the repair, a ligature should be placed around the inferior vena cava above and below the point of injury, The surgeon now proceeds to the completion of the originally planned aortic operation. Postoperatively the patient's legs are raised and he wears full length elastic stockings.

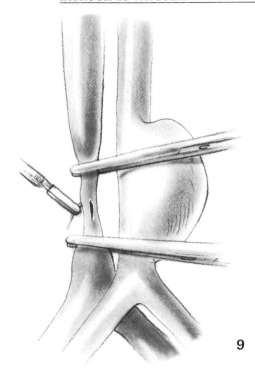

9

CORRECTION OF AN ARTERIOVENOUS FISTULA BETWEEN THE ABDOMINAL AORTA AND THE LEFT COMMON ILIAC VEIN OR INFERIOR VENA CAVA DUE TO LUMBAR DISC OPERATION

This complication was first reported in 1945 by Linton and White. Twenty years later the English language literature contained the reports of at least 27 similar cases. The actual incidence is higher because not all cases are reported. Nevertheless, this is a rare but dangerous complication of lumbar disc surgery. This complication is most likely to occur when the patient is operated upon in the prone position and when the annulus fibrosis is deficient so that the pituitary rongeur used in lumbar disc surgery can slip through the disc space and cause this arteriovenous fistula. A gush of blood follows. This is controlled by packing. Once the diagnosis is considered, careful preparation for a major operation is important. This will include the establishment of a reserve of at least 10 units of blood for transfusion.

10

The incision

An arteriogram should precede the operation so that the exact location of the arteriovenous fistula is known. It is usually between the distal aorta and left common iliac vein. The abdomen is opened through a mid-line abdominal incision, the centre of which should lie over the bifurcation of the abdominal aorta; the position of which will have been shown on the arteriogram. After the usual abdominal exploration, as much as possible of the small intestine is removed from the abdomen and placed in a plastic bag. This will expose the aortic bifurcation together with the iliac veins and inferior vena cava.

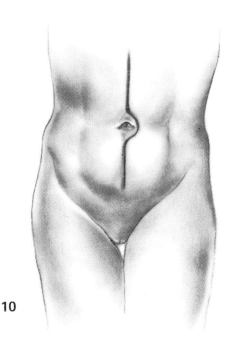

10

11

Isolation of the abdominal aorta and inferior vena cava proximal to the lesion

There may be a retroperitoneal haematoma, but this can be surprisingly small. It is important not to approach the actual arteriovenous communication until the major arteries and veins proximal and distal to the lesion have been controlled. The aorta is isolated just distal to the origin of the inferior mesenteric artery and the inferior vena cava, also isolated at the same level. Any lumbar arteries or veins immediately distal to this point are clamped with bulldog clamps.

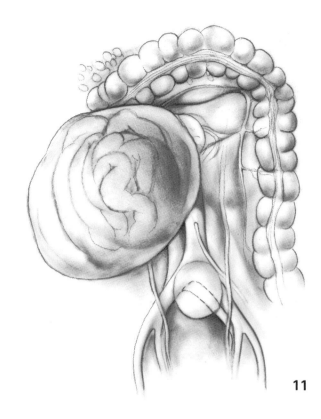

11

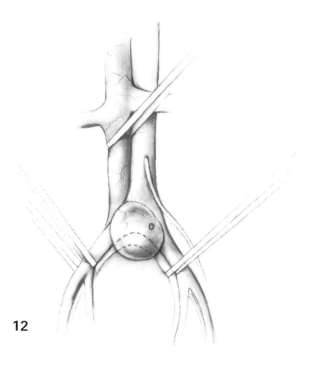

12

12

Isolation of the iliac vessels distal to the lesion

The right and left common iliac arteries and veins are now isolated well away from the lesion and close to the bifurcation of the common iliac artery and the junction of the hypogastric and external iliac veins. The blood flow to the area of the arteriovenous fistula will now be under control except for the middle sacral artery and vein, sometimes a second pair of lumbar arteries and veins closer to the aortic bifurcation and an occasional vessel supplying the ureter. If possible, these vessels are located before opening the vessels and occluded with bulldog clamps, but this step, although desirable, is not essential.

13

Exposure of the arteriovenous fistula

After the anaesthetist has given the patient 50–75 mg of heparin, all the vessels are clamped and the distal abdominal aorta opened opposite the arteriovenous fistula with a longitudinal incision on the anterior aortic wall which may, if necessary, be extended onto one of the common iliac arteries. At this time the surgeon will see the defect in the posterior wall of the distal aorta. If bleeding still occurs, the orifices of the middle sacral or other small vessels should be oversewn with vascular sutures from within the lumen of the aorta. The defect in the left common iliac vein will be seen behind the arterial injury. If bleeding occurs from a branch of this vein, it should be temporarily controlled with a small pack.

14

Ligature of the left common iliac vein

It is a mistake to attempt to repair the left common iliac vein. A ligament or suture is tied around the left common iliac vein proximal and distal to the injury. The fact that this vein has been injured with rongeur or similar forceps means that repair is difficult and ligature is safer and better in most cases. Once this is completed all clamps on the veins involved in the operation are removed.

15

Repair of the arterial injury

The artery is now open on both sides anteriorly because of the surgeon's incision and posteriorly because of the injury which caused the arteriovenous fistula. The posterior defect is closed first. Usually a patch is required. A patch of Dacron velour is sutured to the margins of this defect with a continuous 4/0 Prolene suture from within the lumen of the aorta. The anterior arteriotomy incision is then closed by a simple Prolene suture. But if it appears that this will constrict the lumen, a second patch of Dacron velour may be used. The clamps are now removed. The heparin effect is reversed with protamine sulphate and the abdominal incision closed in the usual manner. Alternatively, the damaged arterial segment may be replaced by a Dacron prosthesis.

If a Dacron patch or prosthesis has been used, we recommend a 5-day course of antibiotics as a prophylactic measure against infection.

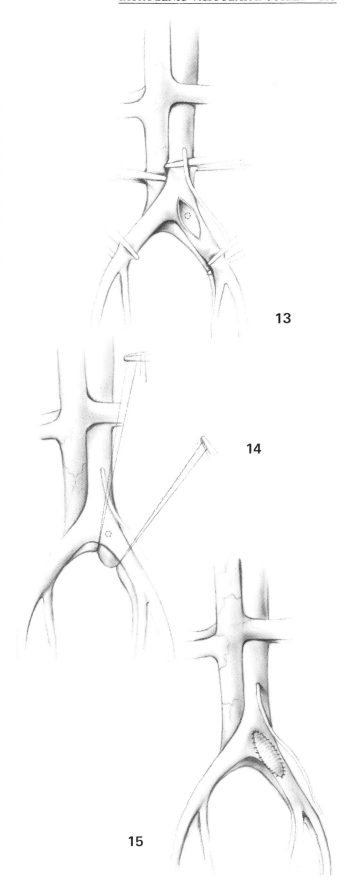

13

14

15

References

Adams, D.F., Fraser, D.B. and Abrams, H.L. (1973). 'The complications of coronary arteriography.' *Circulation* **48**, 609

Collins, J.A. (1974). 'Problems associated with massive transfusion of stored blood.' *Surgery* **75**, 274

Harbison, S.P. (1954). 'Major vascular complications of intervertebral disc surgery.' *Ann. Surg.* **342**, 140

Horton, R.E. (1961). 'Arteriovenous fistula following operation for prolapsed intervertebral disc.' *Br. J. Surg.* **77**, 49

Hunter, W. (1757). 'The history of an aneurysm of the aorta with some remarks on aneurysms in general.' *Med. Obs. Soc. Phys. Lond.* **1**, 323

Hunter, W. (1762). 'Further observations upon a particular species of aneurysm.' *Med. Obs. Soc. Phys. Lond.* **2**, 390

Linton, R.R. and White, P.D. (1945). 'Arteriovenous fistula between the right common iliac artery and inferior vena cava. Report of a case following operation for a ruptured intervertebral disc.' *Archs Surg.* **50**, 6

Sones, F.M. and Shirey, E.K. (1962). 'Cine coronary arteriography.' *Mod. Concepts cardiovasc. Dis.* **31**, 735

[The illustrations for this Chapter on Iatrogenic Vascular Injuries were drawn by Mr. R. Wabnitz.]

Acquired Arteriovenous Fistulas

H. H. G. Eastcott, M.S., F.R.C.S.
Senior Surgeon, St. Mary's Hospital, London

and

A. E. Thompson, M.S., F.R.C.S.
Consultant Surgeon, St. Thomas's Hospital, London

PRE-OPERATIVE

Indications

Acquired arteriovenous fistula is the result of trauma to blood vessels or mycotic aneurysms. Such a connection occasionally occurs as a result of operative trauma or may be surgically created to allow access to the circulation for haemodialysis. Shunting of the blood from the arterial to the venous system produces both general and local effects. The general effects are produced by lowering of the peripheral vascular resistance, resulting in an increased blood volume and progressive enlargement of the left ventricle leading to high output cardiac failure. This may culminate in left ventricular failure. Subacute bacterial endocarditis can occur at the site of the fistula or in the heart.

Local effects depend on the site and size of the fistula. Venous insufficiency and peripheral ischaemia are common if the proximal limb vessels are affected, ulceration of the ankle and calf developing in the lower limbs. These problems are avoided in the arteriovenous fistulas for haemodialysis, by using a small distal fistula in the arm. In pathological fistulas adjacent structures may be compressed by aneurysmal vessels. Buzzing may greatly distress the patient with a carotid-jugular or cavernous sinus fistula.

Primary repair is now the treatment of choice in accessible pathological fistulas.

Contra-indications

Operation should not be lightly undertaken. The cure of this condition presents considerable technical difficulty and if the lesser procedure of proximal arterial ligation has to be performed, drainage of the remaining effective circulation back through the fistula may result in gangrene of a limb.

Small aneurysmal varices need nothing more than an elastic support and regular review for cardiac complications. Very occasionally an arteriovenous fistula closes spontaneously by thrombosis.

Pre-operative preparation

Pre-operative assessment of the patient includes careful examination of the cardiovascular system followed by estimation of the haemoglobin, blood volume and cardiac output. If fever is present repeated blood cultures are made. Preparation must be made for blood transfusion, but it must be remembered that this condition is normally accompanied by a significant increase in blood volume with overloading of the heart. Although some loss of blood is beneficial, blood replacement must be available if profuse bleeding occurs.

Plain radiographs should be taken to localize any suspected metal fragments in the region of the fistula. Arteriography will define the extent of acquired fistulas of this type.

Anaesthesia

General or spinal (epidural) anaesthesia is suitable. Hypotensive agents may be necessary to reduce hypertension when flow through the fistula has been arrested.

THE OPERATION

A wide exposure is essential. It should be centred over the position of the fistula as shown on the arteriogram, or at the point where the bruit is loudest, or where local digital pressure will abolish it, rather than over the region of greatest soft tissue swelling which may be only the partly clotted sac.

Application of tourniquet

1

Pneumatic type

There is much to be said for using a tourniquet: the blood loss is reduced and the preliminary dissection is much simpler. A wide pneumatic type is preferable as it can be released at the stage when the fistula itself is exposed as a test of whether it has been obliterated.

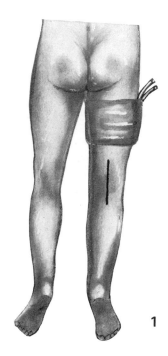

1

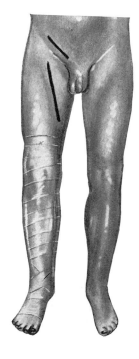

2

2

Esmarch's bandage

If the fistula is large and lies at the root of the limb a separate formal exposure of the main vessels is made proximally. The subclavian artery, the common iliac artery or the external iliac artery is temporarily controlled. If necessary the clavicle can be removed or the inguinal ligament divided. The engorged and hypertrophied limb may be emptied by elevation and by the application of an Esmarch's bandage. It is either taken tightly up to the proximal tourniquet and then removed, or, if no proximal tourniquet is used, as on the higher fistula sites, it is applied much more loosely, up to the lower limit of the sterile field, and is left in place, thus serving to diminish venous bleeding.

3

Superficial dissection

Many dilated superficial veins are encountered in making the long incision. Correct application of the tourniquet will have helped to reduce this difficulty, although if the pressure is not correctly adjusted it may only increase the venous bleeding.

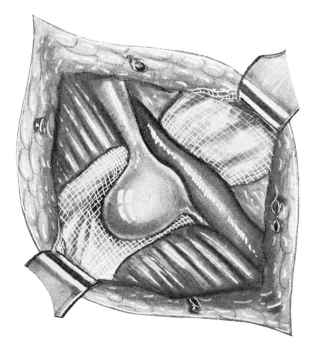

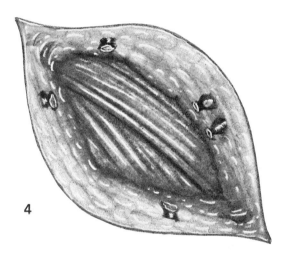

4

The muscle layers

Whenever possible the approach to the deep vessels is by muscle separating or splitting, for many large collaterals course through the bellies.

5

Deep dissection

The dilated afferent artery must first be located, particularly if other means of controlling the blood flow have not been adopted, and a temporary tape ligature or arterial clamp applied. Several medium sized vessels require ligation and division before the main vein can be approached, often along a tributary. Sometimes the sac or fistula itself is the best guide to the main vein which, when found, is temporarily clamped above and below the communication.

6

Exploring the fistula itself

The pulsation and thrill in the communicating region are now abolished by the clamps, and although the sac may still refill slowly after digital compression it should be opened. The source of any remaining branch is seen and can be sutured, or the vessel can be located and tied outside the sac, the operator being guided by the position of its opening within the sac. Any foreign body present is removed. The site and size of the fistula can then be assessed.

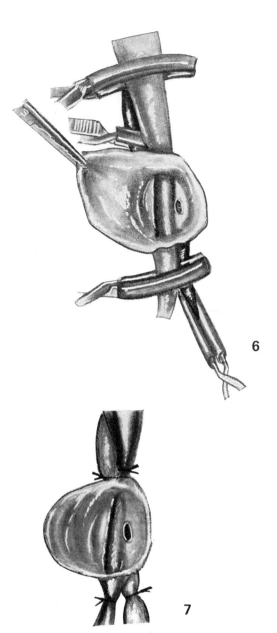

6

7

Quadruple ligation

This simple procedure has been the one most generally used. It carries some risk of producing ischaemia, but it is safer than a complicated repair operation when fibrosis and collateral formation are extensive. The ligatures must be placed between the fistula and the first branch of each vessel, whenever possible, to prevent backward loss through the fistula. More than four ligatures are usually needed. The bruit should be completely abolished at this stage, although a small peripheral pulse may be felt.

7

8

Transvenous repair of fistula

Where the vein is dilated, or forms a sac, the fistula can be explored through it, and repaired with a simple continuous silk suture. The vein is then repaired. It should not be sacrificed to the repair of the artery unless its condition precludes a separate repair, lest venous insufficiency follow. Transvenous repair is best suited to cases with a wide zone of adherence between the artery and the vein around the fistula.

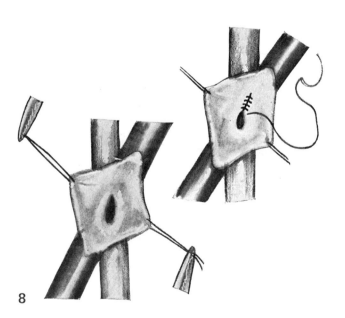

8

9

Simple repair of artery and vein

There is sometimes sufficient varicose aneurysm formation, or increase in the diameters of the artery and vein themselves, to allow tissues to spare for a longitudinal suture of each, without much narrowing of the lumen. A patch graft may be required for the arterial repair.

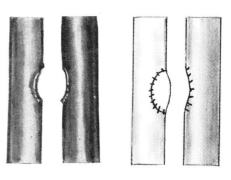

9

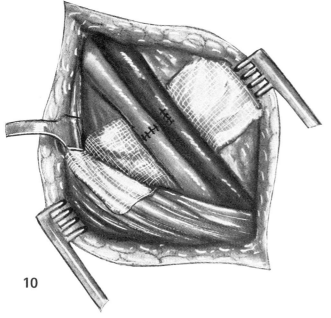

10

10

Repair of artery by excision and anastomosis

The artery wall may be involved in the formation of the sac. Local repair in these circumstances is likely to be followed by recurrence as a simple aneurysm. It is better to excise the damaged segment, which is seldom more than 2·5 cm or so in length, and then to restore the artery by an end-to-end anastomosis. This is the ideal treatment. Tension can be avoided and the gap closed by the use of posture, for example, by raising the shoulder or flexing the knee. The disparity in size between the two ends is overcome by appropriate traction upon the two supporting stitches (*see* page 29). The vein is sutured first, if clotting is thought to be likely, or if it would be obscured by the repaired artery.

11

Repair of artery by excision and grafting

A longer gap in the artery than can be closed by direct anastomosis is an indication for the insertion of an arterial graft. Although only a short length is usually needed it is better not to sacrifice one of the nearby veins for this purpose, for hyperaemia and venous insufficiency are likely sequelae of the reconstruction of the artery. A separate dissection of a vein from another part is permissible, however, and the upper saphenous trunk is very suitable. It must be reversed to avoid obstruction by valves. Alternatively a Dacron graft may be used.

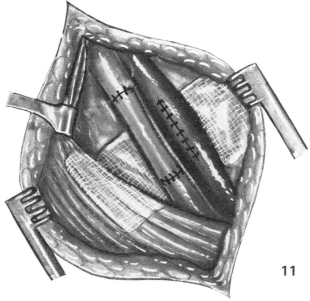

11

POSTOPERATIVE CARE
AND COMPLICATIONS

The restoration of a normal circulation with a pre-existing raised blood volume may cause postoperative complications. Monitoring of the central venous pressure by an indwelling catheter is essential. Direct measurement of the circulating volume may also be helpful. The use of diuretics or venesection will reduce the circulating volume.

Complications

Cardiac failure may follow the repair of a large fistula. Postoperative transfusion should be withheld to avoid precipitating this complication in the presence of an already overloaded circulation. The co-operation of a cardiologist both before and after surgery is valuable.

The use of heparin during the operation and the presence of the numerous high-flow collaterals in this condition increase the risk of postoperative haemorrhage. Suction-drainage and close observation reveal this complication at an early stage. Ischaemia of the extremity occurs more commonly after the multiple ligation procedure and reconstruction is preferable.

Reconstruction is followed by a phase of reactive hyperaemia in the operated extremity. The foot pulses and temperature must be closely watched; any sudden deterioration is an indication for re-exploration.

References

Beall, A. C., Harrington, O. B., Crawford, E. S. and DeBakey, M. E. (1963). *Am. J. Surg.* **106,** 610
Bell, D. and Cockshutt, W. P. (1965). *Clin. Radiol.* **16,** 241
Brown, J. J. Mason (1949). *Br. J. Surg.,* War Surgery Supplement No. 2, 354
Holman, E. (1937). *Arteriovenous Aneurysm.* New York: Macmillan
Ross, J. Paterson (1946). *Br. med. J.* **1,** 1
Sako, Y. and Varco, R. L. (1970). *Surgery* **67,** 40
Treiman, R. L., Cohen, J. L., Gaspard, D. J. and Gaspar, M. R. (1971). *Archs Surg.* **102,** 559

[*The illustrations for this Chapter on Acquired Arteriovenous Fistulas were drawn by Mr. G. Lyth and Mr. F. Price.*]

Congenital Arteriovenous Fistulas

Charles Rob, *M.C.*, M.D., M.Chir., F.R.C.S.
Professor and Chairman of the Department of Surgery,
University of Rochester School of Medicine
and Dentistry, Rochester, New York

PRE-OPERATIVE

It is now thought that a number of haemangiomas and lesions known as haemangiomatous malformations are not tumours but are in fact congenital arterio-venous fistulas. Other names for these lesions include cirsoid aneurysm, pulsating haemangioma, haeman-giectatic hypertrophy and generalized angiomatosis.

Congenital arteriovenous fistulas are of two types—the localized and the generalized. In order to save space the surgery of one example of each type will be discussed on the assumption that, in general, the lines of treatment are applicable to similar lesions in other parts of the body. As an example of the localized type we will take the so-called cirsoid aneurysm of the temporal region of the scalp; for the generalized type we will take the diffuse involvement of the vessels of the lower limb.

Indications

In the localized type the treatment of choice is local excision when possible. In a limb a partial amputation may be necessary. Under these latter circumstances operation should be deferred until either haemorrhage threatens or the local disability is of sufficient severity. The generalized type of lesion should be managed conservatively when possible, but ulceration, haemorr-hage, recurrent cellulitis, recurrent haemarthrosis or the effects on the cardiovascular system may make operation desirable. In addition orthopaedic pro-cedures such as epiphyseal stapling may be required to limit the increased limb length.

Types of operation

The ideal procedure would be to dissect out and ligate all the arteriovenous communications, but this is rarely possible. As stated, the localized fistulas can be excised, but for the generalized type the surgeon must be content with an indirect approach. This may take the form of a synovectomy to prevent recurrent haemarthrosis, epiphyseal stapling to limit the exces-sive growth of the limb, or raising the shoe of the sound leg. Here arterial and venous ligation combined when possible with embolization using muscle, the patient's own clotted blood or small silicone spheres will be described, which is to date the only vascular operation apart from partial excision which may be of value in these patients. In many of these patients multiple operations will be required combined with repeated partial excisions and embolizations. The patient with a generalized type must be told this before surgery is begun.

Anaesthesia

In most patients general anaesthesia is to be preferred but in some with small localized lesions, excision under local anaesthesia is satisfactory.

THE OPERATIONS

LOCALIZED TYPE

1

Ligature of the external carotid artery and facial vein

This is an important preliminary measure which considerably reduces blood loss during the operation. A curved incision about 2·5 inches (6·25 cm) long is made in the line of the skin folds of the neck centred upon the carotid bifurcation. The sternomastoid muscle is retracted backwards, the anterior facial vein tied, and the carotid vessels located. The external carotid artery is distinguished from the internal carotid artery by the fact that it has branches. This vessel is ligated and divided.

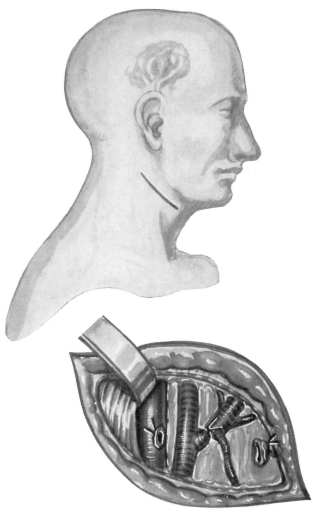

1

2

The scalp flap

These lesions are most easily approached from the deep surface of the scalp. The first step is therefore to turn down a scalp flap containing the fistulas. A curved incision down to the periosteum is made well clear of the lesion and the flap dissected from the skull in the plane just superficial to the periosteum. All large vessels passing to other parts of the scalp are ligated or controlled with sutures and any vessels passing to the bone are coagulated with diathermy. If bleeding from the latter vessels persists, firm pressure by an assistant—if necessary for the remainder of the operation—after application of bone-wax or haemostatic gauze will produce haemostasis.

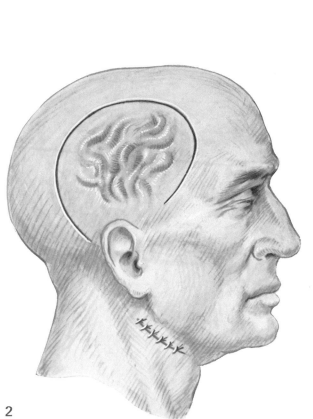

2

3

Removal of the lesion

The large mass of distended blood vessels contained in the scalp flap is now removed by dissection from the inner or deep surface. Each large vessel is separated from the neighbouring connective and muscular tissues and the whole lesion removed. Any bleeding points are ligated or coagulated with diathermy. Care should be taken to avoid injury to the skin.

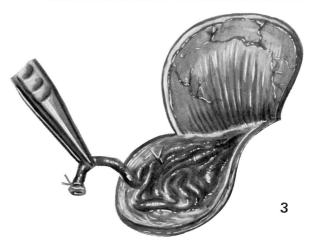

3

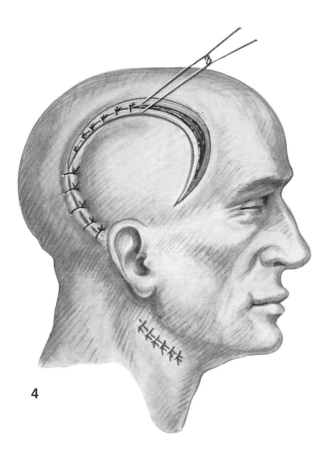

4

4

Wound closure

The galea aponeurotica and then the skin are closed with interrupted sutures. Drainage may be necessary. Several small areas of skin necrosis may appear adjacent to the suture line. These should be allowed to separate, when healing will rapidly occur. Most of the scar will eventually be covered by the patient's hair.

GENERALIZED TYPE

When the skin or mucous membrane over the huge pulsating vessels which may form shows signs of ulceration a severe or fatal haemorrhage is likely. Arterial and venous ligation reduces the risk of this and may be performed at multiple points and combined with partial or even complete excisions when possible, usually as multiple-staged procedures. A useful addition is to embolize and occlude the actual fistulous communications. This is the only technique which may cure these lesions.

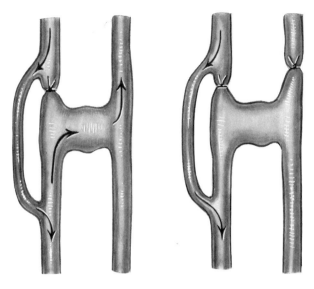

5

5

Proximal arterial and venous ligation

It is essential to ligate both the artery and the vein. Proximal arterial ligation alone in the presence of an arteriovenous fistula can be disastrous and may lead to loss of the limb. The reason, as shown in the accompanying illustrations, is that the viability of the part after arterial ligation depends upon the collateral circulation. After arterial ligation alone most of the collateral flow returns through the fistula to the low-pressure venous system and does not go down the artery to the periphery; gangrene usually follows. Ligation of the accompanying vein abolished this tendency and allows the collateral flow to pass down the arterial tree. This observation is of equal importance in both congenital and acquired arteriovenous fistulas.

6

Embolization of the involved vessels

It is important that the emboli are placed only in the vessels containing the actual fistulas. Embolization of the main arteries is not beneficial. The best way to introduce the emboli is to catheterize the main artery under x-ray control, the catheter is then positioned in the branches of the main artery which feed the fistulas and about 200 silicone spheres of 0·5–1·5 mm in diameter are injected, alternatively muscle or thrombi may be used. The procedure may be repeated at intervals in each of the feeding arteries until all the fistulas are obliterated. In *Illustration 6* the embolization of congenital arteriovenous fistulas involving the internal maxillary artery is shown. It is usually necessary to excise the lesion after embolization has reduced the blood flow but before the lesion has recurred.

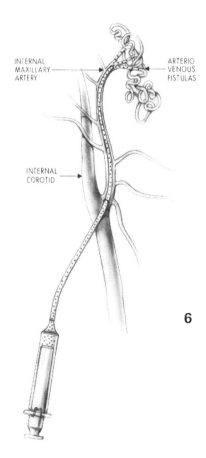

INTERNAL MAXILLARY ARTERY

ARTERIO VENOUS FISTULAS

INTERNAL COROTID

6

References

Bennett, J. E. and Zook, E. G. (1972). *Plastic reconstr. Surg.* **50,** 84
Cunningham, D. S. and Paletta, F. X. (1970). *Plastic reconstr. Surg.* **46,** 305
Holman, E. (1937). *Arteriovenous Aneurysm.* New York: Macmillan
Lin, S. R., LaDow, C. S., Tatoian, J. A. and Go, E. B. (1974). *Neuroradiology* **7,** 201
Longacre, J. J., Benton, C. and Unterthiner, R. A. (1972). *Plastic reconstr. Surg.* **50,** 618
Reid, M. R. (1925). *Archs Surg.* **10,** 997
Robertson, D. J. (1954). *Ann. R. Coll. Surg.* **18,** 73
Robertson, D. J. (1957). *Postgrad. med. J.* **33,** 17

[*Illustrations 1–5 for this Chapter on Congenital Arteriovenous Fistulas were drawn by Mr. R. N. Lane; Illustration 6 was drawn by Mr. R. Wabnitz.*]

Popliteal Artery Entrapment

G. W. Taylor, M.S., F.R.C.S.
Professor of Surgery and Director,
Surgical Professorial Unit,
St. Bartholomew's Hospital, London

and

J. S. P. Lumley, F.R.C.S.
Assistant Director,
Surgical Professorial Unit,
St. Bartholomew's Hospital, London

Aetiology

The popliteal entrapment syndrome (Love and Whelan, 1965) arises when an initially structurally normal popliteal artery is compressed by a local anatomical abnormality. Insua, Young and Humphries (1970) classify the anatomical variants into two types.

1

Type I

The popliteal artery takes an abnormal course and passes medial to, or may pierce, the medial head of the gastrocnemius muscle.

2

Type II

Less commonly the popliteal artery is normal in position but is compressed by an aberrant origin of the gastrocnemius (*illustrated*) or plantaris muscle or by an accessory fibrous band (Haimovici, Sprayregan and Johnson, 1972). In either variety the artery is compressed between the posterior face of the femur and the overlying muscle or aponeurotic band. Initially the compression is incomplete but eventually secondary changes in the arterial wall lead to fibrotic stenosis and thrombosis. Local aneurysm formation has also been reported (Carter and Eban, 1964).

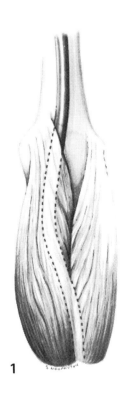

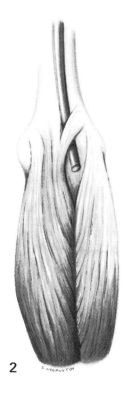

1   2

198

Clinical presentation

The presenting feature is intermittent claudication. The age at onset is usually (but not exclusively) well below that of the typical atherosclerotic patient. Men are affected more commonly than women and the entrapment is unilateral in the majority of patients. In the early stages the pedal pulses are preserved but may be felt to diminish with sustained active plantar flexion against resistance. With thrombosis of the entrapped segment the pedal pulses are absent and pulsation may be detected in collateral vessels particularly on the medial aspect of the knee.

Arteriography

In early cases the only arteriographic abnormality may be a medial deviation of the popliteal artery. When occlusion occurs a normal proximal and distal arterial tree will be seen with a sharp cut-off at the point of obstruction. The termination of the popliteal artery remains patent and distal embolization to the tibial vessels is rare.

OPERATIVE TREATMENT

The popliteal artery may be approached medially as in femoropopliteal bypass, but because of the localized nature of the pathology a direct mid-line approach through the posterior aspect of the popliteal fossa is more satisfactory. With the patient in a lateral position and the affected leg uppermost, access to the popliteal fossa and long saphenous vein is secured from one or other side of the operating table. Alternatively a length of long saphenous vein may be excised before the patient is turned into the prone position for the popliteal approach.

In early cases, without structural change in the artery, simple division of the medial head of gastrocnemius or overlying fascial bands may be all that is necessary. More frequently permanent stenosis or occlusion is encountered. Local repair by patch grafting is unsatisfactory (Darling *et al.,* 1974) and the segment should be bypassed with a length of reversed long saphenous vein. The vein graft should reach comfortably into normal artery above and below the occluded segment. The anastomoses may be made end-to-end or end-to-side. It is easier to judge the tension and lie of the bypass with an end-to-side technique.

References

Carter, A. E. and Eban, R. (1964). 'A case of bilateral developmental abnormality of the popliteal arteries and gastrocnemius muscle.' *Br. J. Surg.* **51,** 518

Darling Clement, R., Buckley, C. J., Abbot, W. M. and Raines, J. K. (1974). 'Intermittent claudication in young athletes.' *J. Trauma* **14,** 543

Haimovici, H., Sprayregen, S. and Johnson, F. (1972). 'Popliteal artery entrapped by fibrous band.' *Surgery* **72,** 789

Insua, J. A., Young, J. R. and Humphries, A. W. (1970). 'Popliteal artery entrapment syndrome.' *Archs Surg.* **101,** 771

Love, J. W. and Whelan, T. J. (1965). 'Popliteal artery entrapment syndrome.' *Am. J. Surg.* **109,** 620

[*The illustrations for this Chapter on Popliteal Artery Entrapment were drawn by Mrs. S. Neophytou.*]

Operations for Varicose Veins

F. B. Cockett, B.Sc.(Lond.), M.S.(Lond.),
F.R.C.S.(Eng.)
Teacher and Examiner in Surgery,
The University of London; and
Consultant Surgeon, St. Thomas's Hospital, London

CLASSIFICATION OF VARICOSE VEINS

The phrase 'varicose veins', as normally used in conversation or writing, embraces a fairly wide spectrum of venous disease. When we talk of 'operations for varicose veins', we must therefore be a good deal more specific as to just what type of varicose vein we are referring to.

In general, 'varicose veins' may be classified as follows.

Primary familial varicose veins

(*1*) Long saphenous incompetence. (*2*) Short saphenous incompetence. (*3*) Primary perforator incompetence.

Secondary varicose veins

(*1*) Secondary to ankle perforating vein incompetence (caused by a previous deep vein thrombosis of the peripheral type), usually leading to ankle ulceration. (*2*) Secondary to a high obstruction of the iliac veins or vena cava (caused by an old iliofemoral thrombosis or iliac compression syndrome, or tumour or mass obstructing these great veins). (*3*) Secondary to pregnancy. (*4*) Secondary to arteriovenous fistula, either congenital or acquired.

Congenital types of venous dilatation

All types of Klippel–Trenaunay syndrome of the lower limb. This embraces many unusual varicose vein presentations on the outer side of the limb.

Internal iliac incompetence

This is usually a sequel of pregnancy and occurs only in women, causing pudendal varicosities and a spray of small aching veins down the internal aspect and back of the thigh which are typically very painful in the premenstrual period.

Venous 'stars' or telangiectases

Athletes hypertrophic veins

From a consideration of this classification two points are immediately evident. These are: (*1*) the first essential in the treatment of varicose veins is an accurate diagnosis and appreciation of exactly what type one is dealing with; (*2*) the management and operative treatment of these various types differ widely.

There is no 'standard operation for varicose veins'.

PRIMARY FAMILIAL VARICOSE VEINS

This chapter describes the operative treatment of this particular group of varicose veins.

Primary familial varicose veins of the long saphenous system and of the short saphenous system are by far the commonest type in the white races. They are much less common in the coloured races.

Indications for operation

The condition is progressive throughout life and, if left, the veins increase in size and number as the patient gets older.

As this condition is almost completely curable by adequate radical surgery in the earlier stages, the presence of this condition and evidence that the veins are increasing in size may be taken as an adequate indication.

The two most common complaints which bring a patient seeking surgical relief are: (1) postural aching pain in the legs on standing; (2) the cosmetic appearance of the veins.

COMPLICATIONS

Further indications for operation

As the veins increase in size and spread over the leg and ankle as age advances, then serious complications may appear.

The four main complications are (1) thrombosis in varicose veins (This may spread into the deep veins, causing thrombo-embolism.); (2) acute bleeding— either external (sometimes threatening life), or subcutaneous, leading to massive bruising; (3) varicose eczema; (4) ulceration at the ankle.

The presence or threat of any of these complications constitutes a much more urgent and definite indication for operation.

THE OPERATIONS

The operations are as follows.

(1) Flush ligation and division of the long saphenous vein at the groin, together with stripping of the main trunk and its major superficial tortuous branches, for long saphenous incompetence.

(2) Flush ligation and division of the short saphenous vein in the popliteal fossa, and stripping of its trunk and major branches, for short saphenous incompetence.

(3) Occasionally exposure and ligation and division of ankle perforating veins if these are enlarged or incompetent.

Note: In this context on the word 'flush' refers to ligature and division of the saphenous flush with the femoral, or popliteal vein, so that the ligature lies proximal to all possible branches, a most important point.

Pre-operative preparation

On admission, a careful physical examination of the patient to confirm the exact diagnosis is done. Routine urine examination, chest x-ray, and examination of the peripheral pulses is performed in every case. The whole of the leg and pubic area is shaved.

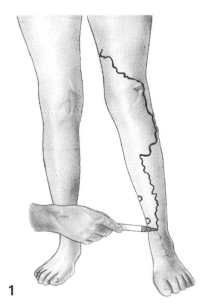

1

The patient is then asked to stand in a good light and the superficial varicosities are marked in carefully with an indelible pencil ('Pentel' pencils are the best.)

Anaesthetic

General anaesthesia is best—but inhalation anaesthetics, such as 'halothane' which cause widespread vasodilatation are best avoided, as excessive bleeding may occur after stripping when they are used. For this same reason an excessively hot theatre should be avoided—bleeding is noticeably less if the leg is cool.

2

Position of patient

For operations on the long saphenous vein the patient is placed in the supine position with feet apart.

For operations on the short saphenous vein the patient is placed in the prone position, feet apart and knees slightly flexed (*see* page 207).

In both cases the table is tilted so that the legs and feet are up and the head and body down to an angle of at least 10°. This is as essential as in this position the venous pressure in the leg drops to zero and bleeding is minimal. The legs are parted with the heels supported on foam cushions.

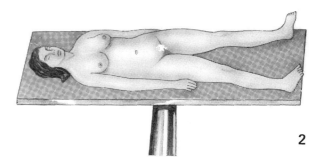

2

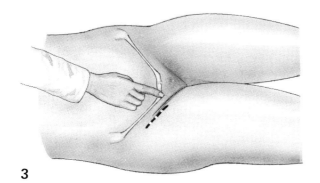

3

OPERATION FOR LONG SAPHENOUS INCOMPETENCE

3

The incision

An oblique incision in the groin about 3 inches (7·5 cm) long. The landmark for the incision is the pubic tubercle, and the left forefinger is placed on this point. The incision is centred on the saphenofemoral junction which lies 1·5–2 inches (3–5 cm) below and lateral to it.

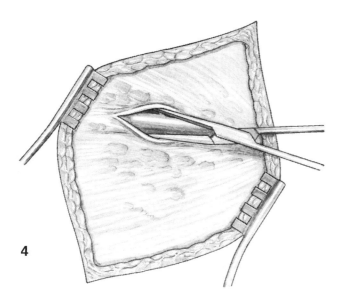

4

4

Division of Scarpa's fascia

The incision is deepened until the deep layer of the superficial fascia is reached. The bluish great saphenous vein can often be seen just deep to this layer. This fascial layer is opened.

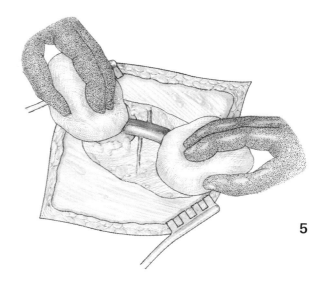

5

5

Exposure of saphenofemoral junction

After opening the deep fascial layer, the sapheno-femoral junction is then exposed by several sweeps of a gauze swab. This method of exposure is clean, easy, quick and does not disturb the lymphatics.

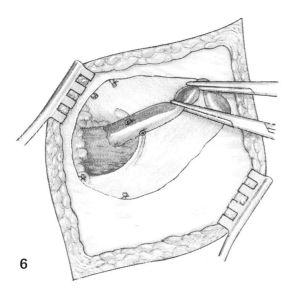

6

6

Division of saphenous vein and juxtafemoral tributaries

The saphenous vein is then lifted up, and divided and all the juxtafemoral tributaries are divided.

7

Exposure of common femoral vein and placing of saphenofemoral ligature

The common femoral vein is then visualized by dissecting the cribriform fascia away by using the points of a blunt Mayo scissors. The saphenofemoral ligature, using thread or silk (unabsorbable) is then placed flush on the side of the femoral vein.

The superficial external pudendal artery usually lies in the lower edge of the fossa ovalis in close relation to the saphenofemoral junction. It occasionally runs over the junctions, and needs division.

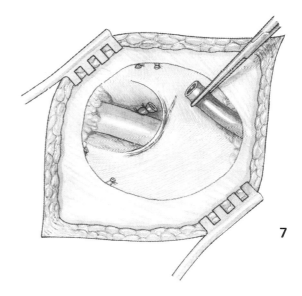

7

8

Introduction of stripper

The stripper is then introduced into the upper end of the saphenous vein and threaded into it downwards towards the knee. It nearly always tends to enter the anteromedial tributary, and must be directed with a finger down into the main saphenous vein.

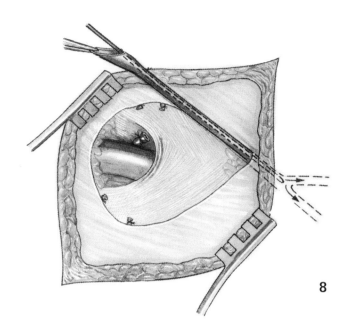

8

9

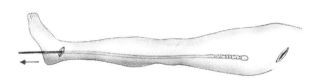

9

Exit of stripper

Below knee or at ankle perforator region

By frequent gentle advancement and withdrawals ('shaking' the stripper), the smooth head of the instrument may be advanced past valve remnants and varicose 'blow-outs' on the wall down as far as just below the knee or as far as the ankle perforator area on the inner side of the ankle.

10

At ankle

Often the stripper can be passed right to the ankle and can be withdrawn through a small transverse incision just below the internal malleolus.

The vein is withdrawn slowly and steadily. When it has been completely withdrawn there should be little bleeding because of the 'feet up' position of the patient. However, if there is bleeding, this is rapidly controlled by holding the leg vertically upwards for a minute or so.

10

11

Relation of saphenous nerve to saphenous vein

As seen in the diagram, the saphenous nerve runs closely applied to the saphenous vein in the leg. About 3 inches (7·5 cm) above the internal malleolus it bifurcates to form a two pronged fork over the saphenous vein at the ankle.

A stripper pulled upwards from the ankle may easily impact in the angle of the fork, and avulsion of whole or part of the saphenous nerve may occur. A stripper pulled *downwards*, however, will not impact and there is thus far less chance of saphenous nerve damage.

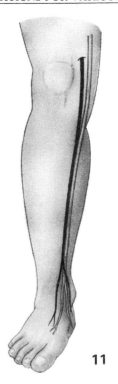

11

12

Stripping upwards

Where the ankle perforator veins have to be explored through a separate incision (when they are judged to be enlarged or incompetent), then the saphenous vein can be stripped upwards towards the groin from this incision.

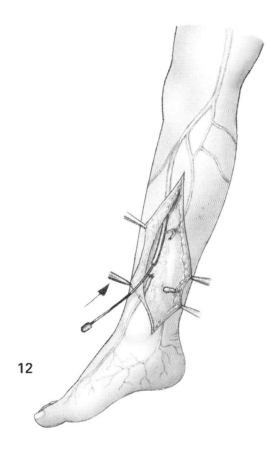

12

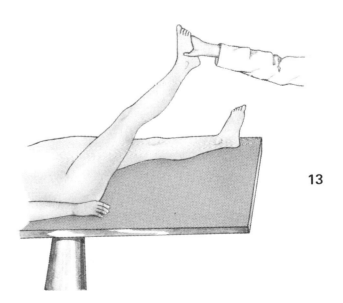

13

13

Elevation of limb

Immediately after stripping, either upwards or downwards, the whole leg is elevated almost vertically for a minute or so. This controls bleeding and prevents haematoma formation in the stripper track better than pressure or any other manoeuvre.

14

Removal of superficial tortuous tributaries

After the main saphenous trunk has been withdrawn on the stripper, the various subsidiary tortuous branches, which have previously been accurately marked, are withdrawn through a series of very small incisions.

The fine artery forceps are plunged into the small incision and opened once or twice to separate the subcutaneous tissue and display the vein. This is then grasped firmly in the tip of the forceps and by a gentle rocking movement quite long segments of these tortuous veins can be withdrawn from these small incisions.

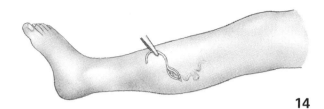

14

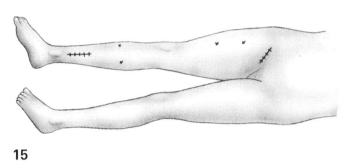

15

15

Closure of wound

The wounds are then closed with fine 0/0 silk. No subcutaneous sutures are necessary.

Just before closing the top wound, the stripper track is given a final massage to express clot from it.

The small subsidiary incisions are closed with one stitch of fine silk.

16

Bandaging

The whole limb is then pressure-bandaged with a crepe bandage.

Heavy webbing elastic bandages (Bisgaard bandages) should never be used on an unconscious patient as they may be inadvertently put on so tight that skin necrosis can occur.

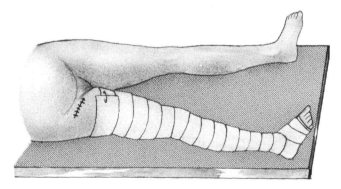

16

OPERATION FOR SHORT SAPHENOUS INCOMPETENCE

17

Position of patient

For short saphenous ligature and stripping the patient lies prone on the table with the knee flexed, so that the structures in the popliteal fossa are relaxed.

The vein is approached by a transverse incision across the middle of the popliteal fossa.

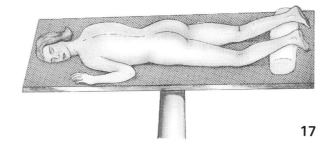

17

18

Exposure of short saphenous vein

The short saphenous vein lies *deep* to the deep fascia in the popliteal space and cannot be found until the deep fascia has been divided by either a transverse or longitudinal incision. It is accompanied by and often fairly closely applied to the sural nerve.

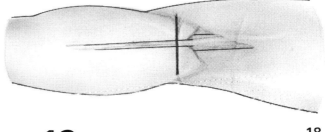

18

19

Flush ligation of short saphenous vein and branches

The vein is lifted up, divided, and its upper end traced down into the popliteal space. Once again flush ligation on the popliteal vein must be achieved. There is usually at least one large branch going upward in the space, which must be divided.

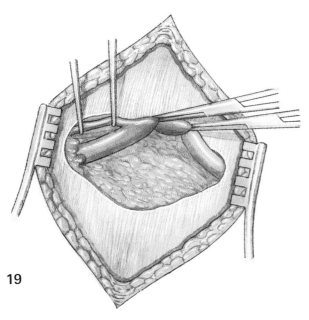

19

20

Stripping to level of external malleolus

The stripper is then inserted into the short saphenous vein in a downward direction and the exit is made by a small transverse incision placed just below the external malleolus.

Occasionally the stripper is held up at mid-calf, by a large branch or a mid-calf perforating vein. The stripper should be cut down upon at this spot, extricated and then re-inserted to complete the strip to the external malleolus.

Note that the sural nerve is in close relation with the vein at the external malleolus.

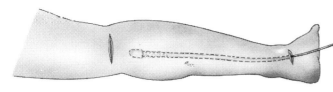

20

RELIGATION FOR RECURRENCE AT SAPHENO-FEMORAL JUNCTION

21

Incision

A longer incision going more medially to explore the femoral vein, is required.

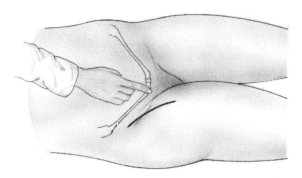

21

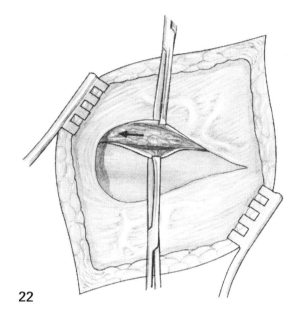

22

22

Opening of femoral sheath and exposure of femoral vein

The femoral sheath is identified well below the scar tissue of the old operation. The femoral artery can be identified by its pulsation, and the sheath is opened just medial to this, to expose the femoral vein.

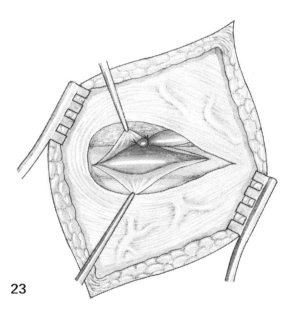

23

23

Dissection upwards to saphenous origin

The dissection is carried upwards on the femoral vein until the saphenous origin is seen. This is then isolated and ligatured. The whole dissection is within the femoral sheath.

POSTOPERATIVE CARE

The immediate postoperative care of patients who have had stripping or ankle perforator ligation is important. Our practice is as follows.

(*1*) The patient has the foot of the bed elevated to give a 'foot up' tilt of about 10°, and no more than two pillows are allowed. This position, which ensures a low venous pressure in the legs and fast venous return, is maintained throughout the first 6 days of the postoperative period. The patient is allowed to sit up for meals only. Once the patient has got used to it, this position is surprisingly comfortable.

(*2*) Throughout the postoperative 6-day period, the patient is allowed out of bed for short active walking periods (5–10 min only). Before getting out, firm webbing elastic bandages are applied from toes to thigh. As the days progress the number and length of walking periods is increased up to five or six a day.

(*3*) Even when lying in bed with the feet up, movement of the legs and ankles is encouraged.

(*4*) The pressure bandages applied at operation are not disturbed until the sixth day when the stitches are removed.

After the sixth day the patient is returned to normal active life, with instruction to wear a supporting bandage (or stocking) for another fortnight, and to be as active as possible with as much intermittent walking exercise as possible.

If this routine is followed, the whole procedure is remarkably painless. There is minimal haematoma and bruising, and the complication of deep-vein thrombosis is almost unknown. Moreover, at the end of the 6-day period, the patient really can return to almost normal life with legs which are comfortable—

with the minimal extra support which is usually necessary for about another 2 weeks.

An indurated line along the course of the stripped vein is usually present for up to 4 weeks after the operation, and may cause the patient some concern unless a prior warning or explanation is given.

Complications arising during operation

The most common difficulty which arises, particularly with an inexperienced surgeon, is massive venous bleeding while dissecting out the saphenofemoral junction.

When this occurs, mild finger or swab pressure on the spot will control the haemorrhage while the table is tilted so that the feet are high. When the finger or swab pressure is then withdrawn after about 2–3 min the bleeding is usually reduced to a trickle and can be accurately controlled either with artery forceps, or by a fine silk stitch, which should be in readiness. Blind clamping with haemostats should never be done as this may lead to serious damage to the femoral vein or even the femoral artery.

Occasionally the stripper may pass into the deep veins via a perforating vein. This is more likely to happen when the stripper is being passed upwards from the ankle, and the subcutaneous position of the stripper must be checked continuously with this in mind.

Excessive sharp dissection in the groin, leading to severance of too many lymphatics in this region, occasionally results in a chronic lymphocele of the wound. Serious lymphatic obstruction however is extremely rare.

[*The illustrations for this Chapter on Operations for Varicose Veins were drawn by Mr. F. Price.*]

Injection Treatment of Varicose Veins

W. G. Fegan, M.Ch., F.R.C.S. (I.)
Research Professor of Surgery,
University College of Dublin,
Trinity College at Sir Patrick Dun's Hospital,
Dublin

PRETREATMENT

Indications

Venous drainage

There is no such thing as venous drainage in the standing, walking or sitting patient. Blood in veins drains only when the bottom of the patient's bed is considerably elevated. Blood will move only from one segment of vein to the next when there is a favourable pressure differential. The haemodynamics of the venous segment of the perfusion arch of the tissues of the lower limb is as active and more complex than is the haemodynamics within an artery. The venous pumping system has to generate with each step a high systolic pressure to overcome gravity and a low diastolic pressure to allow for refilling and the development of a favourable gradient for tissue nutrient exchange.

Variation of flow

Flow in a segment of vein can vary in eight different ways. It can flow in either direction at high pressure or low pressure, quickly or slowly, in a laminar or turbulent manner. Retrograde turbulent flow directed against one side of a vein will give rise to a blow out while failure to develop low pressure in the venules after the commencement of walking will interfere with tissue nutrient exchange.

Pronounced superficial varices are quite common in the symptomless leg (varicose veins). A patient with a leg seriously embarrassed with advanced signs and symptoms of chronic venous insufficiency occasionally has no varices (postphlebitic limb).

The two conditions can co-exist in the same leg. This gives rise to the erroneous idea that they are sequential and that as varicose veins get worse they may lead to the postphlebitic limb, one being a more serious degree of the other. In our opinion this confused thinking is responsible for much of the misunderstanding in the diagnosis and treatment of these conditions.

Dilation

If varicose veins were due to an alteration in the pressure pattern within the vein, the vein would react as a vein transplanted into the arterial tree. The changes in pressure would equally affect all surfaces of the vein resulting in uniform hypertrophy and later, symmetrical dilation. This is not the ultimate derangement in the pathological vein.

Varicosity occurs usually on alternate sides of the vein, but it may also dilate in a 'barber's pole' fashion.

Valvular incompetence

The classic saphenovarix occurs at the apex of a reflux turbulent jet of blood due to valvular incompetence (primary or secondary), at the saphenofemoral junction. Where veins are not supported by Sherman's fascia, varicosity develops sooner. Turbulence is easily detected over these veins. High velocity is necessary for the development of turbulence. Turbulence would appear to be extremely damaging or injurious to the functioning of the muscle fibres and the elastic lamina of the vein wall. The muscle fibres decrease in number and the elastic lamina fragments at the apex of the turbulent jet. The difference in the overall thickness of the veins need not be impressive as the intima at this point thickens considerably. This would appear to be due to organization of layering thrombus due to turbulence. Such evidence leads us to the conclusion that asymmetrical dilatation (varicosity) in varices is a result of high velocity turbulent flow in poorly supported veins (Somerville et al., 1974).

Primary varicose veins

If an accurate history can be elicited it is surprising to find that in the majority of cases the condition started below the knee and ascended.

Incompetent perforating veins

A meticulous surgical dissection of the first group of varices to appear will usually demonstrate one incompetent perforating vein. This is not sufficient to interfere with pump reserve or efficiency, but it is sufficient to cause insidious upward uniform dilation in the related superficial veins. With normal functioning valves in the superficial veins, alterations in pressure patterns due to incompetent perforating valves can only ascend. The superficial dilation due to the inadequate drop in pressure after the commencement of walking gives rise to secondary valvular incompetence in the superficial veins (Fegan et al., 1964) and when it involves a higher perforating vein valve a reverse high velocity circuit is established.

Turbulence

Flow in superficial varices is found to be turbulent when the velocity reaches certain critical points. These are (1) shortly after assuming the erect position and (2) at the high velocity peaks developed after the commencement of walking (Fegan and Kline, 1972).

Postphlebitic syndrome

When treating a patient who has primarily the postphlebitic syndrome (Fegan and Kline, 1972), and in whom the varicose veins are either absent or of little importance, all efforts should be directed towards the restoration of the pump. The signs and symptoms of the postphlebitic syndrome are primarily due to the inability of the pumps to reduce the pressure after the commencement of walking to a point at which nutrient exchange will take place. One or two incompetent perforating veins do not necessarily render the pumps incapacitated because of the very considerable reserve pumping capacity, but the more valves that are damaged, especially in the deep perforating veins, the more the pumping capacity is reduced.

Reversibility

In some cases, if the incompetent perforating veins are tied off, the superficial varices disappear and the superficial veins return to normal, demonstrating the reversibility of secondary valvular incompetence (Quill and Fegan, 1971). Injection compression therapy takes advantage of the ability of superficial veins with secondary valvular incompetence to recover as one can give treatment and observe the effects before giving the next treatment.

Classification

The easiest method for the busy surgeon to distinguish these two patterns from each other, is on the basis of symptoms. Patients with symptomless varices rarely have pump damage. Patients with signs and symptoms of the postphlebitic limb arising from venous derangement always have damage to the valves in the deep and perforating veins despite the presence or absence of varicose veins.

Management

The ideal management of such a patient is, in our opinion, injection, compression and ambulation. The first treatment may be nothing more than compression and ambulation, but with meticulous palpation sites of incompetent perforators come to light which are subsequently injected. A patient with an oedematous fixed dropped foot, a lower leg ulcer of 10 or more years duration and wasting of the calf muscles can be restored to normal. Multiple treatments may be required and it sometimes takes 2 years to relieve the symptoms completely. It should be explained to the patient that there is no known way of replacing their damaged deep valves, but that we can block the leak that is contributing to the impaired efficiency of the pump.

Summary

To summarize there are two basic diseases in this group, one in which you can, with confidence, give the patient a promise of complete cure while in the other you are essentially bringing a dysfunctioning pumping system within its reserve. Therefore, although the second group may appear to be rendered symptom-free and thus clinically cured, they are never fully restored to the degree of normal pumping efficiency which they enjoyed before the first episode of deep-vein thrombosis. This group must be observed periodically and advised to maintain their pump muscles by walking and to remove unnecessary strain to the vein wall and valves by the avoidance of standing. The judicious periodic use of elastic stockings at specially selected times is advisable.

TREATMENT

1

Materials

Stool and couch with swivel trays underneath containing bandages, sorbo rubber pads and lint. A tray, containing 4–6 all glass or disposable syringes with transparent shanks fitted with fine disposable needles and loaded with the sclerosant (0·5 ml of sodium tetra-decyl) is at hand, as after commencing treatment the surgeon cannot move away from the patient.

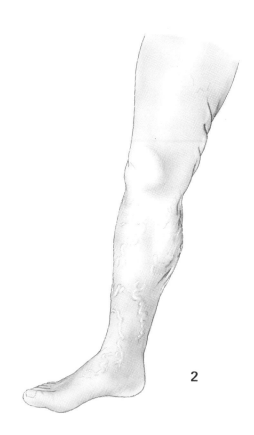

1

2

Varicose veins

Patient standing on stool showing typical varicose veins involving the long saphenous system with some perforator valvular incompetence.

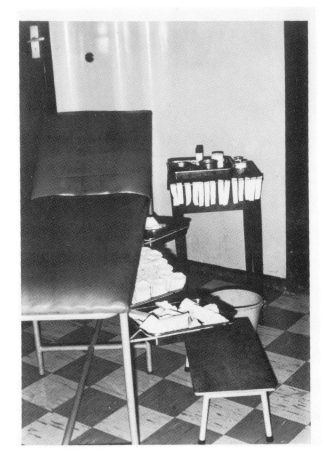

2

3

Inspection and palpation

Veins have been marked by inspection. Percussion of a dilated vein, while the other hand palpates the surface of the limb, will bring still more veins to light and when this mapping process is completed it is sometimes possible to suspect the site of the perforating veins with incompetent valves.

4

Areas of fascial deficiency

The patient is lying down with the heel comfortably supported on the surgeon's shoulder. The limb is palpated with the flat of the hand until the muscles become flaccid. Now the fingers are flexed and the tips should comb the leg in an effort to detect areas of fascial deficiency. These are marked with a grease pencil of a different colour.

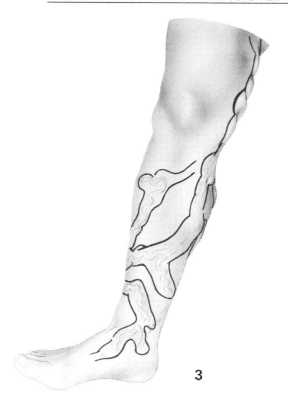

3

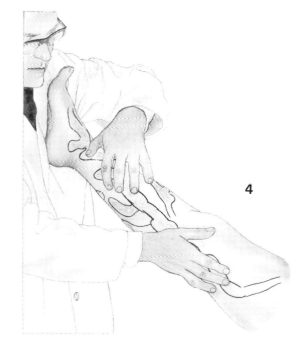

4

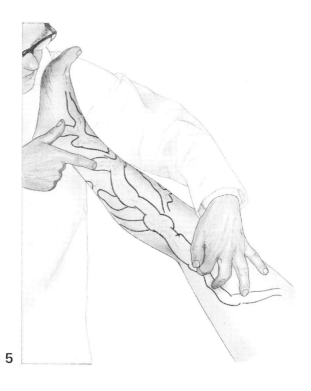

5

5

Likely sites of retrograde filling

The tips of the fingers are pressed into as many as possible of these areas or orifices of fascial weakness.

6

Filling of veins

The patient is now requested to stand and the lower-most fingers are removed first. If filling of the veins in the lower leg does not take place then it is reasonable to assume that there is no incompetent perforator at the site of this apparent fascial weakness and that one is really dealing with an area in which the fat is displaced by a bunch of dilated veins creating the impression of fascial weakness.

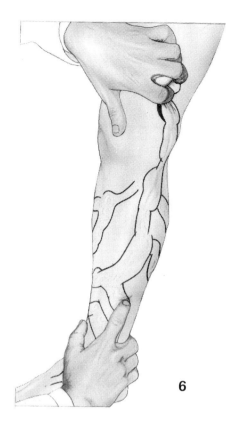

6

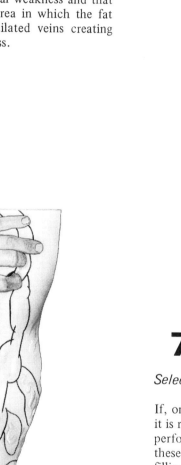

7

7

Selection of sites for injection

If, on the other hand, the veins fill immediately then it is reasonable to suspect that there is an incompetent perforator in this area. It is perhaps wise to consider these the sites at which pressure will control the filling of the superficial system. These we choose as the ideal sites for injection.

8

Removal of pressure

The illustration shows a further distension of the superficial system after removing the pressure from an incompetent Hunterian perforator.

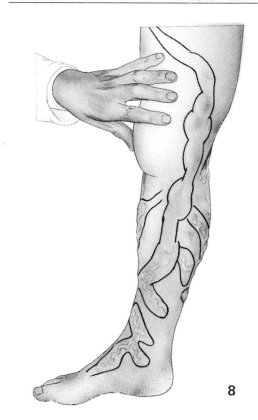

8

9

Insertion of needle

With the patient lying horizontal it is quite easy to enter the vein and withdraw blood (the plunger of the syringe having been tested for freedom of movement). It should be noted here that the blood should not enter the syringe but only the transparent shank of the needle.

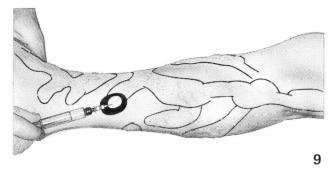

9

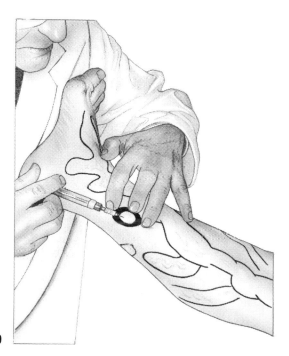

10

10

Injection of the sclerosant

The leg is elevated and placed against the shoulder or upper chest of the surgeon. The injection is given into a segment of vein isolated by the ring and index fingers compressing on either side in an attempt to restrict the sclerosant fluid (sodium tetradecyl) to the selected site. This would appear a pious hope but when the area is examined some weeks or months later the segment of superficial vein involved in the fibrosis matches exactly the gap between the ring and index fingers.

11

Bandaging

The syringe is withdrawn and bandaging above, below and over the site of injection is commenced. It is usually possible to apply one or two turns of the bandage above and below the compressing fingers before removing them.

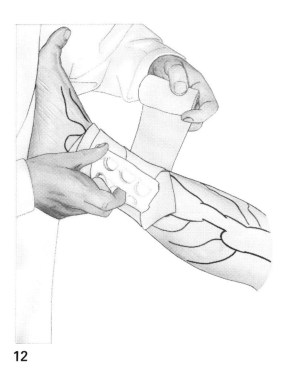

12

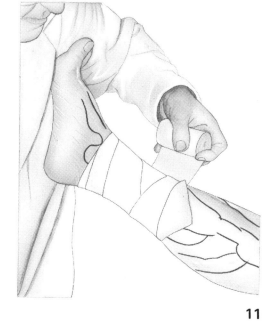

11

12

Sorbo rubber pad

A bevelled sorbo rubber pad is bandaged immediately into position over the site of injection.

13

The importance of bandaging

The remainder of the bandage is applied to the foot excluding the toes. The bandager should not have a preconceived pattern into which he visually forces the bandage. The contour of the patient's leg should determine the pattern of the bandage and the pressure of both borders of the bandages should be exactly the same. Bandaging is much more a sensory art using proprioceptive sensation rather than a visual art. It is the secret of the success of this technique and if the bandages have fallen off or have to be adjusted before the return visit then the surgeon has not mastered the technique and instead of a short segment of hard painless fibrotic veins patients will develop random areas of painful superficial thrombophlebitis which is certainly not the desirable end result.

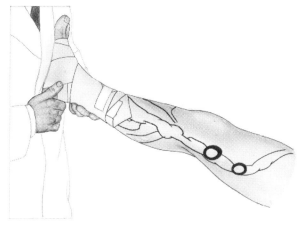

13

14

Prevention of the abrasion of the skin

To prevent the bandage in the region of the knee cutting the skin over the ham-string tendons it is necessary to place a sorbo rubber pad in the popliteal fossa. This becomes an absolute necessity if pressure over the termination of the short saphenous controls the filling in the superficial veins, as this is a common incompetent perforator that is frequently overlooked which responds very well to injection and compression.

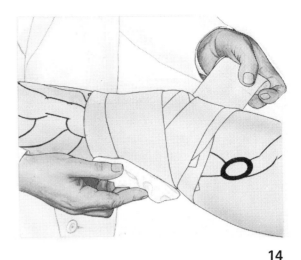

14

15

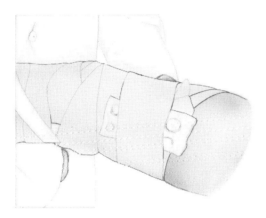

15

Traumatization of the long saphenous vein and thrombophlebitis

Demonstration of a pad placed over an injected superficial vein in the region of the lower Hunterian incompetent perforators. It is important to note that the rubber pad protrudes above the upper edge of the bandage. If the rubber pad does not protrude the bandage will roll down and form a sharp rope-like border which traumatizes the long saphenous vein and gives rise to the complication of ascending thrombophlebitis. This complication is prevented by allowing the long strip of rubber over the vein to protrude. Sometimes it is wise to use adhesive strapping to make sure the bandage does not roll, or the rubber pad slip out.

16

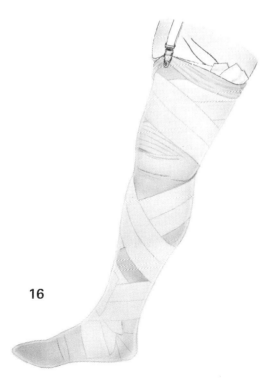

16

The elastic stocking

The elastic stocking is applied immediately after the last bandage is firmly anchored in position. It is of supreme importance that the patient should be able, fit and prepared to walk and should commence walking within seconds after the completion of treatment. Appointments for a return visit in 1–2 weeks should be made prior to commencement of treatment. We are convinced that the lack of complications in our clinic is due to the commencement of walking for 1 hr immediately following injection.

THE ESSENTIALS OF TREATMENT

Clinic

A clinic devoted entirely to the diagnosis and injection treatment of varicose veins is essential to ensure that the technique is carried out to perfection. It should be adequately staffed by the right proportion of experienced nurses, doctors and secretaries for maximum efficiency.

Diagnosis

From the point of view of treatment the patients are classified into three groups.

Group I. Those patients with superficial varices and no symptoms (varicose veins).

Group II. Those patients with signs and symptoms of chronic venous insufficiency, associated with valvular damage by a previous episode of deep-vein thrombosis (postphlebitic limb).

Group III. A combination of groups I and II.

History

A history is taken with particular note of any past injury to the leg, thrombophlebitis or any previous episodes of deep-vein thrombosis. The patient is weighed and if he/she is overweight they are strongly advised to diet. A blood sample is taken for the following tests: blood film, haemoglobin, W.R. Kahn, white cell count and ESR and patients are given written instructions to carry out throughout their treatment.

Varicose veins in pregnant patients

Pregnant patients who have varicose veins are treated routinely as frequently their veins do not return to normal in the puerperium and may continue to deteriorate past the critical point, beyond which recovery in the puerperium is impossible. Initially immediate supportive therapy is provided and any localized incompetent perforations are treated.

Bandaging

The importance of correct bandaging in the technique cannot be overstressed. A surgeon must be competent in the art of bandaging as the best results of the treatment are achieved by excellent bandaging.

Compression is an essential part of the treatment and it is achieved by correct application of the bandages, rubber pads and is completed by the fitting of a full-length two-way stretch elastic stocking.

POST-TREATMENT

Special care

The patient is instructed to walk for 1 hr immediately following injection and to continue to walk as much as possible on the day of injection and thereafter for 3 miles a day. This does not include walking around the house. The most difficult point to get across to the patient is the avoidance of standing. Our patients are warned against the danger of standing and advised if not walking to sit preferably with the legs elevated.

Pain

Pain may occur in the leg and the patient is advised to take analgesics and to increase the amount of walking. If this does not relieve the pain the bandage should be removed and the leg examined.

Superficial thrombophlebitis

Localized superficial thrombophlebitis may occur. This is usually due to failure of the use of the empty vein technique, inadequate compression or excessive use of the sclerosant.

Intra-arterial injection of the sclerosant

The accidental intra-arterial injection of the sclerosant in the hands of the experienced surgeon is a rare but serious complication. If this does occur a procedure of injection of procaine around the artery, local cooling, systemic heparinization and infusion with low molecular weight dextran has been shown to be effective in preventing or minimizing permanent damage to the foot.

Contra-indications

Obesity

Gross obesity is considered to be a contra-indication as it is dificult to maintain adequate compression.

Inability to walk

If a patient is unable or unwilling to undertake the required amount of walking then treatment should not be given.

Allergy

An allergic response to the sclerosant (sodium tetradecyl) is a definite contra-indication to further treatment by this method.

Oral contraceptives

Whilst there is no evidence to suggest that patients taking an oral contraceptive run a higher risk of developing deep-vein thrombosis and pulmonary embolism, treatment is not undertaken until the patient has stopped taking an oral contraceptive for 6 weeks.

ADVANTAGES OF INJECTION COMPRESSION SCLEROTHERAPY

The advantage to the patient of this method of treatment is that they avoid hospitalization and interruption of employment, have no scars and can be treated immediately upon referral to the clinic. The surgeon will avoid an in-patient waiting list and therefore save hospital-bed occupation.

Results

There is no standard method of assessing the results of this method of treatment of varicose veins. In comparison with surgery and injection compression sclerotherapy (Chant *et al.,* 1972; Heslop, 1973) the results of this technique compare favourably with surgery. The patient appears to prefer this method of treatment and provided injection compression sclerotherapy is practised by an expert, it can produce a better end-result in terms of relief of symptoms as well as disappearance of obvious varicosities.

References

Chant, A. D. B., Jones, H. O. and Weddell (1972). *Lancet* **2**, 1188
Fegan, W. G., FitzGerald, D. E. and Beesley, W. H. (1964). *Lancet,* 481
Fegan, W. G. (1967). *Varicose Veins, Compression Sclerotherapy.* London: Heinemann
Fegan, W. G. and Kline, A. L. (1972). *Br. J. Surg.* **59**, 798
Heslop, J. H. (1973). *N. Z. med. J.* **78**, 389
Quill, R. D. and Fegan, W. G. (1971). *Br. J. Surg.* **58**, 389
Somerville, J. J. F., Byrne, P. J. and Fegan, W. G. (1974). *Br. J. Surg.* **61**, 40

[*The illustrations for this Chapter on Injection Treatment of Varicose Veins were drawn by Mr. F. Price.*]

Venous Ulcers

F. B. Cockett, B.Sc.(Lond.), M.S.(Lond.),
F.R.C.S.(Eng.)
Teacher and Examiner in Surgery,
The University of London; and
Consultant Surgeon, St. Thomas's Hospital, London

The treatment of venous ulcers may be divided into three separate stages: (*1*) diagnosis; (*2*) management and pre-operative treatment; and (*3*) surgical treatment.

DIAGNOSIS

First, it must be established that the ulcer is due entirely to a venous cause. Ulcers of infective origin, due to underlying bone disease, trauma of various sorts and arterial ischaemia, also occur in the gaiter area. All these other causes must be excluded before the ulcer is regarded as purely venous in origin.

If entirely venous in origin, there is next a diagnosis as to which group or combination of veins is at fault. It may be entirely due to a long or short saphenous incompetence, but more often the ankle-perforating veins are involved as well.

If the whole limb is swollen and if the patient gives a previous history of white leg or iliofemoral thrombosis there may be a permanent iliac vein obstruction complicating the picture.

Accurate diagnosis is the only key to successful management, either non-surgical or surgical.

MANAGEMENT AND PRE-OPERATIVE TREATMENT

A venous ulcer can always be induced to heal in either of two ways.

1

Elevation of legs

The patient rests with the legs elevated to just above the level of the heart. This drops the venous pressure in the ankle region to nil, and if the ulcer is of purely venous origin it will at once begin to heal. In quite a short time, such as a week or ten days of rest in elevation, there will be a most remarkable difference.

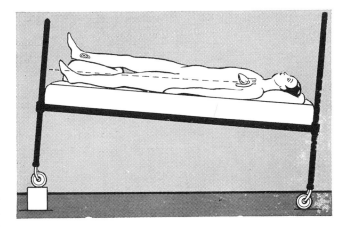

1

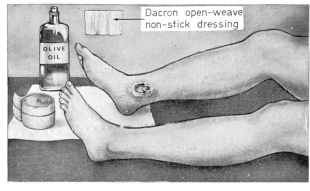

2

2 & 3

Elastic pressure bandaging

Occlusive elastic pressure bandaging is carefully placed from toes to just below the knee with a large gauze or felt pad over the ulcer. The bandage must be a stout elastic webbing one capable of exerting a pressure of at least 100 mmHg under it. Such bandages may be worn while the patient is at work during the day, and removed at night when the patient sleeps with the foot of the bed elevated.

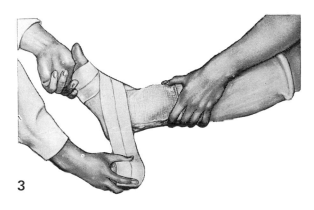

3

Local dressing to ulcer

Nearly all severe eczemas and infections are caused by the skin sensitivity induced by the application of local ointments of various sorts.

On no account should any local application be put on or around a venous ulcer, other than a little olive oil to the skin around it and an inactive Dacron open mesh 'non-stick' type of dry gauze.

All ointments containing antibiotics, cortisone derivatives or antiseptics should be avoided as they cause more trouble than they ever cure.

If surface sepsis of the ulcer is a problem then this should be controlled by systemic administration of antibiotics after culturing the surface.

SURGICAL TREATMENT

Ideally, surgery should take place after the ulcer has been healed or nearly healed by one of the forms of conservative treatment outlined above, and it is directed at eliminating (as far as possible) the incompetent veins which caused the ulcer. Full scale long or short saphenous ligation and stripping, together with full length exploration of the incompetent perforating veins, may be required.

In most cases this will cure the ulcer. However, if the ulcer has been present for many years, or if the limb is chronically swollen due to old iliofemoral thrombosis, then continuous elastic support may be necessary to maintain healing, even after a radical operation.

Local excision of ulcers

Occasionally for long standing ulcers excision of the ulcer and grafting is necessary as an adjunct to vein surgery. It is often necessary for the complete cure of the localized ulcers of the inner side of the ankle near the malleolus which become very indurated and chronic after being present for many years. Skin grafts should never be put on an ulcerated area—the whole of the ulcerated area should be widely excised (full thickness skin) and a split skin graft applied. At least 3 weeks with full elevation of the limb is necessary before the patient is allowed up, and then the skin-grafted area must be supported carefully with a gauze pad and elastic bandage. If this is not done the graft area becomes congested with the high venous pressure, and the whole graft is very liable to break down.

[*The illustrations for this Chapter on Venous Ulcers were drawn by Miss J. Dewe.*]

Ligation of the Ankle-perforating Veins

F. B. Cockett, B.Sc.(Lond.), M.S.(Lond.),
F.R.C.S.(Eng.)
Teacher and Examiner in Surgery,
The University of London; and
Consultant Surgeon, St. Thomas's Hospital, London

PRE-OPERATIVE

Indications

The direct ankle-perforating veins in the lower half of the leg are the main channels of venous drainage of the ankle skin into the deep veins of the calf. In the erect exercising limb nearly all the venous blood from the superficial tissues drains this way. Incompetence or destruction of the valves in one or more of these veins allows a high-pressure reflux from the calf into the ankle skin and subcutaneous tissues, resulting in widespread venular dilatation and ankle swelling. As time goes on, such lesions as eczema, subcutaneous fat necrosis and fibrosis and ulceration may make their appearance (the so-called 'postphlebitic syndrome').

Thus in any case in which these lesions are present round the ankle it is probable that one or more of the ankle-perforating veins are incompetent, and their ligation is indicated. The sites of the incompetent perforators can sometimes be seen on inspection of the leg. In more advanced cases their presence is completely disguised by the indurated oedematous ankle skin overlying them, and their incompetence is only to be suspected because of the presence of the ulcer and induration, and because of the presence of a flare of dilated venules below the internal malleolus (the ankle flare).

The best results of operation are obtained early, either when the pre-ulcer signs only are present, or when an ulcer has just appeared and has been present for a relatively short time (6 months to 2 years). After ulceration has been present unchecked for many years, irreversible local changes in the skin occur, and even radical perforating vein surgery may fail to heal the ulcer permanently.

Pre-operative treatment

This operation must never be done when the leg is oedematous, in the presence of an active eczema, or in the presence of an open infected ulcer. The essential pre-operative treatment is a period of Bisgaard pressure bandaging to control the oedema, and to bring the ulcer into a healing phase. This must usually be supplemented by a few days' rest in bed, with the foot of the bed raised, before operation.

Sepsis is controlled by oral antibiotics, and for local treatment a simple dry gauze dressing or one wrung out in normal saline is used. Strong local antiseptics and preparations containing antibiotics should not be used as local dressings, as they tend to promote a local eczematous reaction.

Position of patient

Operations on the perforating veins should be done with the patient lying flat on the back, with the legs widely apart on a foot board, and the table tilted head down about 20° to reduce the bleeding during the operation. The operator sits at the foot of the table.

THE OPERATION

1

Anatomy of the ankle-perforating veins

On the inner side of the limb there are two main direct perforating veins (*2*) emerging from holes in the deep fascia. They are situated behind the great saphenous vein (*1*). The upper one is approximately half-way up the leg. The lower one is four fingers' breadth above the internal malleolus. Note that the perforating veins communicate by fine venous arches, and also with the great saphenous vein by a large constant posterior arch vein (*3*) arising at knee level.

On the outer side of the limb there is only one constant large perforator (*5*) which communicates directly with the short saphenous vein (*4*). Much less constant is the so-called mid-calf perforating vein (*6*) emerging close to the insertion of the gastrocnemius into the soleus tendon. When present, however, it is often large and important.

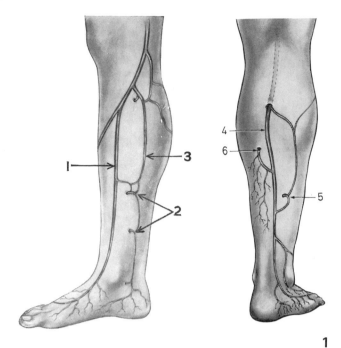

1

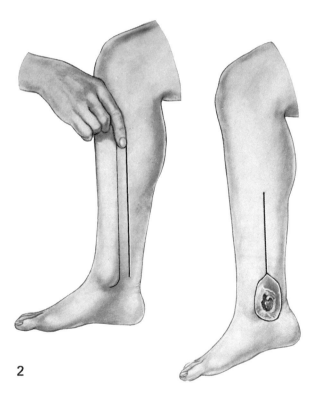

2

2

The incision

The incision starts just above half-way up the leg, one fingers' breadth behind the medial subcutaneous border of the tibia. It is carried straight down to a point half-way between the medial malleolus and the tendo Achillis. The vertical incision must never be dropped beyond the internal malleolus, otherwise the lower part may exhibit delayed healing and a troublesome scar, sometimes with a keloid reaction.

If there is an unhealed ulcer in the ankle region, well localized and of long duration, then this may be completely excised to the full depth of the skin as part of the incision. This defect is then grafted 2 or 3 days later.

3

The extrafascial operation

When the subcutaneous tissues are in good condition, freely mobile, and contain large palpable masses of veins, the extrafascial approach is used. The line of emergence of the perforators is cut down on, carrying the knife straight down the deep fascia. Any large vein in the subcutaneous tissues is then identified and followed up and down—it will lead to one or other of the enlarged perforating veins. Any lateral dissection is carried out mainly by gauze dissection right down on the deep fascia, sweeping the flaps medially and laterally. This is quite safe, but excessive local dissection in the subcutaneous plane may impair the arterial supply of the skin, leading to areas of skin necrosis in the incision, and delayed healing. However, under the anterior flap the great saphenous vein can be identified and used to insert a stripper. Stripping of an incompetent great saphenous vein can thus be combined with ankle-perforator exploration.

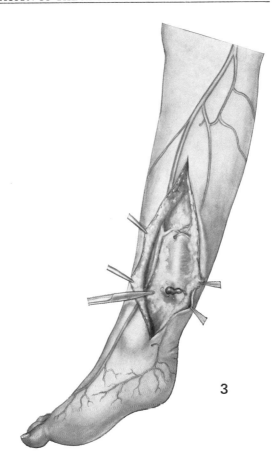

3

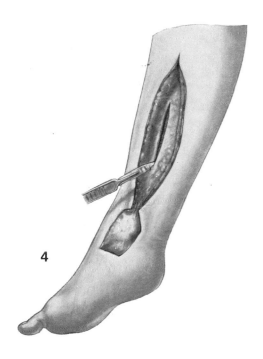

4

4

The subfascial operation

Incision through fascia

This operation is performed through the same incision. It is more suitable for the case with the indurated leg in which the skin has been bound down to the underlying fascia. The knife is carried straight down through the deep fascia, exposing the muscle.

5

Subfascial exploration

A number of artery forceps are then attached to the deep fascia of the anterior aspect and this flap is lifted up and the perforating veins sought as they pass from muscle to deep surface of fascia. In this plane wide lateral and medial dissection can be done without jeopardizing the blood supply of the skin. All ligating should be done with fine catgut—unabsorbable ligatures should never be used.

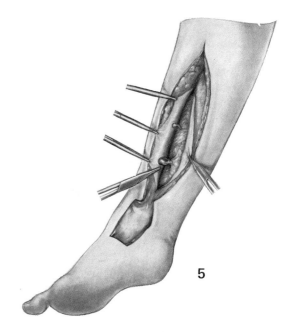

5

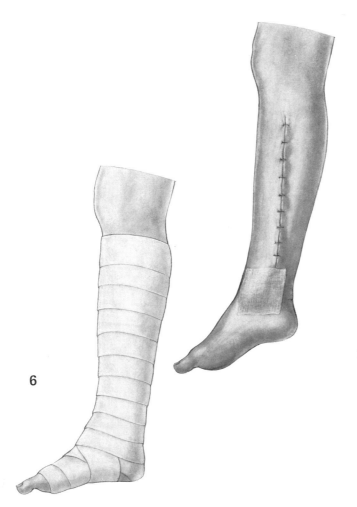

6

6

Closure

A few fine catgut sutures may be placed in the fascial layer to draw it together, but these are not strictly necessary. The skin is best closed by a few mattress sutures of nylon or silk. If the skin of the ankle cannot be closed without tension, it is best left open and the elliptical defect grafted at a later date. The limb is then enclosed in a firm crepe bandage. (Heavy duty webbing elastic bandages should never be put on to an unconscious patient as they are capable of causing skin necrosis if put on too tight.)

The lateral and mid-calf perforating veins may be ligatured through short vertical incisions over them.

POSTOPERATIVE CARE

The limb is elevated while the patient is at rest in bed, and active ankle movements are encouraged.

Ambulation for short walking periods begins on the second or third postoperative day, with a firm webbing bandage for extra support when the patient is up.

Stitches are removed on the tenth postoperative day, and then the patient is fully mobile, but must wear the elastic webbing bandage over foot, ankle and leg for at least a month, all the time during the day. After that it can be either discarded altogether (in most cases) or replaced by a light openwork (lastonet) elastic stocking for a further period.

Reference

Dodd, H. and Cockett, F. B. (1976). *Pathology and Surgery of the Veins of the Lower Limb*. Edinburgh: Churchill Livingstone

[*The illustrations for this Chapter on Ligation of the Ankle-perforating Veins were drawn by Miss J. Dewe.*]

Venous Thrombectomy

James A. DeWeese, M.D., F.A.C.S.
Chairman of the Division of Cardiothoracic Surgery,
University of Rochester Medical Centre, and
Professor and Surgeon, Strong Memorial Hospital,
Rochester, New York

PRE-OPERATIVE

ILIOFEMORAL VENOUS THROMBOSIS

Iliofemoral venous thrombosis is characterized by massive painful oedema of the entire leg which may be accompanied by vasospasm and, in some instances, gangrene. The thrombosis is usually initially localized to the iliac and proximal femoral veins but may also ascend from the calf veins. There is significant early morbidity and death may occur. There is usually late morbidity due to the postphlebitic syndrome.

Indications for thrombectomy

Thrombectomy is indicated in the following situations.

(*1*) When the disease process is less then 10 days old and is still localized to the iliac and femoral veins as demonstrated by phlebography. Patent channels can be re-established immediately and the valves of the femoral and saphenous veins can be maintained. Early and late morbidity can significantly be decreased.

(*2*) When vasospasm or the cyanosis of extreme venous stasis does not respond to conservative treatment. Increased venous drainage from the leg can prevent loss of limb.

Pre-operative management

A phlebogram is obtained to determine the extent of the thrombosis. Patients with only proximal iliofemoral venous thrombosis are taken immediately to the operating theatre. If there is more extensive thrombosis the patient is anticoagulated with heparin, placed in bed with the legs elevated at least 1 foot above the level of the heart, and observed. If cyanosis or arterial pulsations do not improve within 12 hr, the operation is performed.

SUBCLAVIAN VEIN THROMBOSIS

Venous thrombosis of the upper limb classically occurs following unusual exercise of the arm. It is characterized by painful massive oedema of the arm and tenderness along the course of the axillary and subclavian veins. The thrombus is usually initially localized to the subclavian vein between the clavicle and first rib but frequently extends distally to the axillary vein. Pulmonary embolization occasionally occurs. There may be significant early and late morbidity due to the persistent or intermittent pain and oedema.

Indications

The presence of a thrombosis less then 10 days of age, particularly if the patient is young. The risk of the operation is minimal, and early and late morbidity can be significantly decreased.

Pre-operative management

A phlebogram is obtained to determine the extent of the thrombosis. Anticoagulation is not necessary unless the operation is to be delayed for more than 6 hr.

228

THE OPERATIONS

ILIOFEMORAL VENOUS THROMBOSIS

Local anaesthesia is preferred. The groin and upper thigh are prepared. The entire leg is enclosed in sterile stockinette so that it can be manipulated during the procedure.

1

The incision

The incision is made along the inguinal crease from the mid-point of the inguinal ligament to within 1 cm of the pubic tubercle. If necessary it can be extended distally, medial to the course of the femoral vessels.

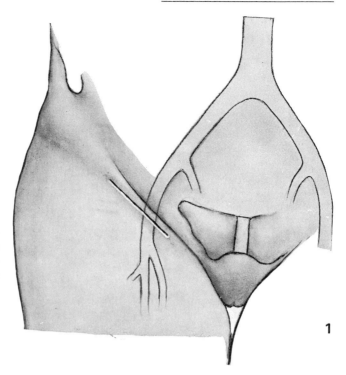

2

Mobilization of vessels

The femoral vein and its branches are carefully mobilized. Particular care is taken to identify and control the posterior branches which otherwise would cause unnecessary bleeding later in the procedure. A tape with its ends slipped through a short segment of rubber tubing is used for proximal and distal control. This allows occlusion of the vessel around intraluminal catheters.

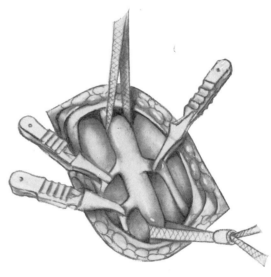

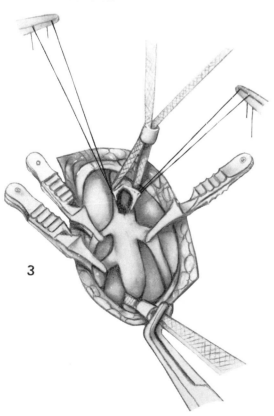

3

Venotomy

A longitudinal venotomy is made in the common femoral vein. Stay sutures are placed in the edges of the incised vein to minimize handling of the vein with instruments. The thrombus bulges forth and as much as possible is gently extracted with forceps. It is rarely possible to completely extract the clot by this method.

Iliac thrombectomy

4

Insertion of Fogarty catheter

A Fogarty venous thrombectomy catheter is carefully passed alongside the thrombus to the level of the inferior vena cava.

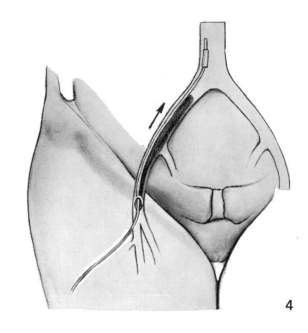

4

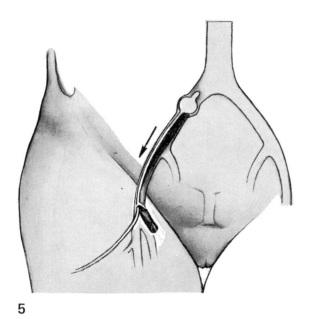

5

5

Inflation of balloon

The balloon on the tip of the Fogarty venous thrombectomy catheter is then inflated and the catheter removed. The thrombus is extruded from the venotomy incision ahead of the baloon.

6

Use of alternative catheter

Older thrombi may be too adherent to the vein wall to be removed with the Fogarty catheter. In that case, a semirigid plastic catheter, which is slightly smaller than the vein and which is attached to a 50-ml syringe, is cautiously introduced until resistance is met and then suction applied to remove the remainder of the thrombus. Unnecessarily vigorous suction such as that provided by a high-power vacuum line should be avoided or the blood loss will be excessive. After the operator believes that all of the thrombus is extracted, a phlebogram of the iliac vein should be obtained to demonstrate patency to the level of the vena cava. Further passages of the catheters may prove necessary.

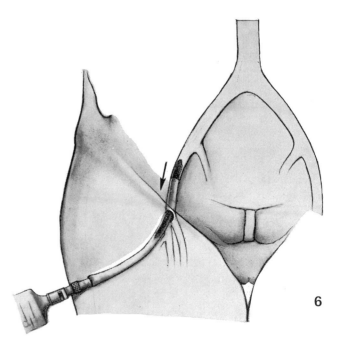

6

7

Femoral thrombectomy

The proximal femoral vein is occluded and the distal clamps removed. The leg is elevated and a tight rubber elastic bandage is wrapped tightly about the leg beginning at the foot and ending just distal to the groin incision. It may be possible to remove all thrombi in this manner and obtain a brisk flow of blood.

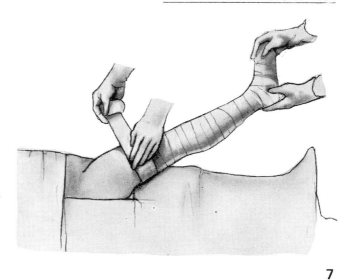

7

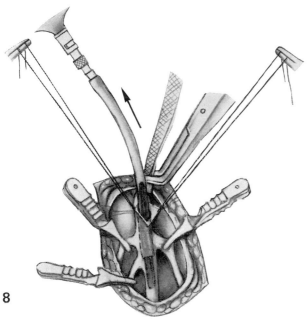

8

8

Passing of catheter

It may be necessary to pass catheters distally to remove all thrombi completely. Fogarty catheters can usually be passed to the level of the knee by gently manipulating the catheter tip through the valves. Plastic catheters can be introduced, if necessary, by intermittently distending the vein with a saline solution as the catheter is inserted.

9

Closure

The venotomy is closed with fine silk or plastic suture on atraumatic needles using stay sutures at each end of the incision and a continuous running stitch. If a satisfactory flow of blood cannot be established from one of the branches it is ligated flush with the femoral vein. The wound is closed with interrupted sutures without drainage.

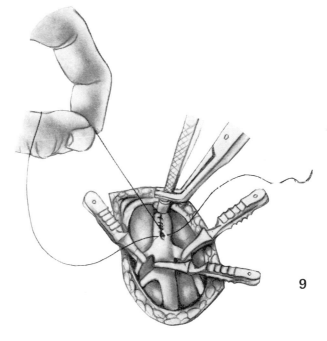

9

SUBCLAVIAN VEIN THROMBOSIS

A general anaesthetic is preferred. The neck and upper chest is prepared and draped.

10

The incision

The incision is begun at the medial head of the clavicle and carried along the clavicle to its mid-point.

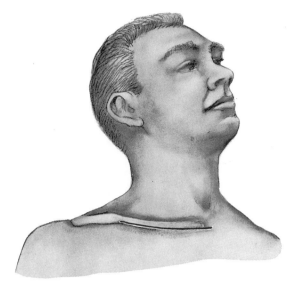

10

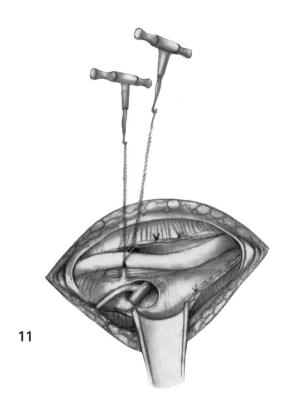

11

11

Excision of medial half of clavicle

Although the operation can be performed without the removal of the clavicle, the exposure is infinitely superior when it is resected. There is surprisingly little deformity or morbidity associated with the absence of the medial half of the clavicle.

The insertion of the sternocleidomastoid muscle into the superior border of the clavicle is incised. The insertion of the pectoral muscle into the inferior border of the clavicle is incised and the muscle retracted inferiorly to expose the clavipectoral fascia and costocoracoid ligament. The clavicle is divided with a Gigli saw just lateral to the junction of the cephalic vein with the axillary vein.

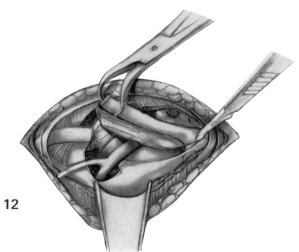

12

12

Division of subclavius and clavipectoral muscles

The subclavius muscle and clavipectoral fascia are divided at the level of the insertion of the cephalic vein. The clavipectoral fascia is incised medially along the inferior border of the costocoracoid ligament to the point where it inserts into the first rib and this insertion is divided. The costoclavicular ligaments and sternoclavicular ligaments are similarly divided. The medial half of the clavicle, subclavius muscle, and clavipectoral fascia are then retracted anteriorly as posterior attachments are divided, including the insertion of the sternohyoid muscle.

13

Exposure of subclavian vein

The entire course of the subclavian vein is now exposed. The internal jugular, innominate, axillary and other significant branches such as the external jugular vein are occluded and the longitudinal incision made in the subclavian vein. The thrombosis is usually surprisingly localized to the subclavian vein beneath the clavicle. Thrombus which has propagated distally can usually be manually expressed through the venotomy. The use of plastic catheters or the Fogarty catheter is rarely necessary.

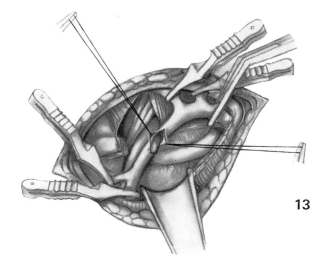

13

14

Closure

The venotomy is closed with fine sutures on atraumatic needles using a continuous stitch between two stay sutures.

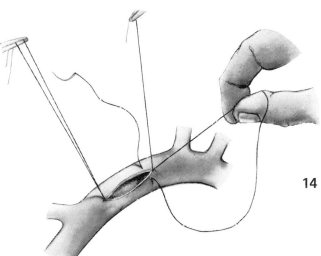

14

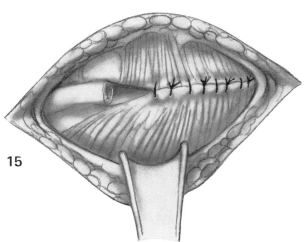

15

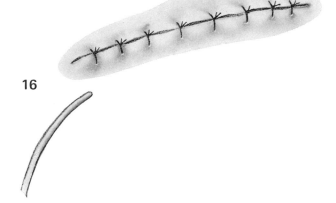

16

15

Approximation of fascia

The fascia of the sternocleidomastoid muscle and the pectoralis major muscle is approximated.

16

Drainage

A small plastic catheter is inserted into the subcutaneous tissue and brought out through a stab wound inferior to the incision for constant suction drainage for a period of 24–72 hr. The arm is elevated on pillows for only 24 hr. Anticoagulation is begun on the second postoperative day and continued for 1 month.

POSTOPERATIVE CARE

ILIOFEMORAL VENOUS THROMBOSIS

The patient remains in bed with the feet elevated 1 foot until the oedema subsides. He is then allowed to get up and walk with elastic support from the toes to the high thigh. He is not allowed to sit for 2 weeks. Elastic support is not necessary after that time if the thrombectomy has been completely successful.

The patient receives 2500 units of concentrated aqueous heparin (20,000 units/ml) every 12 hr for 2 days, and then larger doses are administered to maintain the clotting time at least twice normal for 1 week. Anticoagulation with one of the coumarin drugs is then maintained for 1 month.

References

Adams, J. T., McEvoy, R. K. and De Weese, J. A. (1965). 'Primary deep venous thrombosis of upper extremity.' *Archs Surg.* **91,** 29
DeWeese, J. A. (1964). 'Thrombectomy for acute iliofemoral venous thrombosis.' *J. cardiovasc. Surg.* **5,** 703
DeWeese, J. A., Adams, J. T. and Gaiser, D. L. (1970). 'Subclavian venous thrombectomy.' *Circulation* **41 & 42,** 11
Edwards, W. H., Sawyers, J. L. and Foster, J. H. (1970). 'Iliofemoral venous thrombosis: reappraisal of thrombectomy.' *Ann. Surg.* **171,** 961
Mavor, G. E. and Galloway, J. M. D. (1969). 'Iliofemoral venous thrombosis pathological considerations and surgical management.' *Br. J. Surg.* **56,** 4

[*The illustrations for this Chapter on Venous Thrombectomy were drawn by Mr. R. Wabnitz.*]

Interruptions of the Femoral Veins and Vena Cava

James A. DeWeese, M.D., F.A.C.S.
Chairman of the Division of Cardiothoracic Surgery,
University of Rochester Medical Centre, and
Professor and Surgeon, Strong Memorial Hospital,
Rochester, New York

PRE-OPERATIVE

Indications

Anticoagulation is the treatment of choice for patients with acute deep venous thrombosis with pulmonary embolization. Anticoagulation, however, does not always prevent recurrent pulmonary emboli. In addition, anticoagulants are sometimes contra-indicated such as may occur in a patient with a bleeding duodenal ulcer. The two indications for interruption of the femoral vein or vena cava are therefore: (1) recurrent pulmonary emboli in a patient who is adequately anticoagulated; (2) a single pulmonary embolism in a patient for whom anticoagulants are contra-indicated.

Site of interruption

Interruption of the femoral vein in the groin is the procedure of choice when one can be reasonably certain that the source of the pulmonary emboli are in the deep veins of the lower extremity. Phlebography can be very helpful in identifying the presence of such a thrombosis.

Interruption of the inferior vena cava is indicated when one is reasonably certain that the source of the pulmonary emboli is in the pelvic veins. This source should be suspected if there is clinical or phlebographic evidence of pelvic disease, or if phlebograms of both lower extremities fail to identify the source.

Vena caval interruption is reserved for patients with pelvic vein thrombosis for the following reasons: (1) vena caval procedures require general anaesthesia, whereas femoral vein procedures can be performed under local anaesthesia; (2) anticoagulation must be discontinued for a vena caval interruption but can be continued if the femoral vein is interrupted; (3) the mortality rate in these frequently desperately ill patients is higher with the larger operation of vena caval interruption; (4) the early and late morbidity is greater if the vena cava is interrupted.

Type of interruption

Ligation or ligation and division of the femoral vein or vena cava were formerly the procedures of choice. These procedures, in general, are considered to increase the late morbidity of the post-thrombotic syndrome since propagation of the thrombosis occurs distal to the site of the ligature. During the past few years, several techniques of partial interruption were described. These techniques prevent loose thrombi from reaching the lungs, but do not occlude the vein, thereby decreasing the severity of the post-thrombotic sequelae.

Techniques for partial interruptions include: (1) the creation of a harp-grid filter by passage of sutures across the lumen of the vein, as described by DeWesse and Hunter (1963); (2) compartmentalization of the vein by approximation of the wall of the vein at two or three points, as described by Spencer *et al.* (1962); (3) application of a smooth-edged plastic clip which compresses the vein, as advocated by Moretz, Rhode and Shepherd (1959); (4) the use of a clip with serrated edges which compresses the vein but also compartmentalizes it, as suggested by Miles, Chappell and Renner (1964); (5) the use of a clip with one flat and one serrated edge which also compartmentalizes the vein but is easier to apply, as described by Adams and DeWesse (1966). All of the techniques appear equally capable of catching thrombi without decreasing venous flow. The Adams and DeWeese clip is preferred at the vena cava level because of the ease of application. The harp-grid filter of M. S. DeWeese is preferred at the femoral level since clips do not seat properly in the cramped femoral space, and angulation of the vein occurs. The operations will be described using these newer procedures. Ligation, if preferred, can be performed through the same incisions.

Pre-operative preparation

Patients on anticoagulants are maintained on the medication if a femoral vein interruption is to be used. Anticoagulants are discontinued and their activity reversed with vitamin K or protamine sulphate if the vena cava is to be interrupted. Local anaesthesia is used for the femoral procedure and general anaesthesia for vena caval interruption.

THE OPERATIONS

PARTIAL INTERRUPTION OF FEMORAL VEIN

1

The incision

An incision is made in the skin crease just inferior to the inguinal ligament with the medial extent of the incision at the pubic tubercle.

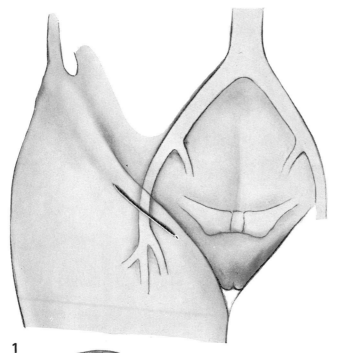

2

Identification of saphenous vein

The saphenous vein is identified and followed to the fossa ovalis. The small superficial external pudendal artery which is usually found beneath the saphenous vein passing medially over the lower margin of the fossa ovalis is ligated and divided. The fascia over the femoral vein is then incised.

3

Mobilization of femoral veins

The superficial femoral and deep femoral veins are mobilized and the superficial femoral vein occluded between two vascular clamps. The upper clamp also partially occludes the deep femoral vein.

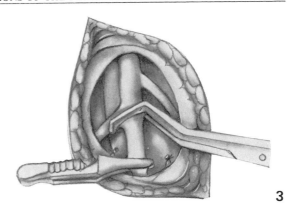

3

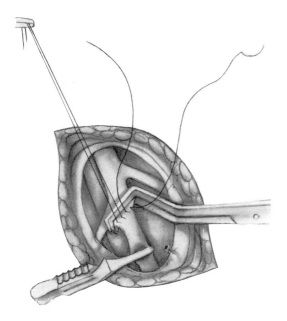

4

Suturing of vein

Mattress sutures are then passed through the vein, keeping the strands 2–3 mm apart; 5/0 arterial silk can be used but sutures of a plastic material are preferred.

5

Removal of clamps

The clamps are removed and the sutures individually tied to provide optimal tension without significantly narrowing the vein. The inset indicates the cross sectional appearance of an ideal filter.

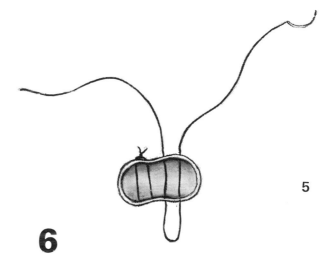

5

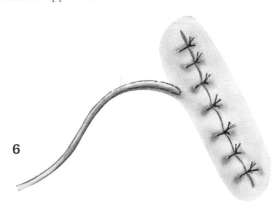

6

6

Closure

The wound is closed in layers after meticulous haemostasis is obtained. A small plastic catheter is brought out of the subcutaneous tissue through a stab wound inferior to the incision. The catheter will be connected to constant low-pressure suction for a period of 24–72 hr.

INTERRUPTION OF INFERIOR VENA CAVA

7

The incision

Either a right subcostal or upper mid-line incision is made with the patient in a supine position.

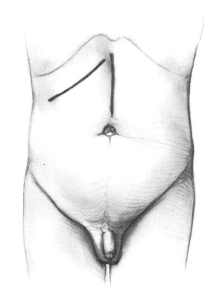

7

8

Division of muscles

The subcostal incision is followed by division of the right rectus muscle and a portion of the external oblique muscle. The internal oblique and transversus abdominis muscles are then split in the direction of their fibres. The peritoneal cavity is entered.

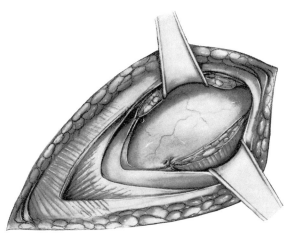

8

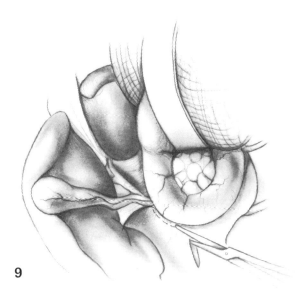

9

9

Exposure of inferior vena cava

The viscera are packed out of the right upper quadrant of the abdomen. The peritoneum lateral to the second portion of the duodenum is incised to enter the retroperitoneal space.

10

Mobilization of inferior vena cava

Using blunt dissection, the duodenum and head of the pancreas are retracted medially to expose the vena cava and both renal veins. A right-angled clamp is cautiously passed around the cava *just* distal to the renal veins taking care to avoid the first lumbar veins and the right spermatic or ovarian vein, which usually enter the cava slightly more distal.

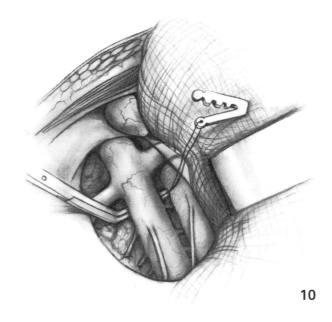

10

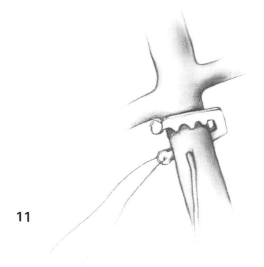

11

11

Passage of clip around the cava

The suture on the posterior smooth limb of the Teflon clip is grasped and the opened clip gently pulled around the cava.

12

Securing of clip

The clip is positioned to lie just distal to the renal veins and the suture tied about the end of its anterior serrated limb. The right and left spermatic or ovarian veins are ligated if pelvic venous thrombosis is present. The wound is closed in layers without drainage.

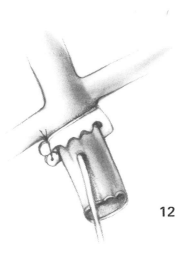

12

POSTOPERATIVE CARE

The patient continues to receive treatment for his deep venous thrombosis consisting of anticoagulants and bed rest with elevation of the feet for 7–10 days. Following that, he is ambulated with elastic stockings but not allowed to sit for a period of 1–4 weeks.

References

Adams, J. T. and DeWeese, J. A. (1966). 'Partial interruption of the inferior vena cava with a new plastic clip.' *Surgery Gynec. Obstet.* **123**, 1087

Adams, J. T., Feingold, B. E. and DeWeese, J. A. (1971). 'Comparative evaluation of ligation and partial interruption of the inferior vena cava.' *Archs Surg.* **103**, 272

DeWeese, J. A. and Rogoff, S. M. (1963). 'Phlebographic patterns of acute deep venous thrombosis of the leg.' *Surgery* **53**, 99

DeWeese, M. S. and Hunter, D. C., Jr. (1963) 'A vena cava filter for the prevention of pulmonary embolism.' *Archs Surg.* **86**, 852

Miles, R. M., Chappell, F. and Renner, O. (1964). 'A partially occluding vena caval clip for prevention of pulmonary embolism.' *Am. Surg.* **30**, 40

Moretz, W. H., Rhode, C. M. and Shepherd, M. H. (1959). 'Prevention of pulmonary emboli by partial occlusion of the inferior vena cava.' *Am. Surg.* **25**, 617

Spencer, F. C., Quattlebaum, J. K., Quattlebaum, J. K., Jr., Sharp, E. H. and Jude, J. R. (1962). 'Plication of the inferior vena cava for pulmonary embolism: A report of 20 cases.' *Ann. Surg.* **155**, 827

[*The illustrations for this Chapter on Interruptions of the Femoral Veins and Vena Cava were drawn by Mr. R. Wabnitz.*]

Operations for Superior Vena Caval Obstruction

James A. DeWeese, M.D., F.A.C.S.
Chairman of the Division of Cardiothoracic Surgery,
University of Rochester Medical Centre, and
Professor and Surgeon, Strong Memorial Hospital
Rochester, New York

and

Charles Rob, *M.C.,* M.D., M.Chir., F.R.C.S.
Professor and Chairman of the Department of Surgery,
University of Rochester School of Medicine and
Dentistry, Rochester, New York

PRE-OPERATIVE

Indications

Localized superior vena caval obstruction due to external compression from benign tumours, aneurysms and chronic mediastinitis, is amenable to surgical therapy. Surgery is rarely if ever indicated for obstruction secondary to malignant invasion with extensive venous thrombosis or untreated granulomatous mediastinitis.

Pre-operative preparation

Malignant or granulomatous causes of a superior vena caval obstruction can generally be excluded with a careful history, appropriate skin tests, evaluation of previous radiography, and bronchoscopy.

In addition, there should be a careful search for the presence of a Horner's syndrome secondary to involvement of the stellate ganglion or vocal cord paralysis from recurrent laryngeal nerve involvement. These signs are more frequently observed in malignant processes but also serve to define the extent of benign processes.

A phlebogram of the superior vena cava should be obtained by the simultaneous injection of radio-opaque material into the median antecubital veins of both arms. In this way the extent of the obstruction can be clearly defined.

Position of patient

The patient is supine on the operating table with the right side and arm elevated 10° with folded blankets.

Choice of operation

The primary aim of treatment is to decompress the veins of the upper body. In other words, some type of conduit between these veins (right and left, innominate, and/or azygos) and the right atrium or inferior vena cava must be established. The preferred operation, when feasible, is the placement of a graft between the extrapericardial and intrapericardial superior vena cava. However, decompression can be and has been achieved in many different ways.

If a graft is necessary the ideal material would be autogenous veins. Readily accessible veins are not large enough for total replacement of the superior vena cava and composite grafts are difficult to fashion. Fortunately, Teflon prostheses or homologous arteries do function well in the superior vena cava and are the preferred material for total replacement. For decompression of individual veins short segments of saphenous vein, external jugular vein, or femoral vein can be used.

THE OPERATION

1

The skin incision

A curvilinear incision is made beneath the right breast from the mid-sternum to the mid-axillary line. The breast tissue is retracted superiorly to expose the muscles over the fourth interspace.

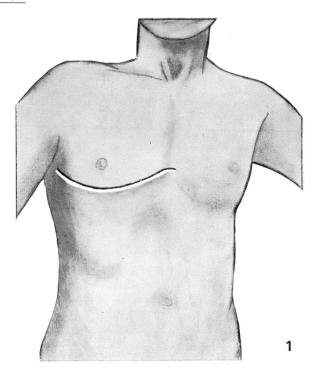

1

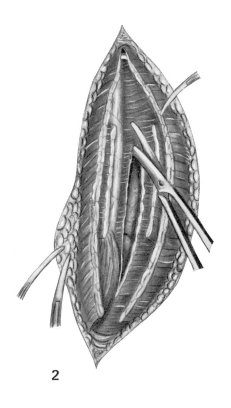

2

2

Thoracotomy

The pectoralis major muscles are incised over the fourth interspace. The serratus anterior muscle is split in the direction of its fibres to beyond the mid-axillary line. The intercostal muscles in the fourth interspace are incised and the pleura opened, care being taken to ligate individually the internal mammary artery and vein. If further exposure is needed the sternum can be divided transversely to enter the opposite thoracic cavity or the sternum can be split longitudinally to the suprasternal notch.

3

Normal anatomy

The lesions producing the superior vena caval obstruction will cause considerable distortion and it is important to be well acquainted with the normal anatomical relationships. The right innominate and left innominate veins join to form the superior vena cava. The azygos vein enters the superior vena cava outside the pericardium. The intrapericardial vena cava, right atrium and right atrial appendage are illustrated. The course of the phrenic nerve should be noted. The right pulmonary artery passes behind the superior vena cava just inside the pericardium and separation of the two structures may be quite difficult in the presence of scarring.

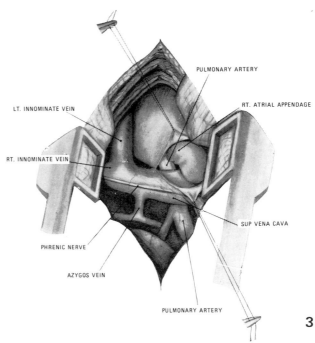

3

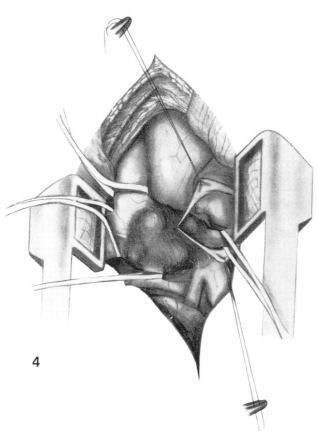

4

4

Typical lesion

The typical mediastinal fibrosis which causes superior vena caval obstruction may be surprisingly localized. The dense fibrous tissue mass distorts and obscures normal landmarks. The innominate veins and azygos vein will be markedly distended, as opposed to the more normal intrapericardial superior vena cava. Tape control of these major veins is obtained.

PREFERRED OPERATION

5

Replacement of superior vena cava

The superior vena cava is divided just below the innominate vein and also within the pericardium. An end-to-end anastomosis has been made between a short Teflon prosthesis and the extrapericardial superior vena cava. A similar end-to-end anastomosis is made between the graft and the intrapericardial vena cava.

Decompression has been achieved by an anastomosis between the intrapericardial and extrapericardial superior vena cava. The obstructing mass of tissue can be, but need not be, removed. The phrenic nerve is preserved if possible. The azygos vein is ligated.

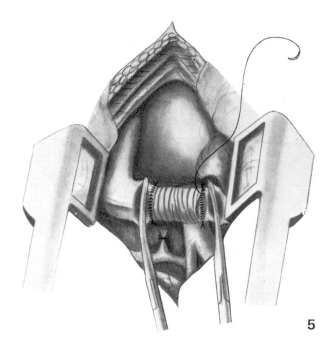

5

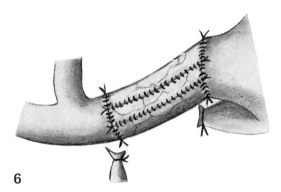

6

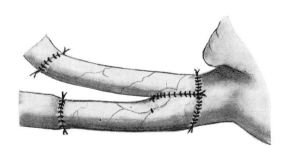

7

OTHER OPERATIONS

6

Superior vena cava to atrial appendage
(Benvenuto *et al.*, 1962)

If the intrapericardial vena cava is involved by the obstructing lesion an anastomosis can be made between the superior vena cava and the atrial appendage. A composite venous graft has been constructed by suturing together short segments of the saphenous vein over a stent.

7

Both innominate veins to superior vena cava
(Hanlon and Danis, 1965)

If the process involves the superior vena cava at the bifurcation of the innominate veins another approach may be necessary. The veins can be decompressed by suturing short venous grafts end-to-end to each vein and then anastomosing the ends of the vein grafts side-to-side. This enlarged end is then anastomosed end-to-end to the intrapericardial superior vena cava.

8

One innominate vein to atrial appendage
(Hanlon and Danis, 1965)

If a cuff of superior vena cava cannot be obtained, but there is still communication between the two innominate veins, another form of decompression is possible. A venous graft is sutured end-to-side to the innominate vein and end-to-end to the atrial appendage or intrapericardial superior vena cava.

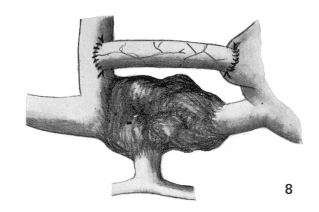

8

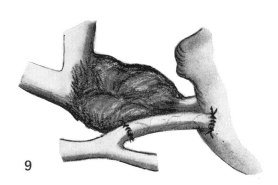

9

9

Azygos vein to right atrium
(Hanlon and Danis, 1965)

In the presence of superior vena caval obstruction the azygos vein becomes an important collateral for drainage of vein from the upper extremities. If the cava is obstructed below the azygos vein, partial decompression of the veins of the upper body can be achieved by providing communication between the azygos vein and the atrium. The azygos vein is divided and a venous graft is sutured end-to-end to the vein. The other end is sutured end-to-side to the right atrium.

10

Azygos vein to inferior vena cava
(Cooley and Hallman, 1964)

There are other ways of decompressing the azygos vein, including drainage into the inferior vena cava. A side-to-side anastomosis can be made between the azygos vein in the lower chest and the inferior vena cava.

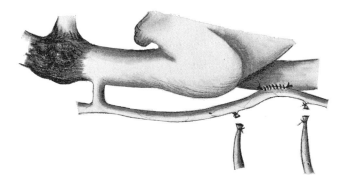

10

11

Jugular vein to femoral vein
(Schramel and Olinde, 1961)

In desperately ill patients, it is possible to provide some decompression of the veins of the upper body without entering the thoracic cavity. The intact saphenous vein is mobilized to below the level of the knee and delivered into the groin incision. The external jugular vein is exposed in the neck. The free end of the saphenous vein is anastomosed end-to-side to the external jugular vein. Blood now flows from the distended jugular vein through the saphenous vein and into the femoral vein in the groin.

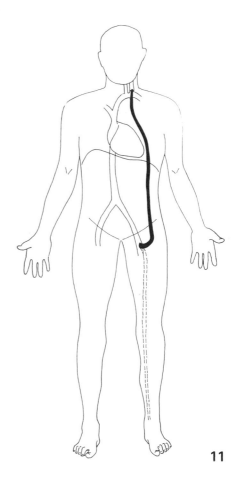

11

12

Endophlebectomy
(Templeton, 1962)

In some patients obstruction of the cava is secondary to localized thrombosis. The wall of the vein may be relatively normal. In these circumstances it may be possible to perform a localized endophlebectomy. The vein is incised longitudinally and a plane between the thrombus and intima or media of the vessel is established. The obstructing core is removed and the venotomy closed with a continuous suture.

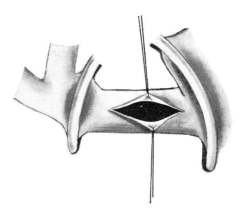

12

POSTOPERATIVE CARE

The patient receives 50 mg of aqueous heparin intravenously a few minutes before the vascular clamps are applied, and 50 mg of protamine sulphate is given intravenously when the vascular anastomoses are completed. No anticoagulation is given in the postoperative period.

References

Benvenuto, R. Rodman, F.S.B., Gilmour, J., Phillips, A.F. and Callaghan, J.C. (1962). 'Composite venous graft for replacement of the superior vena cava.' *Archs Surg.* **84,** 570

Cooley, D.A. and Hallman, G.L. (1964). 'Superior vena caval syndrome treated by azygos vein-inferior vena cava anastomosis: Report of a successful case.' *J. thorac. cardiovasc. Surg.* **47,** 325

Dale, W.A. and Scott, H.W., Jr. (1963). 'Grafts of the venous system.' *Surgery* **53,** 52

Hanlon, C.R. and Danis, R.K. (1965). 'Superior vena caval obstruction: Indications for diagnostic thoracotomy.' *Ann. Surg.* **161,**771

Klassen, K.P., Andrews, N.C. and Curtis, G.M. (1951). 'Diagnosis and treatment of superior vena cava obstruction.' *Archs Surg.* **63,** 311

Schramel, R. and Olinde, H.D.H. (1961). 'A new method of bypassing the obstructed vena cava.' *J. thorac. cardiovasc. Surg.* **41,** 375

Templeton, J.Y. (1962). 'Endvenectomy for the relief of obstruction of the superior vena cava.' *Am. J. Surg.* **104,** 70

[The illustrations for this Chapter on Operations for Superior Vena Caval Obstruction were drawn by Mr. R. Wabnitz and Miss D. Elliott.]

Portal Hypertension

Seymour I. Schwartz, M.D.
Professor of Surgery,
University of Rochester School of Medicine
and Dentistry, Rochester, New York

Portal hypertension is an elevation of pressure, that is, greater than 250 ml of saline in the portal venous system. It is associated with the clinical manifestations of oesophagogastric varices, ascites, hypersplenism, and portal systemic encephalopathy. The causes of portal hypertension may be categorized conveniently as suprahepatic, intrahepatic and infrahepatic in origin. Well over 90 per cent of the cases are due to an intrahepatic block, postsinusoidal in nature, and related to cirrhosis. A presinusoidal block may occur intrahepatically in patients with schistosomiasis or hepatic fibrosis, but is most frequently due to thrombosis or cavernomatous transformation of the portal vein. The rarest of the aetiologic factors occur suprahepatically and are associated with the Budd-Chiari syndrome of endophlebitis of the hepatic veins.

The modern era of clinical application of shunting procedures dates to the reports in 1945 of Whipple, Blakemore and Lord demonstrating the feasibility of an operation. Initially there was increasing enthusiasm and indications for surgical intervention were extended from the therapy for bleeding oesophageal varices to the treatment of ascites and prophylactic shunts for varices which had not bled. As data have been analysed, it is now felt that bleeding oesophageal varices represent the sole indication for a decompressive procedure.

A wide variety of portal systemic shunts have been performed to reduce portal hypertension, and decompress oesophageal varices. The use of either small vessels, or 'make-shift' shunts which employ larger collaterals, is generally regarded as inappropriate since the reduction of portal pressure is relatively insignificant and rarely permanent. The shunting procedures which have significantly and persistently reduced portal pressure include: the end-to-side portacaval shunt, with or without arterialization of the distal portal vein, the side-to-side portacaval shunt, either as a direct anastomosis or employing a graft between the portal vein and the inferior vena cava, the splenorenal shunt using the central end of the splenic vein, the central side-to-side splenorenal shunt, the selective splenorenal shunt using the splenic end of the splenic vein combined with ligation of the coronary vein and devascularization of the stomach, and anastomoses between the inferior vena cava and superior mesenteric vein either as a direct end-to-side anastomosis or with the interposition of an 'H' graft.

Selection of procedure

In most instances, preference for a given surgical procedure is based on personal experience and it is now felt that it is difficult, if not impossible, to select a procedure based on pre-operative haemodynamic studies. With a readily accessible and 'shuntable' portal vein, the end-to-side portacaval shunt is the most commonly performed. It is the easiest shunt to carry out and is generally associated with the lowest incidence of thrombosis. The presence of a large caudate lobe is less compromising to this procedure than to the side-to-side shunt.

In patients with extensive adhesions from previous operations in the right upper quadrant, the splenorenal or mesocaval shunts are generally easier to perform. Thrombosis, with or without recannulization of the portal vein (cavernomatous transformation) generally precludes a portacaval anastomosis and requires either a splenorenal or a mesocaval shunt. The Budd-Chiari syndrome with massive ascites dictates a side-to-side shunt to decompress the liver. To define whether the portal vein is acting as a significant effluent conduit from the liver and therefore requiring a side-to-side shunt to decompress hepatic sinusoids in the patients with cirrhosis, one can determine the portal pressure, apply a vascular clamp, and then remeasure the pressure on the cephalad limb. In the event that the portal vein is serving as a natural decompressive channel for the liver, the portal pressure in the cephalad limb will be significantly increased, but this is extremely rare. In a patient with severe hypersplenism and bleeding varices, a portacaval shunt is generally preferred, but if the platelet count approaches zero, it is reasonable to carry out a splenectomy and a splenorenal shunt in an attempt to obviate significant postoperative bleeding complications. Ascites is no longer considered to be a significant factor in determining the type of shunt to be performed except that it precludes performance of a selective splenorenal shunt. Similarly, whether previous encephalopathy is an important determinant if the decision to shunt has not been resolved. Since it is felt that reduction in total effective hepatic blood flow is an important factor in the development of encephalopathy, arterialization of the distal portal vein has been advised to prevent this complication, as has the selective splenorenal shunt.

Selection of patients

It has long been appreciated that the status of a patient's liver function is a critical factor in his ability to tolerate a portal-systemic decompressive procedure. Ascites which fails to respond to medical therapy, markedly reduced serum albumin, a bilirubin greater than 5, and a prothrombin time which is two and a half times prolonged and does not respond to vitamin K, plus the presence of encephalopathy after a bleeding episode has been controlled, portend poorly for the patient as an operative risk.

Attempts have been made to evaluate the dynamics of hepatic flow and to serve as a method of defining the shunt to be performed. Unfortunately, it remains difficult to determine which patients will tolerate a shunt, or which is the appropriate shunt.

PORTACAVAL SHUNTS

1a, b & c

End-to-side portacaval shunt

The operation is generally performed through a generous right subcostal incision which transects the medial portion of the left rectus, the entire right rectus, and extends around to the right flank. With this incision, the patient is either supine, or the right side may be slightly elevated. The liver is retracted craniad and a Kocher manoeuvre is performed to permit mobilization of the duodenum. Dissection is then begun in the hepatoduodenal ligament, and the portal vein is approached from the posterior aspect. An umbilical tape may be used to provide retraction of the common bile duct, but this is rarely necessary with a posterior approach to the portal vein. The portal vein is dissected free along its entire course from its retropancreatic origin to its bifurcation in the portahepatus. Occasionally a cystic vein and small pyloric veins require ligation, but it is not usual for the entire portal vein to be freed without ligation of any branches. It is extremely important to transect or remove the fibrous and adipose tissue which constitutes the posterior portion of the hepatoduodenal ligament, posterior to the portal vein, in order to avoid angulation of the portal vein by this tissue.

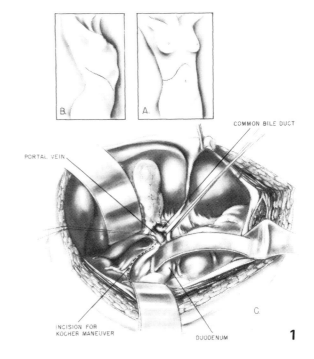

1

1d-j

After the entire length of the portal vein has been freed, attention is directed to dissection of the inferior vena cava. The incision in the retroperitoneum is extended, and the anterior and lateral aspects of the inferior vena cava are exposed from the renal veins to the point where the vessel passes retrohepatically. A partially occlusive vascular clamp is applied to the anterior aspect of the vena cava and the tissue incorporated within the clamp is incised. The length of the incision in the inferior vena cava should be approximately one and a half times as long as the diameter of the portal vein. It is not necessary to remove an ellipse. Vascular clamps or bulldog clamps are applied to the portal vein just above its origin and just below the bifurcation in the portahepatus. The portal vein

is then transected as far craniad as possible, the distal end is oversewn with vascular suture. Two guide sutures are placed in the cut end of the portal vein, which is then turned down to the inferior vena cava. The upper end of the portal vein is then secured to the portion of the inferior vena caval incision. This craniad suture is then passed through the posterior wall of the portal vein into its lumen. The next suture passes from the inside out on the portal vein and outside in on the inferior vena cava, to facilitate the placement of a continuous suture along the posterior aspect of the anastomosis. After this suture has run the entire length of the lumen, it is then passed outside again on the portal vein and tied to the inferior stay suture. The anterior row of the anastomosis is then performed with a continuous suture or interrupted, and tied eventually to the superior stay suture.

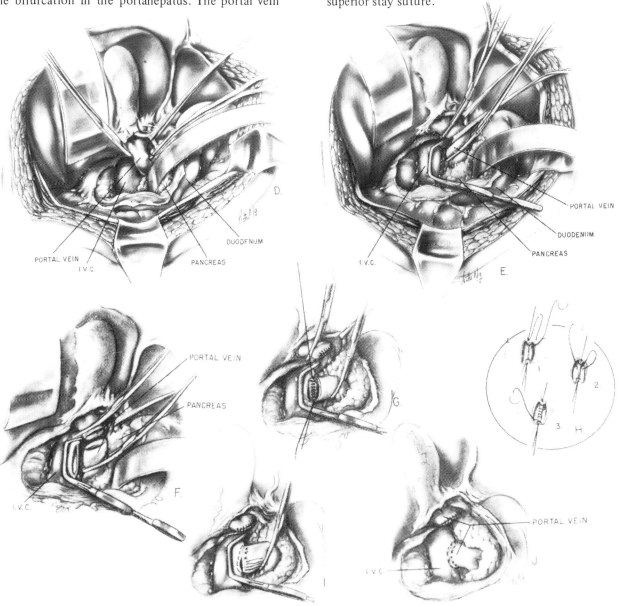

After completion of the anastomosis, the clamp is removed from the inferior vena cava first, followed by removal of the clamp from the portal vein. The pressure is recorded directly from the portal vein to define the efficacy of the shunt. Less than a 5-cm gradient between the portal vein and inferior vena cava should be present.

1k-m

Side-to-side portacaval shunt

The initial stages of the operative procedure are identical to those described for the end-to-side portacaval shunt. A partially occlusive clamp is applied to the anterior medial aspect of the inferior vena cava, and bulldog clamps or occlusive umbilical tapes are applied to the upper and lower end of the portal vein to occlude this structure. A longitudinal incision of equivalent length to that made in the inferior vena cava, that is approximately one and a half times the diameter of the portal vein, is then made in the lateral aspect of the portal vein. An elliptical segment may be excised, but this is not necessary. Non-absorbable 4/0 vascular sutures are placed at the upper and lower ends of the stoma. A continuous technique similar to that described in the end-to-side portacaval anastomosis is employed to the posterior row. After this suture is tied, an anterior continuous suture is placed. The double-barrel shunt is a modification of the side-to-side shunt.

'H' graft interposition between the portal vein and the inferior vena cava

After a partially occlusive clamp has been applied to the inferior vena cava as described above, and bulldog clamps are applied to the upper and lower portion of the portal vein, a No. 19 conduit Dacron tube is sutured first to the inferior vena cava as an

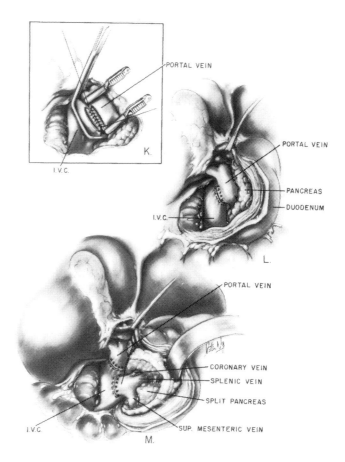

end-to-side shunt, then to the portal vein as an end of prosthesis to side of portal vein shunt. The conduit should be constructed so that the shortest possible length is utilized. It is possible to use jugular vein rather than prosthesis for this shunt. Both apparently work equally well.

2a-h

Central splenorenal shunt

The operation is performed with the patient supine or the left side slightly elevated and a left subcostal incision transecting the medial portion of the right rectus and extending well around to the left flank is employed. The transverse colon and splenic flexure are mobilized and retracted caudad. The short gastric vessels are doubly ligated and transected. Division of the splenophrenic and artery results in the establishment of an ultimate pedicle of splenic vein. This is freed along the course of the pancreas, by entering the avascular plane between the posterior surface of the pancreas and the posterior abdominal wall. In order to perform a central splenorenal shunt, the splenic vein is dissected free to its junction with the superior mesenteric vein. A vascular clamp is applied centrally, and the splenic vein is transected as far distally in the hilum as possible. Stay sutures are placed in the stoma of the splenic vein. The

peritoneum is incised just medial to the hilus of the kidney, and the left renal artery and vein are dissected free. Umbilical tapes are passed around the main renal vein and the major branches in the hilus of the kidney. It is preferable to occlude the renal vein with the umbilical tapes, but a partially occlusive clamp may be utilized. An incision is made on the anterior–superior aspect of the renal vein, measuring approximately one and a half times the diameter of the splenic vein. The renal artery is occluded temporarily with a bulldog clamp prior to this manoeuvre. The cut end of the splenic vein is brought down to the stoma on the anterior–superior aspect of the renal vein. An end-to-side anastomosis is performed by initially securing the two stay sutures and completing the posterior layer in the same fashion as described for the end-to-side portacaval shunt. Anastomosis of the anterior layer is then accomplished with a continuous 5/0 vascular suture. The occluding tapes around the renal vein are released first, and then the central clamp is removed from the splenic vein. Finally the bulldog clamp is removed from the renal artery.

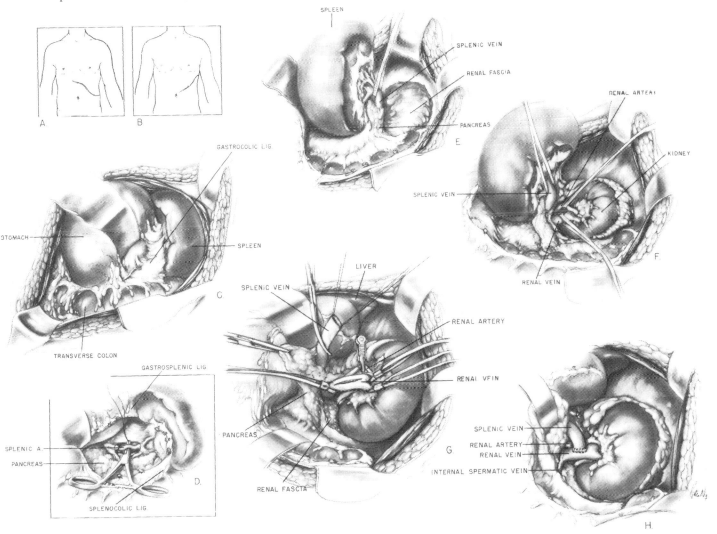

CAVAMESENTERIC SHUNTS

3a & b

End-to-side cavamesenteric shunt

The peritoneal cavity is entered via a mid-line or paramedian incision. Upward traction is exerted on the transverse colon in order to expose the superior mesenteric vessels. The peritoneum is incised in the region of the superior mesenteric arterial pulse and the superior mesenteric vein is identified to the right of the artery. The colic vessels are preserved and the right side of the vein is carefully dissected. Tapes are passed around the mesenteric vein. The lateral reflection of the ascending mesocolon is then incised along its entire length to prevent medial displacement of the transverse colon, ascending colon and medial reflection of the ascending mesocolon. This results in exposure of the inferior vena cava and the third portion of the duodenum.

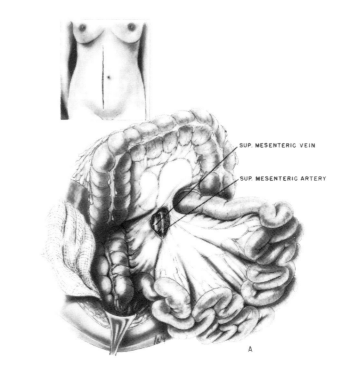

3c & d

The inferior vena cava is mobilized from its origin at the convergence of the two common iliac veins up to the entrance of the right renal vein. In the course of this dissection, the paired lumbar veins are ligated in continuity and transected. After the infrarenal vena cava has been freed along its entire length, a vascular clamp is applied immediately below the renal veins. Generally it is preferable to preserve a segment of the right common iliac vein to achieve added length. Therefore, the left common iliac vein is oversewn, and the right common iliac vein is transected as far distally as possible. In turning the inferior vena cava up, there should be a gentle curve around the caudad portion of the third part of the duodenum. The inferior vena cava is then passed through a window which is created in the small intestinal mesentery between the ileocolic vessels and the origin of the main ileal trunk. This permits approximation of the end of the inferior vena cava to the right posterolateral aspect of the superior mesenteric vein. Anastomosis is usually performed proximal to the right colic vein. A partially occlusive clamp is positioned on the right side of the superior mesenteric vein, and an ellipse is removed from the right posterolateral aspect. This should result in a stoma one and a half times longer than the diameter of the inferior vena cava. The anastomosis is performed with vascular silk, using a continuous suture posteriorly, interrupted at either end, and a continuous suture anteriorly. The opening of the peritoneum at the base of the transverse mesocolon is repaired, the ascending colon is repositioned in its natural location, and the lateral reflection of the ascending colon is sutured back in place.

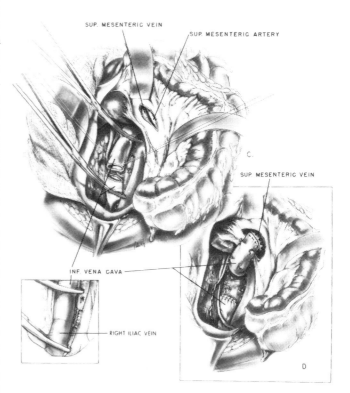

4

'H' graft mesocaval shunt

The superior mesenteric vein is isolated as described above for the classic cavamesenteric shunt. The tunnel is established directly through the right transverse mesocolon to permit visualization of the anterior surface of the inferior vena cava. At this point there is complete mobilization of the third and fourth portions of the duodenum, including the ligament of Treitz, in order to permit the duodenum to be moved craniad and prevent possible obstruction of the low lying duodenum by the graft. The length utilized ranges between 5 and 8 cm and knitted Dacron with a diameter of 19–22 mm is employed. The caval anastomosis is effected first, utilizing a partially occluding atraumatic vascular clamp placed on the anterior surface of the vena cava. A single row of 4/0 vascular suture is used, interrupted at the craniad and caudad ends. The graft is then trimmed to the adequate length to avoid both tension and excessive length. In view of the normal course of the superior mesenteric vein in relation to the inferior vena cava, it is considered advisable to rotate the graft clockwise approximately 20° prior to initiation of the anastomosis of the superior mesenteric vein. A venotomy approximately one and a half times the diameter of the superior mesenteric vein is made after proximal and distal occlusion. A single-layer anastomosis is then affected between the prosthetic conduit and the superior mesenteric vein.

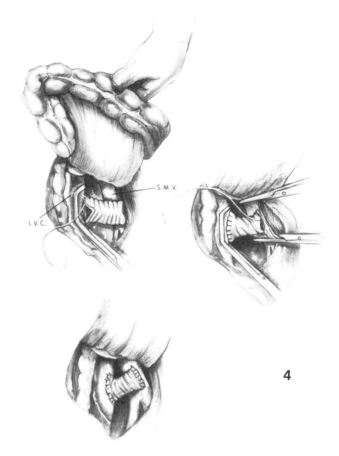

4

PROCEDURES DIRECTED AT PRESERVING PORTAL FLOW

5

Arterialization of the portal vein

Following the establishment of the end-to-side portacaval shunt, arterialization of the stump of the portal vein can be achieved by using the splenic artery turned up as a graft into the portal vein stump, or the gastroduodenal artery. Another approach to achieving arterial flow is direct interposition of a small conduit (8 mm) between the aorta and the portal vein stump.

Selective splenorenal shunt

The operation is performed through the same type of subcostal incision used for a classic splenorenal shunt. The umbilical vein is divided; the greater omentum is divided between the stomach and the colon to provide access to the lesser sac, and the superior mesenteric vein is exposed. The gastro-epiploic vein is then ligated and divided at the pyloric end of the stomach, leaving the gastro-epiploic arch to provide venous drainage from the stomach. The inferior mesenteric vein is doubly ligated and divided at its entrance into the splenic vein. The splenic vein is dissected free from the pancreas, and the junction of the splenic and superior mesenteric vein and the proximal portal vein are cleared. A tape is placed around the splenic vein proximally. An incision is made into the retroperitoneum and the left renal vein is mobilized, and a clamp is applied in a partially occlusive fashion to the anterior aspect. The incision made in the renal vein should measure approximately one and a half times the diameter of the central splenic vein, and an ellipse can be removed, but this is not necessary. The proximal stump of the splenic vein as it joins the inferior mesenteric vein to form the portal vein is oversewn with continuous suture and the splenic vein is divided at its junction with the mesenteric vein to provide maximal length and calibre. Anastomosis is then made between the splenic vein and the renal vein using continuous silk interrupted at two ends. The coronary vein is exposed along the lesser curvature of the stomach and is ligated with some small vessels near the gastro-oesophageal junction.

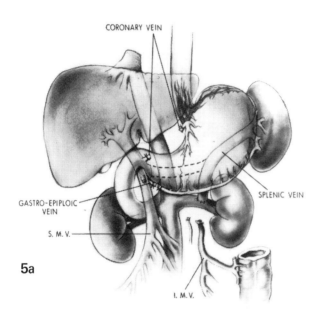

5a

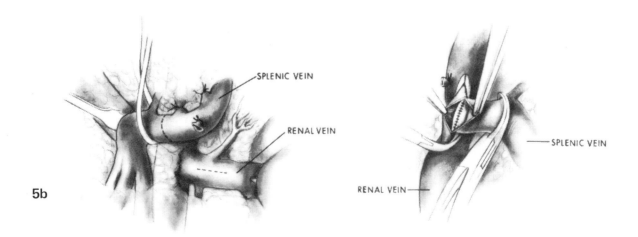

5b

[The illustrations for this Chapter on Portal Hypertension were drawn by Mr. P. Ng.]

Operative Management of Lymphoedema

The Late Harold W. Bales, M.D.
Associate Professor of Plastic Surgery,
University of Rochester, School of Medicine and
Dentistry, Rochester, New York

PRE-OPERATIVE

Lymph is that fraction of extracellular fluid containing large protein molecules and other particles too large to be returned to the intravascular compartment through the capillary membrane. Hence, it requires a separate transport system of capillary tubules—the lymphatic system. These vessels take origin embryologically along with the venous drainage system and parallel the venous systems anatomically. The dermis bears a rich plexus of unvalved vessels which empty into valved superficial trunks lying in the subcutaneous tissue. The distribution in the lower limb corresponds to the greater and lesser saphenous systems while in the upper extremity three drainage routes are recognized, radial, median and ulnar. The subfascial compartments are relatively devoid of lymphatics.

Lymphoedema, the excessive accumulation of proteinaceous extracellular fluid, may appear in numerous pathological states. These have in common an alteration in the dynamics of extracellular fluid formation as enunciated by Starling (1896). Two general types may be recognized:

(1) *Primary lymphoedema.* Lymphangiographic studies by Kinmonth (1955) have shown states of hypoplasia, dilatation or aplasia of lymphatic vessels with dermal back-flow of lymph. Congenital lymphoedema of the lower extremity (sometimes called Milroy's disease) and lymphoedema praecox are the most common examples of this.

(2) *Secondary lymphoedema.* This is an obstructive phenomenon due to mechanical blockage, such as by parasites or tumour or by scarring following infection and radiation.

The types most frequently subjected to and most amenable to surgery are idiopathic lymphoedema of the legs and postoperative lymphoedema of the arm.

The arm lesion is an obstructive one due to damage to the lymphatic trunks either by the operation for clearance of axillary lymph nodes or by subsequent irradiation. Venous obstruction may complicate the condition, in which case the oedema will appear within a few hours of surgery. The pure lymphatic obstruction may take weeks or months to manifest.

Swelling begins in the arm and spreads peripherally to involve the hand. Function is limited by the great weight, the increased bulk and the tension of the tissue. The cosmetic disturbance may be appreciable. Recurrent cellulitis and lymphangitis following the most minor trauma is common, which in turn, leads to further fibrosis and lymphatic obstruction.

Lymphoedema of the lower extremity is usually primary with typical onset at the age of puberty. It may be unilateral and is much more common in the female. Similar to the upper extremity the disability consists of impaired function, cosmetic disturbance and recurrent cellulitis, usually due to beta-haemolytic streptococcus, causing increased fibrosis and further disability. When the process is uncontrolled the skin becomes hyperkeratotic with a loss of skin appendages, thinning of epidermis and increase in dermal collagen.

Treatment

Gratifying response and long-term control may be attained in early cases before skin changes occur, by continuous external compression, scrupulous hygiene and prompt and adequate antibiotic treatment for the least infection. Such an approach should be tried initially in all early and moderate cases. Surgical intervention should be considered when conservative means fail to control the progression of oedema, when recurrent bouts of cellulitis occur, when advanced dermatoses appear and when the bulk of the limb diminishes function. A cosmetic indication also exists but the results in appearance are often disappointing to the patient. A careful explanation is essential.

Two general types of surgical approach have been suggested over the years: (1) an attempt to reconstruct or substitute an adequate lymphatic system; and (2) excision of the diseased lymphatics and their host tissue and fascia. This latter approach has enjoyed most widespread use and confidence.

Efforts to establish a flow of fluid from diseased vessels into the central system have included buried strips of dermis, silk threads, fine tubes of various materials, reversed tube pedicles and omental grafts. These have been generally disappointing since most lower limb lymphoedema is due to diffuse destruction or aplasia of channels rather than a band-like obstruction.

Kondoleon (1912) attempted to establish communication between the diseased lymphatics and the deep muscle compartment by excising strips of fascia as windows into the muscle compartment. This operation is often cited but poor results have made it obsolete.

Charles (1912) advocated excision of the diseased skin and subcutaneous tissue down to fascia and resurfacing by split thickness skin grafts. Grafts may be obtained from excised skin if it is of good quality, but are usually secured from a remote donor site. This procedure is very effective in reducing the bulk of the limb and is the procedure of choice in advanced cases. Weeping of lymph through the established grafts and subsequent hyperkeratotic changes in the toes are two late problems encountered in this procedure.

Thompson (1962) has extended Kondoleon's plan and incorporated principles of Sistrunk's flap operation to produce an effective procedure, the buried dermis flap. This involves denuding a posteriorly-based skin flap of its epithelium, a generous excision of diseased subcutaneous tissue and insertion of the resulting dermis flap through the incised fascia into the muscle compartment in the proximity of the vessels. Thus, the bulk of the leg is reduced by the excision and the egress of lymph felt to be improved as evidenced by improved clearance of tagged albumin. This procedure has enjoyed increasing popularity in the past few years and appears to be the most effective technique for dealing with moderately advanced problems.

Pre-operative preparation

Pre-operative preparation includes 3–4 days of preliminary hospitalization for optimum control of oedema by strict bed rest and elevation. Reduction in size is substantial. Lymphangiography may be useful if the aetiology is not clear on clinical grounds. However, at present it is primarily an investigative tool. Antibiotic coverage should be established during this period. Selection of the drug is based on control of the flora of any open wound plus B haemolytic streptococcus which is frequently present in the lymphatic lakes and blind channels. Skin hygiene is attended to by frequent washes with surgical soap. Although a tourniquet is used during the procedure, blood must be available for transfusion.

EXCISION PROCEDURE

1

The incision

The limb may be suspended by a tongs or calcaneal pin. Incisions are made as noted to remove the skin in one piece.

2

Removal of subcutaneous tissue

All subcutaneous tissue and the fascia, if it appears diseased, is removed. Margins of subcutaneous tissue are tapered. Some subcutaneous tissue is left over the Achilles tendon and over the fibular head.

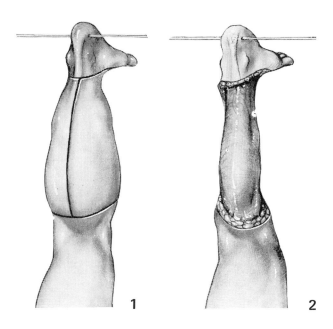

1   2

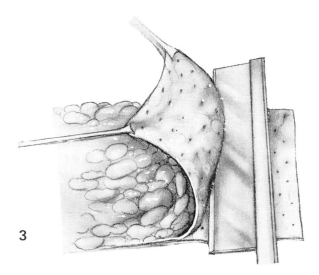

3

3

Replacement of skin

If disease changes in the skin are not marked, the skin is returned as a free graft. The specimen is pinned to a board or glued to a firm surface. The tissue is thinned with a free hand knife to 0·015—0·018 inches. If local skin has significant change, split skin grafts are obtained from a distant source.

4

Closure

The skin graft is returned in one piece using a posterior or medial suture line. If haemostasis is not satisfactory the wound may be dressed snugly and the skin stored in a moist sponge at 4°C for application in 2—3 days.

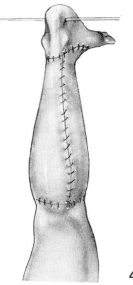

4

BURIED DERMIS FLAP (THOMPSON PROCEDURE)

5

The incision

These flaps are formed on either side of the leg with a posterior base. The dermis is denuded of the epidermis with a dermatome.

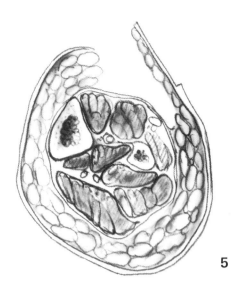

5

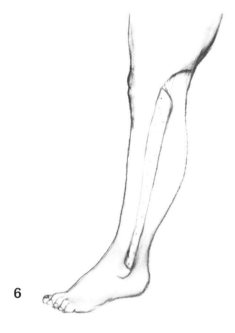

6

6

Formation of the flap

A generous amount of diseased subcutaneous tissue is excised to form the dermis flap and to reduce the bulk of the limb

7

Positioning of the flap

The dermis flap is introduced through the fascia into the muscle compartment in proximity to the vessels and the skin reconstituted by suturing to the base of the flap.

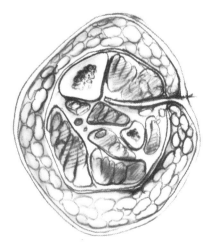

7

POSTOPERATIVE CARE

A bulky dressing incorporating a posterior splint from toes to mid-thigh is applied and left in place for 10–14 days. Bed rest and limb elevation are essential during this period. Ambulation is begun after 2 weeks. Elastic support is necessary for many months when the limb is dependent. Scrupulous skin care must be observed indefinitely.

References

Allen, E. V. (1934). 'Lymphedema of the extremities: classification, etiology and differential diagnosis: a study of 300 cases.' *Archs intern. Med.* **54**, 606

Blocker, T. G. (1949). 'Surgical treatment of elephantiasis of the lower extremities.' *Plastic reconstr. Surg.* **4**, 407

Charles, H. (1912). In *A System of Treatment,* Vol. 3, Ed. by A. Latham and T. C. English. London: Churchill

Homans, J. (1936). 'The treatment of elephantiasis of the legs–a preliminary report.' *New Engl. J. Med.* **215**, 1099

Kinmonth, J. B. (1955). Lymphangiography in man–a method of outlining lymphatic trunks in operation.' *Clin. Sci.* **11**, 13

Kondoleon, E. (1912). 'Die operative Behandlung der elephantiastischen Odeme.' *Zentbl. Chir.* **39**, 1022

Macey, H. B. (1948). 'A surgical procedure for lymphoedema of the extremities.' *J. Bone Jt Surg.* **30**, 339

Milroy, W. F. (1928). 'Chronic hereditary edema: Milroy's disease.' *J. Am. med. Ass.* **91**, 1172

Sistrunk, W. D. (1918). 'Elephantiasis treated by Kondoleon operation.' *Surgery Gynec. Obstet.* **26**, 388

Thompson, N. (1962). 'Surgical treatment of chronic lymphoedema of the lower limb.' *Br. med. J.* **2**, 1566

[*The illustrations for this Chapter on Operative Management of Lymphoedema were drawn by Mr. R. Wabnitz.*]

Sympathetic Ganglion Block

Alastair J. Gillies, M.D.
Professor and Chairman, Department of
Anesthesiology, Professor of Pharmacology
and Toxicology, University of Rochester School
of Medicine and Dentistry, Rochester, New York

and

Charles Rob, *M.C.,* M.D., M.Chir., F.R.C.S.
Professor and Chairman of the Department of Surgery,
University of Rochester School of Medicine
and Dentistry, Rochester, New York

PRE-OPERATIVE

Principles

The sympathetic ganglia may be temporarily blocked by the injection of lignocaine or another local anaesthetic agent. The injection may be made at a number of sites, of which the most usual are the stellate (inferior cervical) ganglion, the upper thoracic ganglia, the splanchnic nerves and adjacent ganglia, and the lumbar ganglia. Semipermanent interruption of the lumbar ganglia may be obtained with the injection of phenol. Complications have followed the injection of alcohol and phenol at other sites and we do not recommend their use except in the lumbar chain.

Indications

These are similar to those listed for the appropriate sympathectomy. Sympathetic block is done to estimate the benefit which is likely to result from a surgical sympathectomy and to differentiate the varieties of vasospastic diseases. In addition, sympathetic ganglion block is useful in the treatment of post-traumatic dystrophies and acute arterial dysfuction, secondary to emboli, thromboses, and crush injuries. Relief of pain, due to carcinoma of the pancreas, acute pancreatitis and various causalgias may be obtained from appropriate sympathetic block. Selected patients may find relief from the pain of angina pectoris by blocking the upper five thoracic ganglia (White and Bland, 1948). Phenol block has also been employed as an alternative to lumbar sympathectomy (Haxton, 1949) in poor risk patients.

Premedication

None is required, yet the occasional apprehensive patient may benefit from intramuscular pethidine (Demerol) 100 mg as a sedative 1 hr before block.

Apparatus

Thin lumbar puncture needles, or long No. 22-gauge needles preferably graduated in centimetres, are satisfactory for the main injection.

Position of patient

Stellate or inferior ganglion block

The route may be anterior, lateral or posterior; the anterior is preferred. The patient lies flat on his back with his arms by his sides and the head in line with the trunk. The neck and head are extended.

Upper thoracic ganglion block

The patient is placed on his side with the head, hips and knees flexed as for a lumbar puncture, the head being supported on a pillow so that the spine is in a straight line.

Lumbar ganglion block

The patient lies face downwards with a pillow beneath the abdomen to reduce the lumbar lordosis.

Posterior splanchnic block

The patient is placed in a semiprone position with the side to be injected turned upwards.

THE OPERATION

Stellate or inferior cervical ganglion block

1

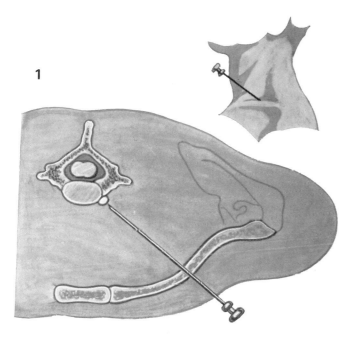

Lateral approach

The mid-point of the clavicle is marked and the skin and deeper structures above the medial to this point anaesthetized with 0·5 per cent lignocaine. A lumbar puncture needle or a No. 22-gauge needle at least 8 cm long is then introduced at an angle of 45° to the sagittal plane towards the body of the seventh cervical vertebra and advanced until the point strikes this bone.

A syringe is applied and aspirated to ensure that the needle is not in either the subarachnoid space or a blood vessel; 10 ml of 0·5 per cent lignocaine are injected. It is unwise to attempt the injection of this ganglion with alcohol or phenol. A successful injection produces a temporary Horner's syndrome as well as the desired diagnostic or therapeutic response.

2

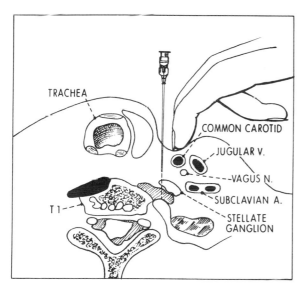

Anterior approach

The patient is positioned supine with the head and neck extended. A skin wheal is raised approximately 1·5 cm lateral and 1·5 cm superior to the suprasternal notch. A 6-cm needle is directed posteriorly between the trachea and the carotid sheath to the lateral aspect of the vertebral body. The needle is redirected to miss the vertebral body and contact the transverse process. At this point the needle is withdrawn 0·5 cm to place the tip in the correct fascial plane. Ten millilitres of 0·5 per cent lignocaine are injected. As above, successful injection produces a temporary Horner's syndrome.

3

Upper thoracic ganglion block

The spines of the upper four thoracic vertebrae are located and the injections made in line with these 4 cm from the mid-line. After infiltration of the skin and deeper structures with 0·5 per cent lignocaine, 10-cm long lumbar puncture needles are introduced at right angles to the skin until the point strikes the transverse process. Each needle is manipulated until it lies at the lower edge of this bone. It is now angled to about 20° to the sagittal plane and advanced until the point strikes the body of the vertebra.

The sympathetic chain lies at an average depth of 3 cm from the transverse process against the side of the vertebral body. If possible the needle should be marked in centimetres so that it can be placed in this position after these two bony points have been located by the needle point.

If aspiration produces neither blood, cerebrospinal fluid nor air, then the injection can be made for a diagnostic block; 5 ml of 0·5 per cent lignocaine are injected into each of the upper four thoracic ganglia.

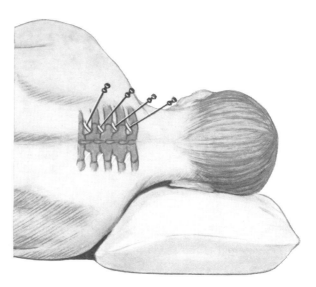

3

4

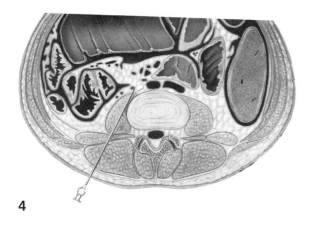

4

Lumbar ganglion block

The injection is made 3 cm from the mid-line at the level halfway between the second and third spinous processes. After infiltration of the skin and deeper structures with 0·5 per cent lignocaine, a 10-cm lumbar puncture needle is inserted and advanced until it strikes the transverse process of the appropriate lumbar vertebra. It is then manipulated until it passes just above or below this bone.

It is now angled so that the point is directed medially towards the body of the vertebra. As soon as it strikes this bone it is carefully aspirated and if neither blood nor cerebrospinal fluid is withdrawn the injection is made; 30 ml of 0·5 per cent lignocaine for a temporary block, 10 ml of 10 per cent phenol in water for a semipermanent denervation. A rise in the skin temperature of the appropriate foot and toes indicates a satisfactory nerve block.

5

Posterior splanchnic block

This procedure will induce a block of the coeliac plexus in front of the first lumbar vertebra which in turn will affect the visceral autonomic nerve fibres in the coeliac ganglia. The injection is made four fingers' breadth from the mid-line at the level of the first lumbar spine, or four fingers' breadth from the mid-line immediately below the twelfth rib.

A 12-cm short bevelled needle is inserted at an angle of 70° through the erector spinae to strike the body of the first lumbar vertebra. The needle is withdrawn for 3 cm and redirected forwards—at about 80°--passing the vertebra and into the retroperitoneal space. Aspiration will confirm that the needle is not in a blood vessel or the subarachnoid space and then about 40 ml of a 0·5 per cent lignocaine solution are injected and will anaesthetize both sides from one injection.

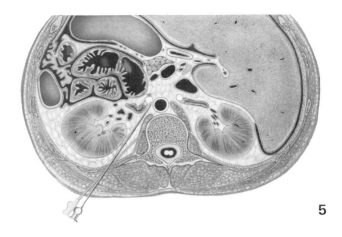

5

References

Haxton, H. A. (1949). *Br. med. J.* **1**, 1026
Moore, D. (1962). *Regional Block*. Springfield, Illinois: Thomas
White, J. C. and Bland, E. F. (1948). *Medicine* **27**, 1

[*Illustrations 1 and 3 for this Chapter on Sympathetic Ganglion Block were drawn by Mr. R. N. Lane. Illustrations 4 and 5 were drawn by Miss J. Akister and Illustration 2 was drawn by Mrs. V. Grasso.*]

Upper Thoracic and Cervical Sympathetic Ganglionectomy

Charles Rob, *M.C.,* M.D., M.Chir., F.R.C.S.
Professor and Chairman of the Department of Surgery,
University of Rochester School of Medicine
and Dentistry, Rochester, New York

PRE-OPERATIVE

Removal of the lower portion of the stellate or inferior cervical ganglion and the second and third thoracic ganglia produces a sympathetic denervation of the whole upper limb and most of the axilla (provided the rami communicantes from the first thoracic nerve to the stellate ganglion are left intact a Horner's syndrome does not develop). This operation also denervates to an undetermined extent the thoracic viscera. Removal of the fourth and fifth thoracic ganglia completes the denervation of the axilla, a wise addition if the operation is for hyperidrosis, and removal of the whole of the stellate ganglion denervates the head and neck with the production of a Horner's syndrome, an abnormality which may be avoided by the standard operation.

This portion of the sympathetic chain may be approached by one of the four routes – the cervical, axillary, anterior thoracic or posterior. The cervical is the best because it causes the patient less inconvenience than any of the others but from the surgeon's point of view it is the most difficult. The axillary route is to be preferred when the ganglionectomy should be taken below the level of the third thoracic ganglion as in hyperidrosis. The anterior thoracic provides excellent exposure but means a thoracotomy (Kirtley *et al.,* 1967) and the posterior route has largely been abandoned.

In the past there has been some argument as to whether a preganglionic section or a ganglionectomy should be performed. Surgical thought was well summarized by Kinmonth and Hadfield (1952) when they stated that in the the treatment of Raynaud's phenomenon the results of each of these methods were similar. Ganglionectomy has the advantage that it is more likely to result in a complete denervation.

Regeneration

We agree with Lee McGregor (1955) that this does occur, but a more frequent cause of relapse or recurrence is an incomplete primary operation.

Indications

The following are some of the diseases for which this operation may be advised when the disability is sufficiently severe and medical measures have failed; hyperidrosis, acrocyanosis, erythrocyanosis, primary Raynaud's phenomenon, secondary Raynaud's phenomenon (provided the cause is also treated), arterial occlusion (atherosclerosis, thrombo-angiitis obliterans, arterial injuries and embolism), causalgia and sometimes painful phantom limbs, certain autonomic nerve dystrophies, and reflex arterial spasm. When there is doubt as to the value of the procedure in a particular patient a diagnostic ganglion block is the best single method of reaching a correct conclusion.

Position of patient

For the cervical or anterior operation the patient is placed flat on his back with the operating table tilted so that the head is raised sufficiently to prevent venous engorgement. The axillary operation is performed with the shoulder abducted and externally rotated and elbow flexed each to a right angle. The posterior operation is performed with the patient prone on his face and with a pillow beneath the centre of the chest so that the shoulders fall forward.

THE OPERATIONS

CERVICAL APPROACH

1

The incision

The patient's head is first rotated to the opposite side and the arms placed by the side of the body. The incision is then made in line with the skin folds of the neck about 0·5 inches (1·25 cm) above the inner third of the clavicle. The incision is about 3 inches (7·5 cm) long and is carried down through the platysma muscle when skin towels may be placed in position.

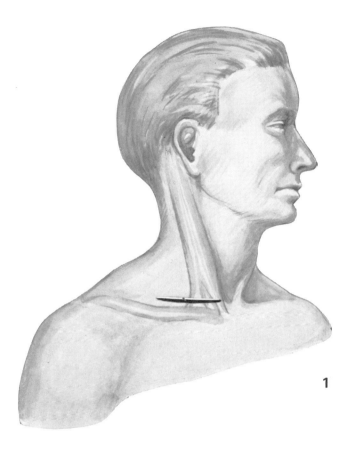

1

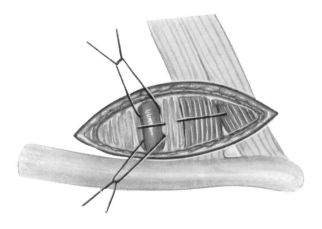

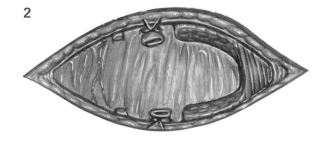

2

2

Partial division or retraction of the sterno-mastoid muscle

The external jugular vein is divided between ligatures and the supraclavicular cutaneous nerves are preserved if possible. The sternomastoid muscle is now exposed and its outer border defined. This muscle may now be retracted medially but in our view it is better to divide the whole of the clavicular head of the sternomastoid muscle because the exposure is more satisfactory and, provided it is sutured at the conclusion of the operation, little disability follows even a bilateral operation.

3

Exposure of the scalenus anterior muscle

The dissection is now carried down through a layer of fibrofatty tissue. The surgeon will encounter the omohyoid muscle, which is divided, and a number of small vessels. Retractors are placed at the inner end of the wound to expose the deeper tissues and protect the internal jugular vein. The dissection is deepened until the scalenus anterior muscle is found; this is identified by the presence of the phrenic nerve lying deep to the fascia which crosses this muscle. This nerve is retracted medially with the internal jugular vein.

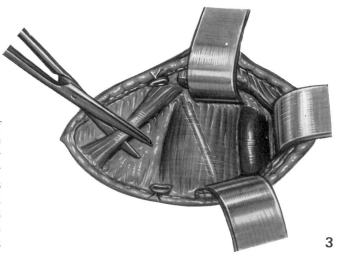

3

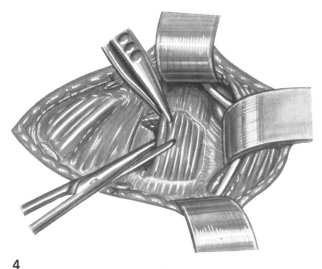

4

4

Division of the scalenus anterior muscle

This is the key to the operation. The muscle is clearly defined for a distance of about 1 inch (2·5 cm), its outer, anterior and medial borders being identified. It is then carefully divided, a few fibres at a time, by picking them up with dissecting forceps and cutting them with scissors. This method avoids damage to the surrounding structures which may follow a dissection completely round this muscle before division.

5

Exposure of the brachial plexus, subclavian artery and the dome of the pleura

Careful dissection will now locate the lower margin of the brachial plexus; this need only be identified. The subclavian artery is next exposed and retracted downwards. In many patients it is unnecessary to divide any of its branches, but in others the costo-cervical artery and sometimes one or two small vessels which leave the upper side of the subclavian artery in this region may need division to complete the exposure of the dome of the pleura as it lies beneath the suprapleural membrane (Sibson's fascia). Some surgeons prefer to retract the subclavian artery upwards.

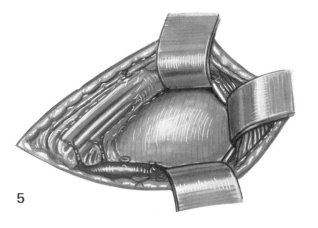

5

6

Mobilization of the pleura

This is best carried out with the finger. The supra-pleural membrane is divided on the inner side of the triangle bounded by the brachial plexus, subclavian artery and internal jugular vein, and a finger introduced so that the pleura may be pushed downwards, forwards and outwards. The pleura is stripped from the side of the vertebral column and posterior portions of the ribs to the level of the fourth rib and held down with a deep retractor which is preferably illuminated. Opening the pleura adds to the difficulty of the operation and for this reason should be avoided if possible.

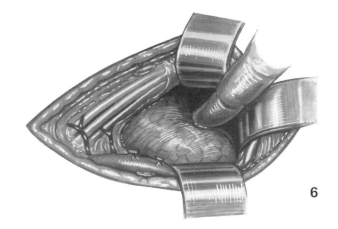

6

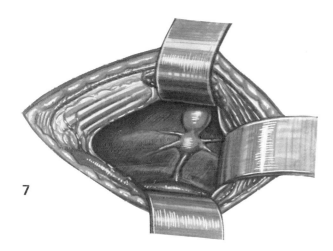

7

7

Identification of the sympathetic chain

The sympathetic chain is most easily identified by palpation. Sympathetic nerves are easily felt as thick cords and the ganglia as enlargements of this cord. After identification of the sympathetic chain by palpation the lower portion of the stellate ganglion is dissected free and its identity confirmed visually. Gentle dissection with a small gauze pad on a long holder will expose the second and third ganglia as they lie on the heads or necks of the appropriate ribs.

8

The sympathectomy

The sympathetic chain between the stellate and second thoracic ganglia is picked up with a nerve hook. The stellate ganglion consists of a large upper portion and a smaller lower portion which is in fact the first thoracic ganglion. This lower portion receives the rami communicantes from the first thoracic nerve. The ganglion is cut across below the point where these join it and the second and third ganglia freed. The sympathetic chain is then divided below the third ganglion and this segment removed. Great care should be taken during this portion of the dissection to avoid injury to the numerous veins which lie near to the sympathetic chain. Should bleeding start firm pressure should be applied for 5 min with a small swab on a long holder and the bleeding point then sealed with a Cushing–Mackenzie haemostatic clip.

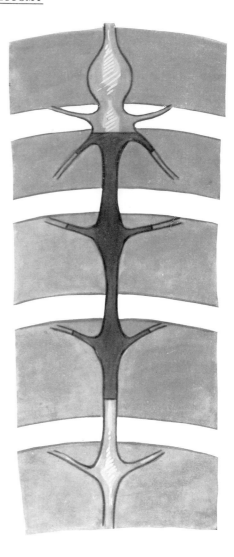

8

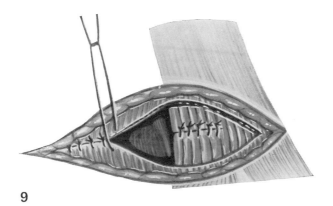

9

9

Closure

The anaesthetist inflates the lung, filling the wound with the pleura if this is intact. If the pleura has been opened it is not closed but the lung must be fully inflated and held so until the skin has been completely sutured. The divided portion of the sternomastoid muscle is united and the platysma layer sutured with fine catgut. The scalenus anterior and omohyoid muscles are not united.

AXILLARY APPROACH

This is a transpleural operation and is therefore contra-indicated if there is evidence that the patient has many adhesions between the visceral and parietal pleura in the region of the apex of the lung.

10

The incision

The incision is made in the axilla and follows the line of the third rib. It passes downwards and forwards across the thoracic wall of the axilla from the posterior to the anterior axillary fold and is usually about 6 inches (15 cm) long. In women the incision should stop at least 1 inch (2·5 cm) before the anterior axillary fold is reached because a major reason for using this approach is the production of a less obvious scar.

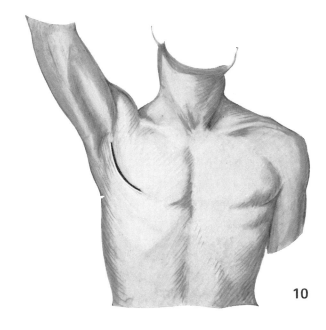

10

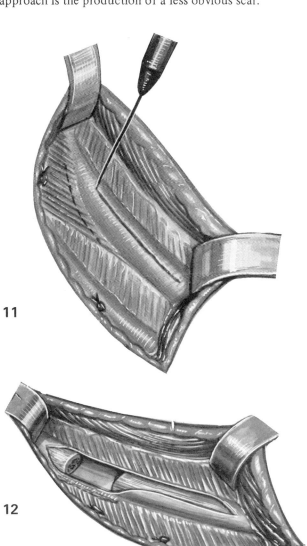

11

11

Exposure of the third rib

After the attachment of skin towels the incision is carried down to the periosteum of the third rib. The pectoral muscles and breast are retracted well forward and the latissimus dorsi, teres major and subscapularis muscles backwards. The long thoracic nerve is identified and placed under the posterior retractor. The lateral thoracic artery usually appears in the posterior portion of the wound and requires division. The third rib is exposed by incising the overlying fibrofatty tissue of the axilla and removing the serratus anterior from its attachment to this bone.

12

Exposure of the pleura

The periosteum on the rib is incised with a diathermy knife throughout the full length of the wound and then separated from the upper surface of the rib and from the back of the rib on its upper part. In large patients the incision can be purely intercostal; for others it is necessary to remove a variable length of the third rib to produce sufficient exposure.

12

13

Opening the thorax

The pleura is opened through the periosteum in the upper part of the bed of the third rib. This avoids damage to the intercostal vessels and nerve and this zone is relatively avascular. A rib spreader is now inserted and the thorax opened to a width of about 4 inches (10 cm). This usually provides sufficient exposure but if it does not the rib above may be divided subperiosteally and about 1 inch (2·5 cm) resected.

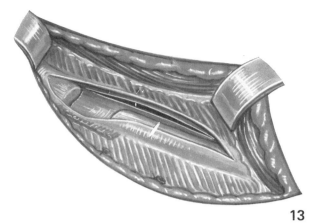

13

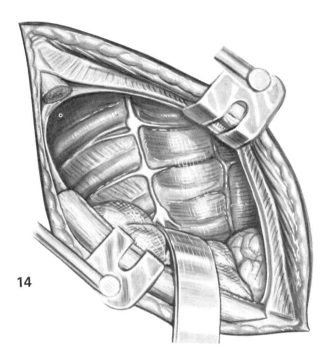

14

14

Exposure of the sympathetic chain

A large gauze pack is placed in the chest and the lung retracted downwards. This exposes the dome of the pleura and the upper part of the mediastinal pleura covering the bodies of the upper five thoracic vertebrae and the posterior portions of the corresponding ribs. The sympathetic chain can easily be seen beneath the pleura as it lies on the heads and necks of these ribs.

15

Mobilization of the sympathetic chain

The parietal pleura is opened with scissors as it lies over the sympathetic chain and swept back for a short distance on each side with a gauze swab on a long holder. The chain is then lifted up with a nerve hook below the fifth thoracic ganglion and divided. Traction is now applied to the chain and the rami communicantes divided between the second and fifth ganglia and the corresponding segmental nerves. The chain is then divided above the second ganglion and removed. It is not possible to remove the whole of the stellate ganglion with safety through an axillary incision, but the inferior portion can often be excised.

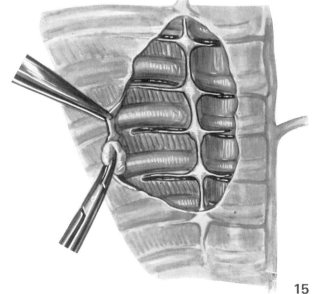

15

16

Control of haemorrhage

Great care should be used in dissection to prevent bleeding, which, should it occur, may be difficult to control. A small gauze swab on a long holder, preferably a dental roll held in a long straight artery forceps, should be pressed firmly on the bleeding point for 5 min; it can then be picked up with a long artery forceps and coagulated with diathermy or controlled with a Cushing-Mackenzie haemostatic clip. As the bleeding usually comes from an intercostal artery or vein, a meticulous technique should be employed otherwise the accompanying nerve may be damaged and painful neuralgia may follow.

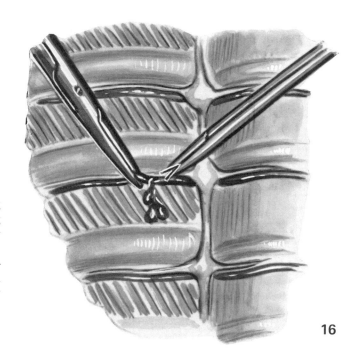

16

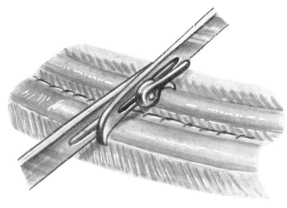

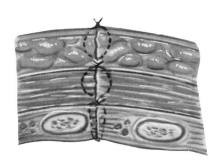

17

17

Wound closure

Once a dry field has been obtained the lung can be inflated and the wound closed. The pleura overlying the bed of the sympathetic chain is not sutured. The ribs are approximated and the periosteum and pleura in the rib bed closed with a continuous catgut suture. The fascia is then sutured and the skin closed. The anaesthetist keeps the lung fully inflated until the last skin suture has been inserted. It is not necessary to drain the chest if haemostasis is satisfactory. It is unwise to perform the axillary operation on both sides at the same operation.

ANTERIOR LATERAL THORACIC APPROACH

This approach provides excellent exposure of the sympathetic chain. It leaves a larger and more obvious scar than the axillary approach. On the other hand it usually causes less pain and provides better exposure than the posterior approach.

18

The incision

The patient lies supine with the arm elevated and supported as shown with the shoulder and elbow joints each flexed to 90°. The incision begins in the intercostal space at the margin of the sternum and is carried laterally between the ribs to the lateral point of the chest wall in the axilla. This long incision provides excellent exposure. In the female it should curve below the breast which is then retracted upwards.

19

Opening the chest

The pectoralis major muscle is incised in the line of the muscle fibres and the third intercostal space exposed. The intercostal muscles and pleura are then incised. A rib spreader is now inserted and the lung retracted downwards. Pleuropulmonary adhesions if present are divided. If further exposure is required the third costal cartilage may be divided in the upper and medial part of the incision.

20

The sympathetic ganglionectomy

The sympathetic chain can be seen under the parietal pleura as it lies on the necks and heads of the ribs. The pleura is incised over the chain and the incision continued from at least the first to the fifth ribs. The sympathetic chain is then removed in the manner shown in *Illustration 15* for the axillary operation. But as this anterior exposure is more adequate, haemorrhage if it occurs can be more easily controlled. The wound is then closed in the manner shown in *Illustration 17*. Chest tube drainage is not necessary.

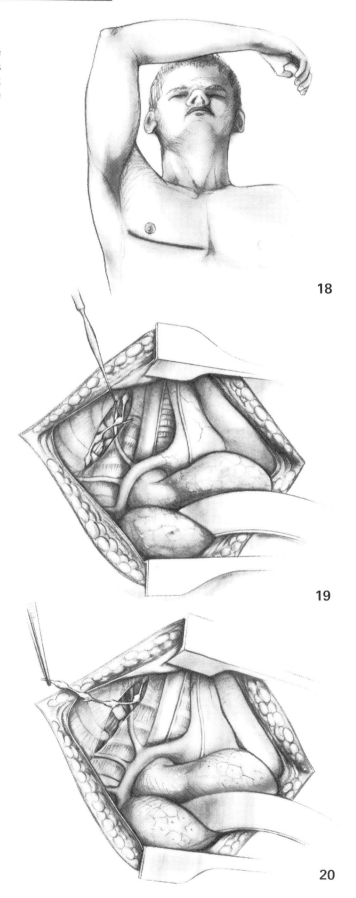

18

19

20

POSTERIOR APPROACH

21

The incision

When bilateral, a long transverse incision across the back at the level of the third thoracic spinous process gives good exposure. For a unilateral operation a vertical incision about 6 inches (15 cm) long centred on the third opinous process is more usual. This is placed about half-way between the mid-line and the inner border of the blade of the scapula.

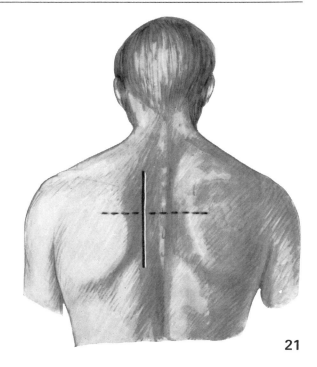

21

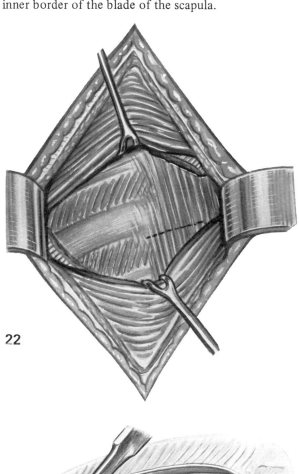

22

22

Division of the muscles

The trapezius muscle is divided throughout the length of the incision. The next step is to insert a finger into the wound and carefully count the ribs to identify the third. This step is important if the standard Smithwick procedure is to be performed. A preliminary radiograph will have excluded a cervical rib and the third rib must be identified with certainty. The major rhomboid muscle is now split in the line of the long axis of the third rib and the serratus posterior in the line of the incision. This exposes the erector spinae muscle, the attachments of which to the third rib are now divided.

23

Resection of the rib

The third rib is now exposed on its upper border and the periosteum over this bone from the neck of the rib to just beyond the angle is incised with a diathermy knife. The periosteum is now removed from the rib and about 1·5 inches (3·8 cm) in the region of the angle removed. The pleura is now depressed with a finger and the neck of the rib and transverse process of the third dorsal vertebra are removed with bone-nibbling forceps. An adequate amount of bone should be removed otherwise the exposure will be insufficient.

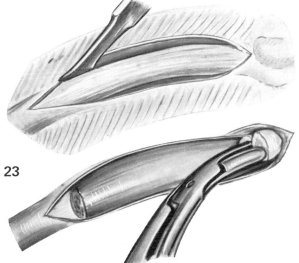

23

24

Identification of the sympathetic chain

The pleura is gently stripped with the finger from the backs of the second and fourth ribs and the sides of the bodies of the vertebrae. The third thoracic nerve is identified and the third ganglion and sympathetic chain isolated as it lies on the anterior surface of this nerve in line with the heads of the ribs. The second and fourth ganglia with the intervening chain are now found. A light introduced into the wound is of considerable help at this stage, because the exposure although adequate for the second and third ganglia is limited above and below this level.

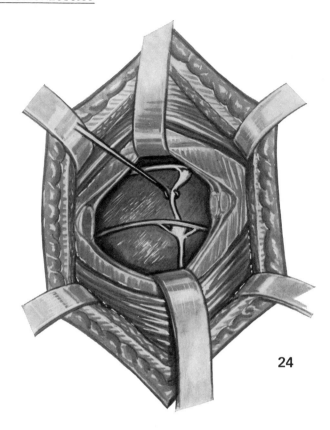

24

25

The sympathectomy

In the Smithwick procedure the third thoracic nerve is divided lateral to the sympathetic ganglion and then followed medially into the intervertebral foramen so that the anterior and posterior nerve routes can be sectioned. The second thoracic nerve is then treated in the same way. After this the sympathetic chain is sectioned below the fourth ganglion, the rami of the second, third and fourth ganglia are divided and this portion of the chain placed in a silk bag and swung upwards and backwards where it is fixed in the erector spinae muscle mass. This procedure produces a satisfactory preganglionic section and little disability follows the sacrifice of the second and third thoracic nerves. However, most surgeons today preserve the second and third nerves and do a sympathetic ganglionectomy, removing the second, third and fourth ganglia. The reason for placing the chain in a silk bag is that in the preganglionic procedure it is not removed and covering by the bag is designed to prevent regeneration. In our opinion a ganglionectomy is a more certain and a better procedure.

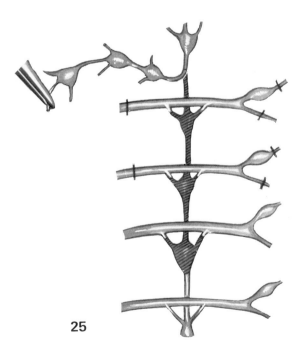

25

26

Wound closure

It is rarely possible to suture the erector spinae or the serratus posterior muscle, which is therefore allowed to fall into the rib bed. The rhomboid muscle is sutured but forms only a weak layer. The main strength of the closure is provided by the trapezius muscle which is carefully sutured, preferably with interrupted stitches. The skin is then closed.

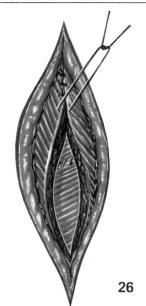

26

SPECIAL POSTOPERATIVE COMPLICATIONS

Sympathectomy

A Horner's syndrome follows removal or the division of the rami from the first thoracic nerve to the stellate (inferior cervical) ganglion. The main complaints are ptosis and the abnormalities of the pupil particularly if unilateral. This syndrome should only occur when the surgeon desires a sympathetic denervation of the head and neck. This syndrome may increase nasal obstruction by causing hyperaemia of the nasal mucosa. It has also been blamed for detachment of the retina in the elderly by reducing intra-ocular pressure.

Excessive dryness of the hands may be noticed. This can be prevented by rubbing the hands daily with an ointment consisting of equal parts of lanoline, glycerin and white Vaseline with rose water.

Cervical approach

Gentle retraction, particularly in the region of the brachial plexus, is essential otherwise a temporary nerve palsy may follow.

On the left side the thoracic duct may be injured. This is recognized by an escape of lymph. The treatment is careful ligation of the duct with transfixion sutures. The advantage of this route is that both the hospital stay and period of disability are shorter than with the other procedures.

Axillary approaches

A moderate degree of surgical emphysema often follows this procedure; it is often present following operation by either of the other routes if the pleura is opened but it rapidly absorbs.

Anterior thoracic approach

Posterior approach

The main disadvantage of this route is that severe and persistent pains may occur in the region of the scar. Although uncommon these may be a serious disability.

References

Atkins, H.B.J. (1949). *Lancet* **2,** 1152
Kinmonth, J.B. and Hadfield, G.I. (1952). *Br. med. J.* **1,** 1377
Kirtley, J.A., Riddell, D.H., Stoney, W.S. and Wright, J.W. (1967). *Ann. Surg.* **165,** 869
Lee McGregor, A. (1955). *Surgery of the Sympathetic.* Bristol: John Wright
Telford, E.D. (1935). *Br. J. Surg.* **23,** 448
White, J.C., Smithwick, R.H. and Simeone, F.A. (1952). *The Autonomic Nervous System,* 3rd Edn. London: Kimpton

[*The illustrations for this Chapter on Upper Thoracic and Cervical Sympathetic Ganglionectomy were drawn by Mr. R. N. Lane and Mr. R. Wabnitz.*]

Lumbodorsal Sympathectomy and Splanchnicectomy; Presacral Neurectomy

Charles Rob, *M.C.,* M.D., M.Chir., F.R.C.S.
Professor and Chairman of the Department of Surgery,
University of Rochester School of Medicine and
Dentistry, Rochester, New York

PRE-OPERATIVE

Indications

Very few patients with malignant or essential hypertension benefit from lumbodorsal sympathectomy and splanchnicectomy especially if the patient's condition worsens in spite of adequate medical treatment or if this treatment is not tolerated. Selection of patients for this operation is difficult. In the past we and others performed this operation quite often. But in recent years the operation has been used very much less frequently in the treatment of hypertension because medical management has so greatly improved; we have only performed the procedures once in the past 10 years.

The position was well summarized by Pickering (1955) when he stated that 'sympathectomy has a strikingly beneficial effect on a few patients, a good effect on some and perhaps no effect on others. It is a major operation with a low mortality in experienced hands, but with some postoperative sequelae, such as severe pain of a causalgic type and giddiness and palpitations on standing and on effort. The major difficulty which has not yet been solved is to determine in advance which patients will react well and which badly'.

This operation has also been used in the treatment of the severe pain associated with chronic relapsing pancreatitis and some other chronic intra-abdominal pain-producing lesions.

Contra-indications

Significant impairment of renal function and uncorrected cardiac failure contra-indicate this operation.

Stages

The operation is a two-stage procedure with an interval of about 2 weeks between each side.

Anaesthesia

General anaesthesia with an endotracheal tube is satisfactory, and we have found hypotensive anaesthesia (Gillies, 1949) using a high spinal, both safe and convenient for these patients.

Approach

This may be via a lateral thoracic incision but the Smithwick operation, a thoraco-abdominal procedure, is the more usual method.

LATERAL THORACIC APPROACH

Lying on the opposite side to that which is to be incised the patient is placed with the trunk rotated backwards towards the surgeon through 30° and the head and feet lowered to extend the operation site.

THE OPERATION

1

The incision

The incision is along the line of the eighth intercostal space from the anterior tip of the rib to a point about 2 inches (5 cm) from the vertebral column. The intercostal muscles and pleura are incised in the eighth intercostal space or the periosteum of the rib is incised and a length of rib removed. If further exposure is needed, 1 inch (2·5 cm) of the posterior part of the rib above may be removed as well.

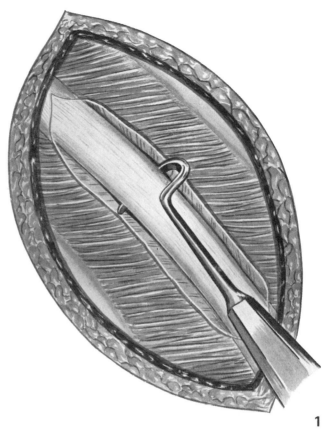

1

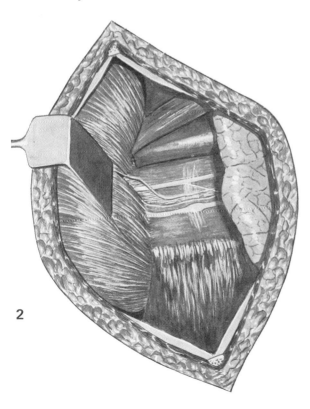

2

2

Exposure of the sympathetic chain and splanchnic nerves

The incision is opened wide by rib spreaders, the diaphragm retracted downwards by a Deaver retractor and the lung collapsed and held upwards by a large pack and another retractor. The great splanchnic nerve and sympathetic chain can be seen through the parietal pleura on the posterior chest wall. This pleura is incised longitudinally between the splanchnic nerves and sympathetic chain. The incision in the pleura is carried upwards to the level of the fifth rib or higher and the flaps dissected back to expose the sympathetic chain and splanchnic nerves from as high as possible in the thorax to the diaphragm.

3

Splitting the crus of the diaphragm and the division of the splanchnic nerves

The diaphragm is split where the splanchnic nerves and the sympathetic chain enter the crus and the hole widened by introducing a finger. A long, flat malleable retractor can now be introduced through the crus of diaphragm to lift up the abdominal viscera. The splanchnic nerves are cut off from the coeliac ganglion, which is easily seen, and dissected upwards to the point where they join the ganglionated sympathetic trunk. This is carefully dissected off the intercostal vessels and nerves to the level of the fourth thoracic ganglion or higher if possible.

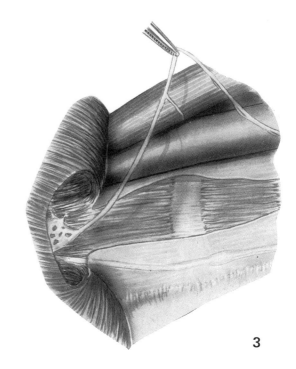

3

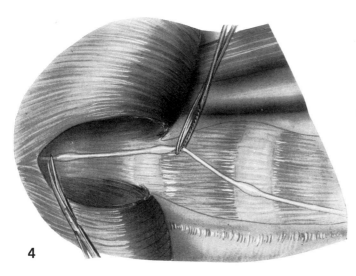

4

4

Removal of the first and second lumbar ganglia

The dissection is continued and the whole sympathetic chain from at least the fourth thoracic to the second lumbar ganglion removed together with the three splanchnic nerves.

The suprarenal gland and kidney can be easily palpated and inspected; by enlarging the incision in the diaphragm if necessary a renal biopsy may be taken.

5

Closure of the diaphragm

Any damaged intercostal vessels are secured with Cushing-Mackenzie clips. The crus of the diaphragm is closed by sutures between the edges of the incision. The pleura over the diaphragm is sutured but the posterior parietal pleura over the bed of the sympathetic chain is not closed.

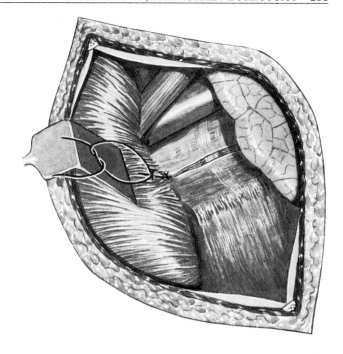

5

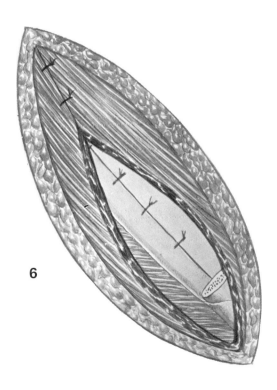

6

6

Wound closure

The wound is closed in layers of interrupted sutures and the lung fully expanded as the pleura is closed.

The skin is sutured, a chest tube drain is not inserted.

THORACO-ABDOMINAL OPERATION

The patient lies on his side in the nephrectomy position. The table should be broken or the bridge elevated so that the region of the twelfth dorsal vertebra is raised. The operation is made easier if the lateral tilt on the table is varied during the procedure to give adequate illumination for the upper thoracic and lower abdominal parts of the operation.

THE OPERATION

7

The incision

This follows the line of the last large rib, usually the eleventh, from the outer margin of the sheath of the rectus abdominis to the sacrospinalis muscle. The rib is resected and the rib bed incised. Sometimes it is necessary to divide the posterior portions of the ribs above and below.

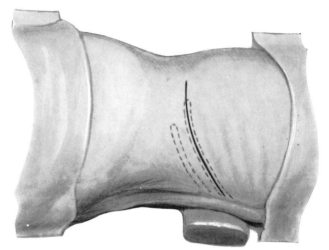

7

8

Stripping the pleura

The thoracic part of this procedure is performed extrapleurally if possible. In the posterior part of the incision the pleura is carefully detached and dissected off the posterior chest wall by blunt dissection; this extends upwards and medially to expose the thoracic sympathetic chain and splanchnic nerves at least as high as the eighth segment and preferably higher.

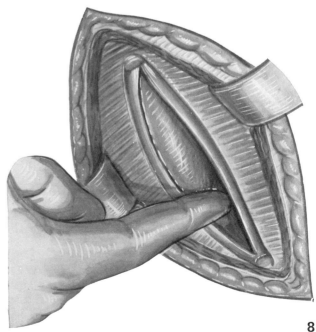

8

9

Incising the diaphragm

The abdominal part of this procedure is performed extrapleurally. The anterior portion of the incision is opened by retracting the peritoneum forwards and medially. The diaphragm is then divided with scissors from its attachments to the ribs. Care must be taken to leave sufficient of this muscle at the peripheral or posterior side of this opening for its suture at the conclusion of the operation. This division of the diaphragm is carried as far as the point where it is pierced by the sympathetic chain. The kidney and adrenal are now examined to exclude an undiagnosed primary cause for the hypertension. A renal biopsy may be performed if necessary.

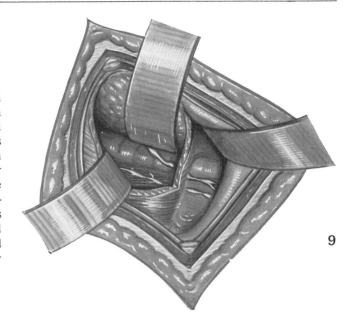

9

10

The sympathectomy and splanchnicectomy

This is a combination of the thoracic sympathectomy and splanchnicectomy described earlier in this chapter and the high lumbar sympathectomy described in the Chapter on 'Lumbar Sympathetic Ganglionectomy' pages 286 –291. The surgeon removes the sympathetic chain from the eighth thoracic to the third lumbar ganglion inclusive and over a longer length if possible. He also removes the three splanchnic nerves, these being divided close to the coeliac ganglion.

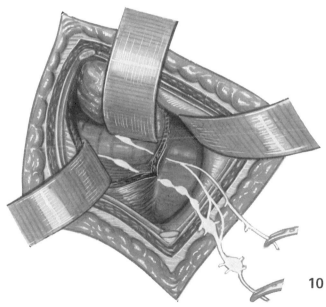

10

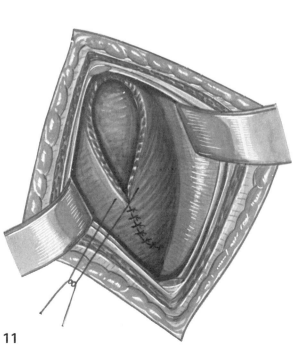

11

11

Wound closure

After haemostasis has been secured and after a renal biopsy has been taken, if this is thought necessary, the wound is closed. First the diaphragm is united and then the lung is inflated. If the pleura has been opened it is usually impossible to close it; under these circumstances the anaesthetist keeps the lung fully inflated until the skin closure is complete. A small suction catheter may be left in until the last suture is tied. Drainage is not necessary.

PRESACRAL NEURECTOMY

This operation has been used with benefit in certain cases of dysmenorrhoea and painful bladder following chronic cystitis, particularly when there is evidence that the pain is associated with spasm of the internal sphincter.

THE OPERATION

12

The incision

The patient is placed in a supine posture with a moderate Trendelenburg tilt. A transverse suprapubic skin incision with vertical mid-line incision opening the linea alba and peritoneum is satisfactory. Alternatively the surgeon may employ any of the other standard lower abdominal incisions such as the paramedian, mid-line, or anterolateral oblique.

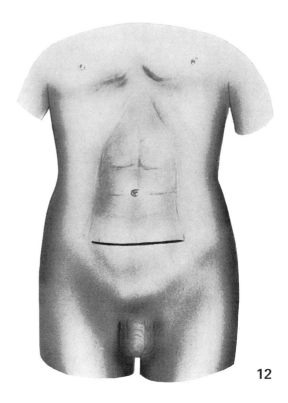

12

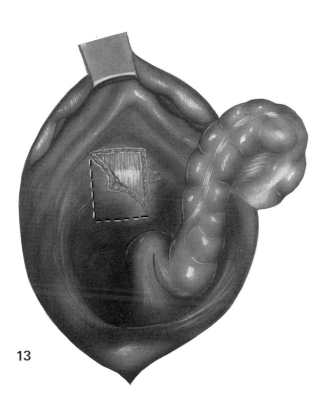

13

13

The neurectomy

The intestines are packed out of the way to expose the posterior abdominal wall. The peritoneum between the iliac arteries is incised transversely and dissected out of the posterior abdominal wall by blunt dissection. A block of tissue is removed down to the fifth lumbar and first sacral vertebral bodies. The presacral 'nerve' consists of a variable plexus in this region.

The posterior peritoneum should be sutured before abdominal closure.

SPECIAL POSTOPERATIVE CARE AND COMPLICATIONS

There are usually few complications after the first side of a thoraco-abdominal sympathectomy. After the second side the patient should be nursed with the foot of the bed raised and, if the pulse rate rises and blood pressure falls the lower limbs should be bandaged and the angle of tilt of the bed increased. Very occasionally when the blood pressure falls to an alarmingly low level, an intravenous infusion of glucose–saline solution containing noradrenaline 2 ml/litre may be given at a sufficient rate to maintain an adequate blood pressure.

If the patient suffers from postural hypertension when he leaves his bed, the legs should be bandaged and a fairly tight abdominal binder applied.

This is an unduly painful operation and most patients require adequate doses of analgesic drugs for the first 3 or 4 days at least—pethidine (Demerol) 100 mg 4-hourly if necessary. Some patients suffer from their worst pain between the fifth and tenth postoperative days when adequate analgesics may be needed.

A small pleural effusion may develop and if this increases in size, it should be aspirated.

References

Gillies, J. (1949). 'Anaesthesia for the surgical treatment of hypertension.' *Proc. R. Soc. Med.* **42,** 295
Pickering, G. W. (1955). *High Blood Pressure.* London: Churchill
White, J. C., Smithwick, R. P. and Simeone, F. A. (1952). *The Autonomic Nervous System.* 3rd edn. London: Kimpton

[The illustrations for this Chapter on Lumbodorsal Sympathectomy and Splanchnicectomy; Presacral Neurectomy were drawn by Mr. R. N. Lane.]

Lumbar Sympathetic Ganglionectomy

Charles Rob, *M.C.,* M.D., M.Chir., F.R.C.S.
Professor and Chairman of the Department of Surgery,
University of Rochester School of Medicine and
Dentistry, Rochester, New York

PRE-OPERATIVE

Indications

The principal indication for lumbar sympathetic ganglionectomy is arterial insufficiency in the lower limb due to atherosclerosis with severe stenosis or thrombosis, thrombo-angiitis obliterans, an embolus or an injury. Under these circumstances the level of denervation should be planned to denervate the area where the artery is occluded so that the collateral circulation around the occlusion may be improved. Thus, removal of the second and third ganglia denervates the limb as measured by skin-sweating tests from the lower third of the thigh distally, inclusion of the first lumbar ganglion carries the denervation to the groin, and the lower two thoracic ganglia must be removed as well if the buttock is to be included. Other indications include hyperidrosis of the feet, acrocyanosis, erythrocyanosis, Raynaud's phenomenon, the cryopathies, old poliomyelitis, causalgia, sympathetic dystrophies, and traumatic arterial spasm. In cases of doubt a preliminary lumbar ganglion block (*see* page 264) is the best method of judging the likely response to operation. It is important to remember that diabetes mellitus may produce a sympathectomy effect by causing neuritis and destruction of these autonomic nerves. These patients can be recognized clinically because they have dry and sometimes warm feet. Surgical sympathectomy is not indicated in these patients.

Effect on sexual function

Bilateral removal of the first lumbar ganglion in many patients results in interference with the function of ejaculation. Therefore, in young men, this ganglion should be preserved on one side if possible. Resection of the pre-aortic autonomic nerves but not the sympathetic chain may cause retrograde ejaculation (May *et al.*, 1969).

Anaesthesia

General anaesthesia is satisfactory.

Approach and position of patient

This will depend upon which portion of the sympathetic chain is to be removed. For removal of the second and third lumbar ganglia a transverse anterior abdominal incision, bilateral if necessary, provides good exposure. For this operation the patient lies on his back and a small sandbag may be placed under the buttock of the same side as that to be operated on.

Removal of the first lumbar ganglion is not always possible through this anterior incision and it is wise, when this ganglion is to be removed, to employ a posterolateral incision through the bed of the twelfth rib with the patient in the lateral position used for nephrectomy.

The removal of the lumbar chain with the lower thoracic ganglia has been described in the Chapter on 'Lumbodorsal Sympathectomy' (*see* pages 278–285).

THE OPERATIONS

ANTERIOR APPROACH

This is the best route of approach to the second and third lumbar ganglia and the intervening chain.

1

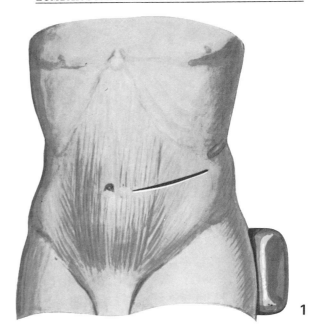

The incision

A slightly curved incision, bilateral if necessary, is made in the line of the skin creases of the abdominal wall. Laterally the incision starts about 2 inches (5 cm) beyond the lateral edge of the sheath of the rectus abdominus muscle. Medially it ends about 1 inch (2·5 cm) from the mid-line at the level of the umbilicus. The incision should be about 6 inches (15 cm) long and the approach is extraperitoneal.

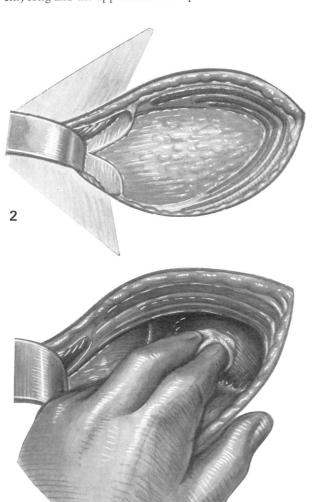

2

Muscle incision

The lateral portion of the sheath of the rectus abdominis muscle is divided in the line of the incision and the external oblique tendon and muscle incised as far as the posterior end of the incision. The internal oblique and transversus muscles are then incised to expose the peritoneum and extraperitoneal fat. The rectus abdominus muscle is retracted medially and the lateral part of the posterior sheath of this muscle opened in the line of the incision. It is important to identify the segmental nerves at the outer edge of the rectus abdominus muscle. These nerves and the corresponding vessels should be preserved. The muscles and fascial incision being parallel to but between these neurovascular bundles.

3

Extraperitoneal dissection

Starting in the lateral part of the wound the peritoneum is stripped by digital and gauze dissection from the lateral, anterior and finally the posterior abdominal wall. Deep retractors are now inserted and the peritoneum displaced medially to expose the psoas muscle. The ureter is lifted up with the peritoneum. If the peritoneum is opened in error it should be sutured at once and the dissection continued in the extraperitoneal plane.

4

Exposure of the sympathetic chain

The sympathetic chain lies just medial to the psoas muscle on the front of the vertebral bodies. On the right side it is covered by the inferior vena cava; on the left it lies close to the side of the aorta. After gentle retraction of the inferior vena cava or the aorta, the sympathetic chain is identified by palpation. The only structures likely to be confused with it are the genitofemoral nerve, which lies about 1 inch (2·5 cm) to the outer side of the sympathetic chain and is not ganglionated, and the lymph nodes. Once located the sympathetic chain is exposed by gauze and scissor dissection and its identity confirmed visually.

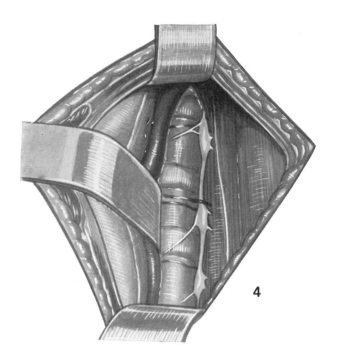

4

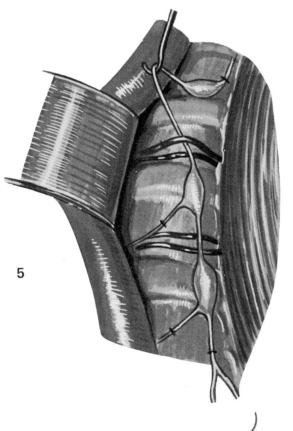

5

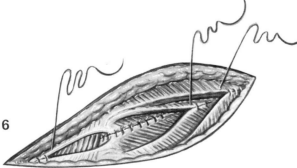

6

5

The sympathectomy

The sympathetic chain is picked up with a nerve hook and the second and third ganglia freed from their attachments including the rami communicantes. The chain is then divided above the second and third ganglion and removed. During this dissection great care should be taken to avoid injury to the lumbar veins. These pass behind the sympathetic chain, but occasionally one or more of these veins passes anterior to the chain, when they must either be divided or the chain carefully threaded out from behind them.

6

Wound closure

Once haemostasis is secured the retractors are removed and the wound closed in layers. First the transversus abdominus muscle and the posterior sheath of the rectus abdominus muscle are united, then the internal oblique muscle and lastly, the external oblique muscle and the anterior sheath of the rectus abdominis muscle. It is important to avoid the inclusion of the segmental nerves by these sutures.

THE POSTEROLATERAL APPROACH

The patient is placed on his side in the lateral or nephrectomy position. This approach allows the removal of the first lumbar and lower thoracic ganglia in addition to the main lumbar sympathetic chain.

7

The incision

The incision follows the line of the twelfth rib. It starts behind at the outer border of the sacrospinalis muscle and is carried forwards for a distance of 6–8 inches (15–20 cm). The latissimus dorsi muscle is divided in the line of the incision which exposes the anterior portion of the twelfth rib. The periosteum on the exposed portion of this bone is incised with a diathermy knife and skin towels applied.

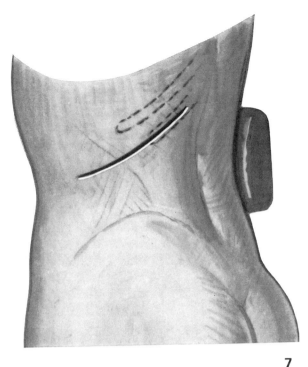

7

8

Resection of the twelfth rib

The periosteum covering the anterior portion of the twelfth rib is stripped away and the rib divided close to the lateral margin of the sacrospinalis muscle, care being taken to avoid injury to either the pleura or the twelfth thoracic nerve or vessels. The anterior portion of the twelfth rib is now lifted up with bone-holding forceps and its removal completed by dissecting the tip of this rib away from its attached muscles and costal cartilage if present.

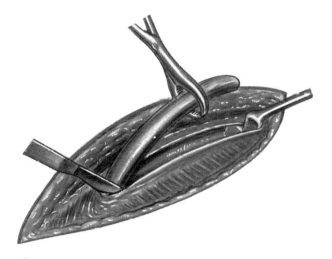

8

9

Division of the abdominal muscles

A finger is now introduced into the wound at the anterior end of the rib bed and passed forwards in the line of the incision between the abdominal muscles and the peritoneum. These muscles are then divided with scissors in the line of the incision. If careful attention is paid to the position and direction of the twelfth thoracic neurovascular bundle, it is possible not only to avoid injury to the twelfth thoracic nerve but also to minimize bleeding from the division of this fairly large muscle mass.

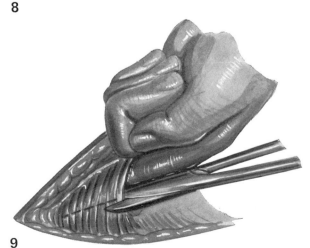

9

10

Exposure and identification of the sympathetic chain

The peritoneum is now stripped away from the posterior and lateral sides of the abdominal wall and held well forwards with deep retractors. The ureter remains adherent to the peritoneum and strips with it. The sympathetic chain is now identified by palpation with lower part of the operation at the level of the second and third lumbar ganglia as it lies on the side of the vertebral column at the inner edge of the psoas muscle, behind the inferior vena cava on the right and by the side of the aorta on the left. The chain is divided below the third ganglion and the second and third ganglia are mobilized from their attachments.

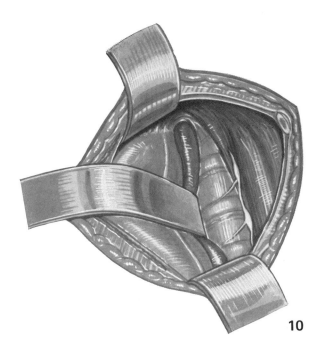

10

11

The sympathectomy

The sympathetic chain is now held up in forceps and the dissection carried upwards from the second ganglion. The chain is followed into the crus of the diaphragm. First the lumbocostal arch and then the crus are split to expose the first lumbar ganglion. This is freed from its attachments and the sympathetic chain, from the first to third lumbar segment, removed. If the surgeon wishes to include the lower thoracic ganglia in this removal then the incision is similar and the ganglia are reached by stripping the pleura and dividing the diaphragm in the manner described on pages 279–280.

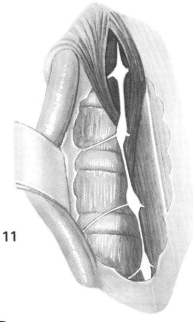

11

12

Wound closure

The retractors are removed and the peritoneum is allowed to fall back. The transversus abdominis muscle is then sutured and after it the internal oblique muscle. The periosteum in the rib bed is not repaired but the tendinous and muscular attachments to the tip of the first rib are united. It is important to avoid including the XIIth nerve in any of these stitches. The external oblique and latissimus dorsi muscles are now sutured and the skin closed. If the pleura has been opened the lung is kept fully expanded until the completion of the skin closure.

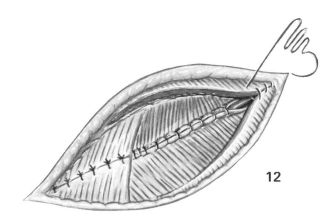

12

POSTOPERATIVE CARE

After the anterior or posterior operation paralytic ileus may occur, although in each case the procedure has been extraperitoneal. This ileus is usually mild and rarely requires active treatment. Should it be severe the treatment is by gastric aspiration, intravenous fluid and electrolyte replacement. Post-sympathectomy pain develops 1—3 weeks after the operation and is usually felt on the lateral surface of the buttock and thigh. Treatment is with analgesics. Fortunately this pain subsides in 2—3 months (Tracy and Cockett, 1961).

References

Leriche, R. and Fontaine, R. (1933). *Presse méd.* **41**, 1819
McGregor, A.L. (1955). *Surgery of the Sympathetic.* Bristol: John Wright
May, A.G., DeWeese, J.A. and Rob, C.G. (1969). 'Changes in sexual function following operation on the abdominal aorta.' *Surgery* **65**, 41
Royle, N.D. (1924). *Surgery Gynec. Obstet.* **39**, 701
Tracy, G.D. and Cockett, F.G. (1961). 'Pain in the lower limb after sympathectomy.' *Lancet* **1**, 12
White, J.C., Smithwick R.P. and Simeone, F.A. (1952). *The Autonomic Nervous System,* 3rd edn. London: Kimpton

[*The illustrations for this Chapter on Lumbar Sympathetic Ganglionectomy were drawn by Mr. R.N. Lane.*]

Amputations in Patients with Peripheral Vascular Disease

Charles Rob, *M.C.,* M.D., M.Chir., F.R.C.S.
Professor and Chairman of the Department of Surgery,
University of Rochester School of Medicine and
Dentistry, Rochester, New York

and

Robert D. Schrock, Jr., M.D.
Clinical Assistant Professor of Orthopaedic Surgery,
University of Rochester School of Medicine and
Dentistry, Rochester, New York

Only four levels are important when amputations of the lower limb for peripheral vascular disease are considered. The above-knee, the below-knee, the transmetatarsal and the local removal of toes and metatarsals. In the upper limb only amputations of the digits will be considered. Other amputations, though the forearm or arm resemble above- or below-knee amputations in the lower limb, will not be discussed separately.

PRE-OPERATIVE

Indications

The usual indications are gangrene, severe rest pain, spreading or intractable infection when associated with diabetes or ischaemia and, in the case of acute irreversible arterial occlusion, preserving life and the patient's renal functions by removing a large mass of necrotic muscle. In the USA ischaemia is the reason for 80 per cent of all amputations. The first essential is to prevent the amputation by an arterial reconstruction or other procedure, but when an amputation becomes inevitable, the correct selection of the level of the amputation is crucial. On this decision rests the future quality of the patient's life.

The level of the amputation

If the patient has at least one palpable ankle pulse, then the local exision of tissue, a transmetatarsal amputation or the amputation of a toe and a metatarsal head will heal. These patients are often diabetic with infective and neuropathic gangrene in whom ischaemia plays a lesser role. It is frequently wise to amputate all the toes in such patients. A good general rule for diabetic patients with palpable ankle pulses and gangrene of the great toe is to amputate all the toes at the first operation. This produces a foot which can easily fit into a slightly modified shoe and the smaller toes do not present a threat of future gangrene. On the other hand if only one of the four smaller toes is gangrenous and the great toe is normal, only the gangrenous small toes need to be removed.

In patients with peripheral arterial disease the transmetatarsal amputation is in our opinion rarely indicated. It is usually better to amputate all the toes and the metatarsal heads separately. This leaves a series of natural skin bridges between the digits which hold the skin together and assist healing. In some patients the dorsal skin over the distal foot is necrotic and then a transmetatarsal amputation with a plantar flap is preferred. In our opinion it is usually a mistake to do a transmetatarsal amputation unless at least one ankle pulse is palpable.

When gangrene or severe ischaemia extends proximal to the mid-foot, amputation at the level of the leg or the thigh becomes indicated. It is now firmly established that wound healing is routinely attainable at the below-knee level leaving a 10—12-cm stump when the skin of the proximal calf is free of trophic changes (Committee on Rehabilitation of the Amputee, 1972; Kendrick, 1957). The presence of palpable pulses and the use of oscillometrics are misleading in determining the level of amputation (Burgess *et al.*, 1971; Condon and Jordan, 1969; Cranley *et al.*, 1969; Kihn, Warren and Beebe, 1972; Wray, Still, Jr. and Moretz, 1972). The patency of the profunda femoris has been considered by many as essential for healing of the below-knee amputation (Wray, Still, Jr. and Moretz, 1972) but there is increasing evidence that in many patients adequate collateral circulation can be present even without this (Burgess *et al.*, 1971; Condon and Jordan, 1969; Cranley *et al.*, 1969; Moore, 1973). Arteriography, while essential to making a decision regarding vascular reconstruction, can be misleading in selection of amputation level (Burgess *et al.*, 1971; Moore, 1973; Murdoch, 1967). Similarly the absence of bleeding at the time of the incision or during the surgery is not necessarily an indication for a higher level of amputation (Burgess *et al.*, 1971; Cranley *et al.*, 1969; Kendrick, 1957; Moore, 1973).

This means that it is possible to obtain sound healing of a below-knee amputation in the majority of patients if there are no trophic skin changes at the level of the incision and if a meticulous technique is used. The following are some of the key factors in performing a technically good above- or below-knee amputation in a patient with peripheral vascular disease.

(*1*) A modern amputation in no way resembles the classic procedures of the past. The surgeon should operate gently and carefully and he should not hurry.

(*2*) The skin must not be traumatized. The only instruments which should touch the skin are the knife and the needle. It should not be picked up with forceps.

(*3*) Haemostasis should be complete.

(*4*) The skin flaps should be under no tension.

(*5*) If the wound is to be sutured, a two-layer closure is essential — a closure of the deep fascia and of the skin.

(*6*) Haemovac suction-drainage should be employed in most patients.

(*7*) The stump should be placed in a plaster-of-Paris cast in most above-knee and in all below-knee amputations.

An open or a closed wound

In general, amputations of the toes and the local excision of tissue for ischaemia are best left open whilst other amputations for ischaemia can be closed.

This means that most amputations for infected or neuropathic gangrene in diabetic patients should not be sutured.

In some patients, particularly those with transmetatarsal amputations, a compromise may be tried. The stump wound is not sutured but it is closed with an adhesive dressing. Steri-strips are satisfactory, but a better method is to use a wide strip of Elastoplast. Elastoplast can be autoclaved if it is placed with the adhesive side on a sheet of glass before or during sterilization.

THE OPERATIONS

AMPUTATION OF ONE TOE FOR GANGRENE

1

The incision

The incision is circular and is made around the proximal phalanx. It is important to stress that the skin will not be sutured unless the blood supply is excellent and this is rarely the case. The skin incision is made about 1 cm distal to the base of the proximal phalanx so that the skin will be loose and fall together over the defect. The tendons are then divided as high as possible and the digit removed through the metatarsophalangeal joint. Any bleeding points are now secured and the head of the metatarsal bone removed with rongeurs. A formal resection of the metatarsal head requires an extension of the circular incision and because this may compromise the blood supply of the skin, it should be avoided.

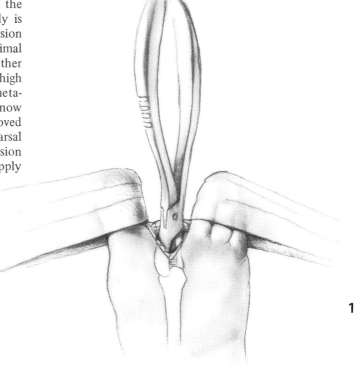

1

2

2

Removal of the distal metatarsal

A small pair of rongeur forceps are now introduced into the wound and the head of the metatarsal bone together with the distal 2 or 3 cm of the shaft is removed piece by piece. Multiple small bites are taken until this portion of the bone has been removed, and the cut end of the shaft of the metatarsal is smooth. Loose fragments of tendon or fascia are now trimmed with scissors and the wound irrigated with saline. It is now dressed by placing a light absorbative dressing across the surface and securing it loosely with a Kling bandage. It is important not to pack the wound. This will lead to skin necrosis and delay or prevent healing.

AMPUTATION OF A TOE AND THE METATARSAL BONE

In some patients with infective or neuropathic gangrene it may be possible to excise the toe and metatarsal bone leaving the rest of the foot. As a good blood supply is essential for healing, this procedure is not indicated if the foot is ischaemic. In addition the infected tendons and fascia are excised.

3

The incision

An incision is made around the base of the toe and extended along the plantar surface of the foot. It is deepened to expose the flexor tendons of the involved toe and the metatarsal bone.

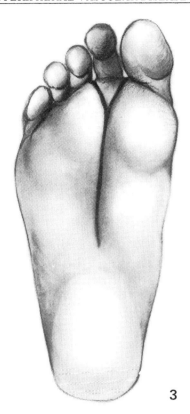

3

4

Removal of the toe and metatarsal

The infected flexor tendons and fascia are divided as far proximal as possible and the base of the metatarsal bone disarticulated. The metatarsal bone and extensor tendon is then freed from the dorsal skin. The wound is now irrigated with saline and any additional necrotic tissue removed with scissors. The wound is not sutured. A Kling bandage is applied to approximate the remaining toes.

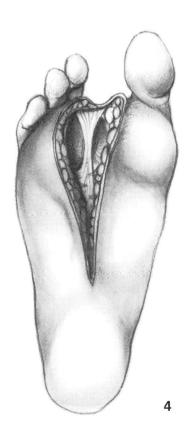

4

AMPUTATION OF ALL THE TOES

5

We believe that this procedure is superior to a trans-metatarsal amputation and should be used when the condition of the skin permits. It should also be used in most diabetic patients with ischaemic, neuropathic or infective gangrene of the great toe even though the other four toes are still viable. Once the great toe has been removed in a patient with this type of gangrene, there is considerable risk that the other toes will soon become gangrenous. The procedure is the same as that described for the amputation of one toe. Again it is stressed that the skin incision is circular and about 1 cm distal to the base of the proximal phalanx. The toe is removed through the metatarsophalangeal joint and then the head and distal shaft of each metatarsal is removed piece by piece with a small pair of rongeurs; the skin incisions are neither sutured nor packed. The skin is dressed with a light absorbative dressing so that the edges are approximated and the bridges of skin between the toes are carefully preserved. These skin bridges anchor together the dorsal and plantar skin.

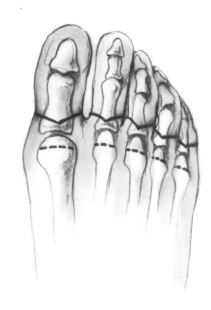

5

POSTOPERATIVE CARE

The wounds should be dressed as infrequently as possible. They should never be packed. If there was pre-operative infection, the appropriate antibiotic drugs should be administered systemically for 5 days beginning 12 hr before the operation.

In general these patients should rest in bed for the first week, and after that when possible keep the leg horizontal, but not elevated above the heart until healing is well advanced. During the period of bedrest ankle, knee and hip excercises should be encouraged.

Associated diabetes mellitus, cardiac and other abnormalities must also be actively treated.

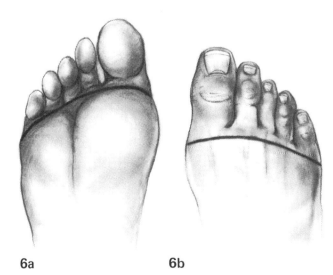

6a   6b

THE TRANSMETATARSAL AMPUTATION

6a & b

The incision

We prefer to amputate the toes and distal meta-tarsals individually so that the skin bridges between the toes aid healing. But if the skin of the distal part of the dorsum of the foot between the toes is gangrenous, a transmetatarsal amputation is indicated. The plantar skin incision is made as close to the digits as possible and the dorsal incision crosses the foot about 3 cm from the base of the toes. The plantar flap is now fashioned by cutting as close as possible to the metatarsals and the plantar tendons, thereby producing a thick but hopefully viable plantar flap. The flexor tendons are then divided individually.

7

Division of the metatarsals

Each metatarsal is now identified from the plantar surface and the shaft divided with bone-cutting forceps or a wire saw about 2 cm from its base. After all five metatarsals have been transected, the tendons and other soft tissues are divided with scissors or a knife and the amputated specimen removed. All bleeding points are now secured. Any redundant portions of fascia or tendon are removed and the whole area irrigated with saline.

8

The skin closure

The skin flaps should be loose and under no tension. The skin must be treated very gently. It should not be picked up with forceps. When possible the deep fascia is closed with interrupted absorbable sutures. Drainage usually through a small stab incision in the plantar flap is recommended. Sometimes it is possible to close the skin with steri-strips or Elastoplast as recommended in the introduction to this chapter. Otherwise interrupted skin sutures will be required. The wound is now dressed with a light absorbative dressing or gauze dressing held in place with a Kling bandage or it can be placed in a plaster-of-Paris cast extending to the tibial tubercle.

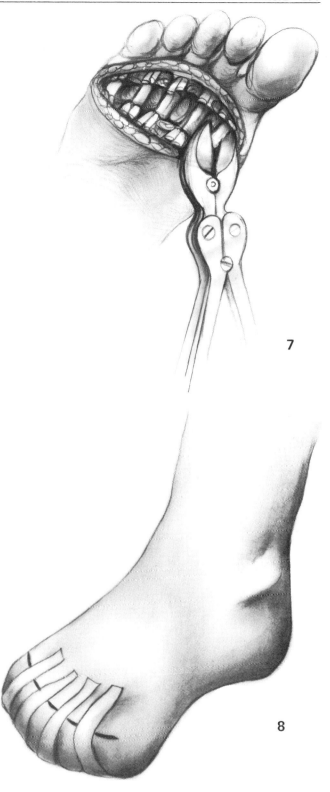

7

8

POSTOPERATIVE CARE

If the toes were infected, the patient should be treated with the appropriate antibiotics. The drain is removed on the fifth postoperative day.

After a transmetatarsal amputation, bedrest is recommended for 5–7 days. Full hip, knee and ankle exercises are encouraged but early ambulation or early weight-bearing may delay healing and should be avoided unless a plaster-of-Paris cast has been applied.

The advantage of a transmetatarsal amputation is that, when ambulation begins, the patient can soon wear an ordinary boot or shoe with the space in the front filled with a soft sponge pad. A prosthesis is not required.

THE BELOW-KNEE AMPUTATION

Patients with lower-limb ischaemia often have serious cardiorespiratory problems. For this reason we prefer to perform this procedure with the patient lying on his back rather than in the face down position.

9

The incision

Equal anterior–posterior flaps may be cut, but a long posterior flap containing part of the calf muscles is preferred. The best level of bone sections is 10–12 cm distal to the medial joint line. The anterior skin incision should be placed about 2 cm distal to the level of the bone section and is taken directly through the deep fascia except over the tibia where it is taken through the periosteum. The posterior flap is cut about 14 cm distal to the level of bone section and the incision goes through the deep fascia into the calf muscles.

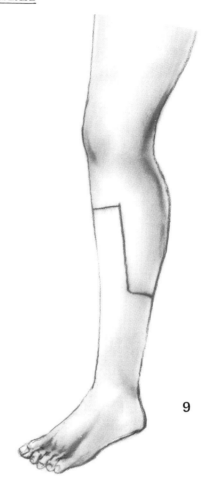

9

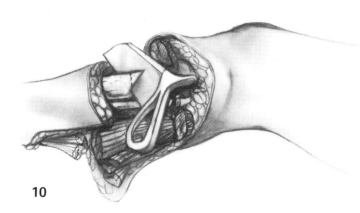

10

10

Division of the muscles and other soft tissues

The periosteum is now raised with a periosteal elevator from the anteromedial surface of the tibia for a distance of 2–3 cm. The deep fascia is also retracted upwards at this time. The surgeon now divides the calf muscles obliquely so that a thick muscular cutaneous posterior flap is fashioned. The other muscles are divided transversely. In amputations for ischaemia it is better not to use a tourniquet so all bleeding points must be secured at this time. The nerves and tendons should be divided clearly and allowed to retract.

11

Division of the bones

The fibula is freed with a periosteal elevator and divided with heavy bone forceps about 2 cm proximal to the proposed level of section of the tibia. The skin flaps and soft tissues are now gently retracted and the tibia divided so that the anterior surface or tibial crest is bevelled. The first saw cut is angled obliquely, distally and posteriorly so that it will meet the next vertical cut at an angle of 45°. The initial cut is then made and the anterior fragment removed to provide a smooth anterior surface to the tibial stump. Any irregularities of the bone end should now be removed with a bone file or rongeurs.

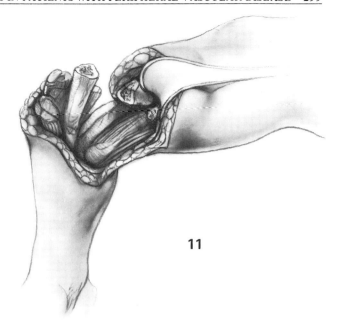

11

12

Drainage and closure of the deep fascia and periosteum

The wound is now thoroughly irrigated with saline and loose fragments of tendon muscle or fascia excised and a final check made to confirm that haemostasis is complete. A Haemovac suction drain is now introduced through the skin above the level of the knee joint and usually on the lateral side of the limb, the suction tube being passed into the wound beneath the deep fascia. This fascia is now closed with a series of interrupted catgut sutures. This is an important step and must be performed gently so that the fascia, subcutaneous tissues and skin are not contused or otherwise damaged. The central part of the anterior layer of this closure consists of the periosteum of the tibia which has previously been freed for this purpose.

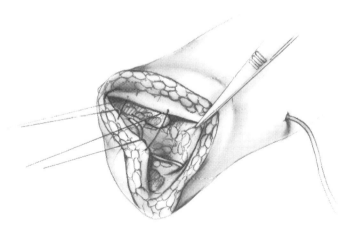

12

13a, b & c

The skin closure

Gentleness is essential whenever the skin is touched. Skin healing is important and in patients with vascular disease, a simple step such as picking up the skin edge with forceps may cause sufficient injury to delay or prevent healing. We believe that only two instruments should touch the skin in these patients: the knife when the incision is made, and the needle when it is closed. The skin should not be touched with dissecting or other forceps. When the skin closure is complete, a dressing is applied and the Haemovac drain or suction adjusted to its final position.

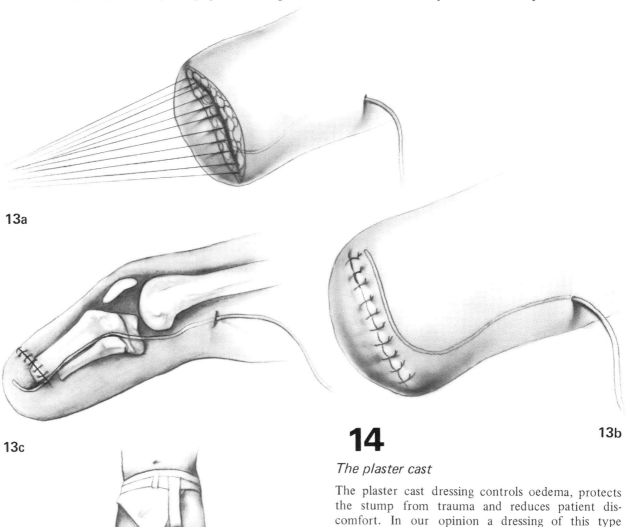

13a

13c

13b

14

The plaster cast

The plaster cast dressing controls oedema, protects the stump from trauma and reduces patient discomfort. In our opinion a dressing of this type should be applied to every below-knee amputation.

The cast can be applied as shown here or according to the method described by Burgess, Romano and Zettl (1969). We have not advised early weight-bearing but there is increasing experience which suggests that early partial weight-bearing on a properly applied postoperative prosthesis is not harmful (Burgess, Roman and Zettl, 1969; Burgess *et al.*, 1971; Committee on the Rehabilitation of the Amputee, 1972; Condon and Jordan, 1969). In this system of management full weight-bearing on the amputation stump is not allowed until the permanent prosthesis has been applied. Early ambulation as contrasted with early weight-bearing is recommended in every patient.

14

POSTOPERATIVE CARE

The patient is encouraged to stand by his bed on the evening of the operation or, at the latest, 24 hr later. This is coupled with physiotherapy in the physiotherapy department as soon as possible including limb excercises and walking between parallel bars on the first day if possible and then with a walker.

Antibiotics and analgesic drugs are given if necessary and associated conditions such as diabetes mellitus and cardiac problems are treated. The Haemovac drain is removed on the fifth postoperative day. The plaster cast is removed and the sutures removed from the wound. The plaster-of-Paris cast is then immediately re-applied and the prosthesis fitted so that the patient can begin weight-bearing as soon as the plaster has dried. Even if healing is not complete, the cast must be re-applied. The rigid protection aids healing even if the wound is partially open and infected. In such patients weight-bearing may await the more complete healing of the wound.

It is important to stress the role of rehabilitation in patients who have a below-knee amputation. The aim is to rehabilitate these patients so that they can walk at least with a cane and hopefully without one. This is often possible in patients aged 75 years or over.

THE ABOVE-KNEE AMPUTATION

The patient is supine and general anaesthesia is preferred. A tourniquet is not used if the amputation is for ischaemia.

15

The skin incision

The skin flaps must be loose and under no tension when closed. A common error is for them to be too short. To avoid this the skin flaps are equal, that is, the amputation is almost circular and the anterior incision is placed at the level of the proximal or superior border of the patella. The skin incision should pass through deep fascia. At this time the long saphenous vein may need ligating. It is stressed that the skin must not be traumatized during the operation. The skin and deep fascia are then dissected proximally for a distance of about 4 cm in the plane just below the deep fascia.

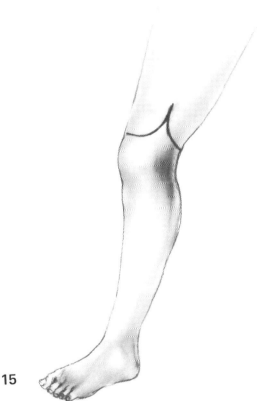

15

16

Division of the soft tissues

The muscles are divided circumferentially at a level 2–3 cm proximal to the level of the skin and fascial section, The femoral artery and veins are clamped and divided. The artery is usually occluded and the vein is usually open. The sciatic nerve is gently pulled down and divided. Frequently it is accompanied by a small vessel which requires a ligature. Posteriorly and laterally there may be several small terminal branches of the profunda femoral artery which require ligature.

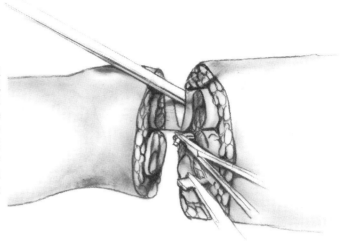

16

17

Division of the bone

The periosteum is now divided circumferentially and it is elevated proximally with a periosteal elevator. Along the linea aspera of the femur there may be some difficulty in elevating the periosteum but the surgeon should persist until the optimum level of bone section 22–28 cm distal to the tip of the great trochanter is reached. The muscles are then protected with a gauze pack or preferably a stump retractor and the bone is divided with a saw and the limb removed.

17

18

Checking for haemostasis and drainage

The wound is now thoroughly irrigated with saline to remove all debris. It is carefully inspected and all residual bleeding points are secured. At the same time any loose tags of muscle or fascia are removed. When haemostasis is complete a Haemovac drain is placed across the wound. This is introduced high on the outside of the thigh so that it can be removed without disturbing the dressing.

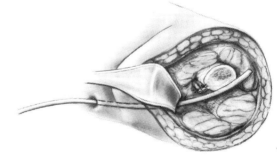

18

19a & b

Closure of the wound

The deep fascia is now closed with interrupted sutures of chromic catgut. It is not necessary to suture the muscles. This fascial closure is important and should be performed with care. As with the below-knee amputation, the skin should only be touched with the needle and the knife. It should not be picked up with dissecting forceps. When the closure is complete, the wound is dressed with a light absorbative dressing and a Kling-type gauze bandage applied. We recommend that unless complications develop, this dressing is not changed for 2 weeks when the sutures are removed. In our opinion this is best achieved by applying a plaster-of-Paris cast shaped as a cap over the stump. This adds protection as well as rigidity.

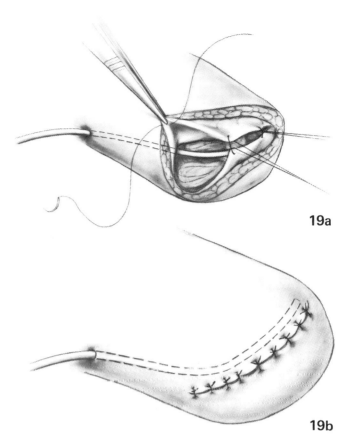

19a

19b

POSTOPERATIVE CARE

The aim is early ambulation and this applies especially to the older patients. Within 24 hr of the conclusion of the operation, the patient should be standing by his bed on his sound limb. The rehabilitation will include early walking between parallel bars, with a walker, and with crutches. Stump exercises are begun immediately and a temporary prosthesis is fitted as soon as possible. This makes it easier for the patient to balance and adds a feeling of security. We do not recommend full weight-bearing until after the sutures are removed, usually on the four-teenth day. Before this, protected weight-bearing between parallel bars can be initiated in favourable cases.

If there is excessive stump pain or evidence of a wound infection, the dressing must be removed and the stump examined. The Haemovac drain is removed on the fifth day without disturbing the cast or dressings.

After the sutures are removed and a temporary limb fitted, exercises and ambulation should be supervised by the physiotherapists. The patient must be taught to bandage his stump. As soon as this has shrunk sufficiently, the permanent pros-thesis is fitted.

Patients with an above-knee amputation often gain weight. The patient should be kept on a diet so that he does not exceed his pre-operative weight. This important point will require active control and supervision for the rest of the patient's life.

AMPUTATION OF A FINGER, PART OF A FINGER OR THE THUMB

Ischaemia in the hand differs from ischaemia in the foot. Vasospastic diseases such as Raynaud's phenomenon may lead to thrombosis of the digital arteries and gangrene of a digit. Embolization of the digital arteries may also be secondary to a cervical rib. In lesions of these types the wrist pulses may be normal and the ischaemic problem confined to the digits. This means that most of these amputations can be closed with sutures in contrast to amputation of the toes which are usually left open.

In the case of the hand the preservation of tissue is of special importance. This applies particularly to the thumb.

For ischaemia of the fingers regional or general anaesthesia is preferred, local digital nerve block may be harmful. It is stressed that healing rather than the cosmetic result is the essential element in amputations of ischaemic digits.

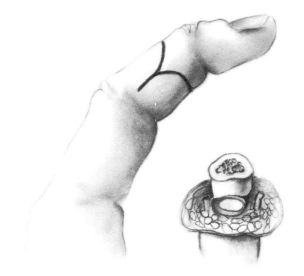

20

20

The incision: amputation through the middle phalanx

Almost equal flaps are fashioned, the palmar being slightly longer than the dorsal. The superficial tissues and extensor tendons are divided. The palmar flap is then fashioned and the flexor digitorum profundus tendon is divided. The middle phalanx is then divided just distal to the attachment of the flexor digitorum sublimis tendon.

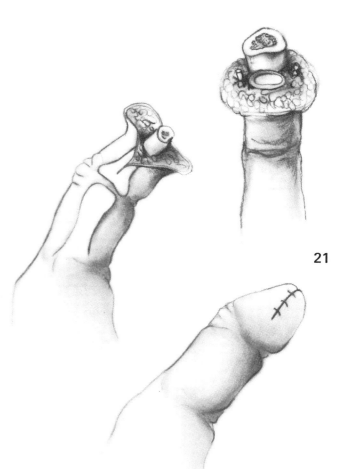

21

21

Haemostasis and closure

Bleeding points are now secured, and the incision closed with a series of interrupted skin sutures. A dressing is next applied.

AMPUTATION DISTAL TO THE METACARPO-PHALANGEAL JOINT

22

The incision

A circular incision is made at the level of the skin web between the fingers. This is carried down to the bone circumferentially. Bleeding points are secured and the divided tendons allowed to retract. The shaft of the proximal phalanx is divided with bone forceps and the finger removed. The proximal portion of the phalanx is then removed with rongeur forceps.

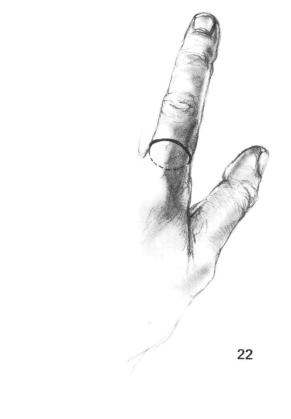

22

23

Closure

The wound is irrigated with saline and any loose tags of tendon or fascia are excised. The wound is now closed with interrupted skin sutures.

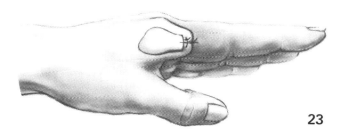

23

POSTOPERATIVE CARE

The problem is wound healing in patients in whom the reason for amputation was ischaemia. This means that the hand should be kept at rest for the first 3 or 4 days. It is wise to inspect the wound daily and to remove the sutures if the blood supply appears to be in doubt.

References

Burgess, E. M., Romano, R. L. and Zettl, J. H. (1969). *The Management of Lower Extremity Amputations,* (TR10-6 available for 7.50 dollars from Superintendent of Documents, U. S. Government Printing Office, Washington, D. C. 20402)
Burgess, E. M., Romano, R. L., Zettl, J. H. and Schrock, R. D. (1971). 'Amputations of the leg for peripheral vascular insufficiency.' *J. Bone Jt Surg.* 53A, 874
Committee on Rehabilitation of the Amputee (1972). *Circulation* 46, A293
Condon, R. E. and Jordan, P. H., Jr. (1969). 'Immediate postoperative prosthesis in vascular amputations.' *Ann. Surg.* 170, 435
Cranley, J. J., Krause, R. J., Strasser, E. S. and Hafner, C. D. (1969). 'Below the knee amputation for arteriosclerosis obliterans.' *Archs Surg.* 98, 77
Kendrick, R. R. (1957). 'Below knee amputation in arteriosclerotic gangrene.' *Br. J. Surg.* 44, 13
Kihn, R. B., Warren, R. and Beebe, G. W. (1972). 'The "geriatric" amputee.' *Ann. Surg.* 176, 305
Moore, W. S. (1973). 'Determination of amputational level.' *Archs Surg.* 107, 798
Murdoch, G. (1967). 'Level of amputation and limiting factors.' *Ann. R. Coll. Surg.* 40, 204
Wray, C. H., Still, J. M., Jr. and Moretz, W. H. (1972). 'Present management of amputations for peripheral vascular disease.' *Am. Surg.* 38, 87

[*The illustrations for this Chapter on Amputations in Patients with Peripheral Vascular Disease were drawn by Mr. R. Wabnitz.*]

Fasciotomy

James A. DeWeese, M.D., F.A.C.S.
Chairman of the Division of Cardiothoracic Surgery,
University of Rochester Medical Centre, and
Professor and Surgeon, Strong Memorial Hospital,
Rochester, New York

and

Charles Rob, *M.C.,* M.D., M.Chir., F.R.C.S.
Professor and Chairman of the Department of Surgery,
University of Rochester School of Medicine and
Dentistry, Rochester, New York

PRE-OPERATIVE

Indications

Painful swelling of the muscles in the compartments
of the lower leg may occur following active exercise,
fractures, crush injuries, revascularization of an
ischaemic limb and acute deep venous thrombosis or
ligation of a major deep vein. The diagnosis should be
considered whenever severe pain occurs in the above
circumstances. It can be confirmed by redness and
glossiness of the skin over the involved compartment
and tender swelling. If untreated at this stage distal
hypaesthesia, loss of arterial pulses and muscle
necrosis occurs. The anterior compartment containing the tibialis anticus, extensor digitorum longus,
extensor hallucis longus and the peroneus tertius
muscle is most frequently involved but the lateral
or posterior compartments may also be affected.

The late changes with anterior compartment involvement are anaesthesia over the medial dorsum of the
foot, loss of dorsalis pedis arterial pulsations and
foot drop.

Pre-operative preparation

If the diagnosis is suspected casts or dressings should
be removed and careful examination repeated until
the diagnosis is confirmed or disproved. Operation
should be performed prior to the development of
neuromuscular or arterial deficits.

Elevation and regional asymptomatic blockade
have little to offer.

A general or spinal anaesthetic is preferred.

THE OPERATION

ANTERIOR COMPARTMENT

1

The incision

A 2-inch (5-cm) longitudinal incision is made two fingers' breadth lateral to the tibia beginning two fingers' breadth distal to the tibial head. Performance of the fasciotomy through such a short incision is preferable to a long incision. It was difficult to close the longer incision and delayed wound healing was frequent.

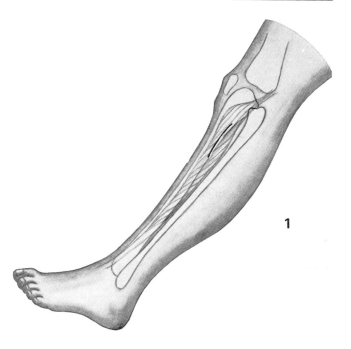

1

2

Fascial incision

A short incision is made in the deep fascia and the muscle inspected. Bulging of the muscle through the fascia further confirms the diagnosis. Grey or brown muscle may be found late but should not be excised.

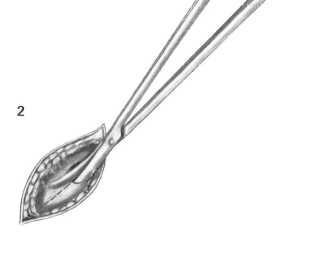

2

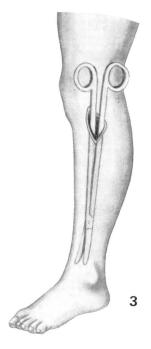

3

3

Splitting of fascia

Using long scissors the muscle is split to ankle level. Fasciotomy knives are available but long scissors inserted subcutaneously are just as satisfactory. The subcutaneous tissue is not approximated. The skin is closed with interrupted sutures.

LATERAL COMPARTMENT

4

Exposure

Involvement of the lateral compartment may be confused with involvement of the anterior compartment because of their close proximity. Therefore, this compartment should be decompressed whenever primary involvement is suspected, or whenever exploration of the anterior compartment reveals normal muscle. The lateral compartment can be reached by lateral retraction of the incision made for the anterior compartment fasciotomy until the fascia over the peroneus muscle is identified.

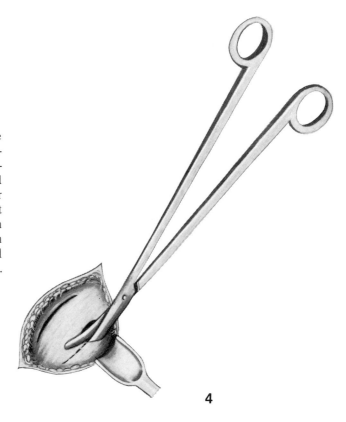

4

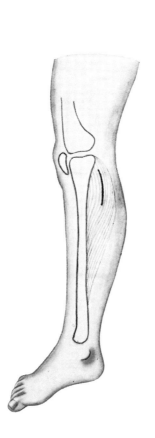

5

POSTERIOR COMPARTMENT

5

The incision

Decompression of the posterior compartment is rarely necessary. Usually two incisions are necessary. They are again made as 2-inch (5-cm) longitudinal incisions over the bulging gastrocnemius muscles on the medial and lateral posterior leg. Scissors are used to divide the fascia proximally and distally.

POSTOPERATIVE CARE

The leg is elevated. If a foot drop has already occurred, a posterior split is applied to maintain dorsiflexion of the foot. Active and passive exercises are begun early but the patient is kept at bed rest until the swelling has disappeared.

References

Dennis, G. (1945). 'Disaster following femoral vein ligation for thrombophlebitis; relief by fasciotomy.' *Surgery* **17**, 264

Leach, R. E., Zohn, D. A. and Stryker, W. S. (1964). 'Anterior tibial compartment syndrome.' *Archs Surg.* **88**, 187

Moretz, W. H. (1953). 'The anterior compartment (anterior tibial) ischaemia syndrome.' *Am. Surg.* **19**, 728

Patman, D. R. and Thompson, J. E. (1970). 'Fasciotomy in peripheral vascular surgery: report of 164 patients.' *Archs Surg.* **101**, 663

Reszel, P. A., Janes, J. M. and Spittel, J. A., Jr. (1963). 'Ischemic necrosis of the peroneal musculature, a lateral compartment syndrome: report of case.' *Proc. Staff Meet. Mayo Clin.* **38**, 130

Rosato, F. E., Barker, C. F., Roberts, B. and Danielson, G. K. (1966). 'Subcutaneous fasciotomy—description of a new technique and instrument.' *Surgery* **59**, 383

Watson, D. C. (1955). 'Anterior tibial syndrome following arterial embolism.' *Br. med. J.* **1**, 1412

[*The illustrations for this Chapter on Fasciotomy were drawn by Miss D. Elliott.*]

Achilles Tenotomy

R.P. Jepson, F.R.C.S.
Honorary Consultant Surgeon,
The Royal Adelaide Hospital, South Australia

PRE-OPERATIVE

Indications; results of operation

Intermittent claudication is the characteristic symptom of relative muscle ischaemia developed by excercise and is most commonly associated with an athersclerotic thrombosis of a major limb artery. Many patients can exist comfortably with the handicap of the claudication and others will derive benefit from direct vascular surgery or sympathectomy. In a selected group in which other treatment is contra-indicated the limitations imposed by severe intermittent claudication may be most harassing and it is in these patients that achilles tenotomy may be employed.

This operation is designed to decrease the power of contraction and work performed by the gastro-soleus group of muscles. The blood supply to the weakened muscle during excercise is therefore more able to satisfy the metabolic demands and the 'claudication distance' is thereby increased.

Before this procedure is carried out it must be ascertained that the exercise pain is in fact restricted to the gastrosoleus group. If claudication pain is felt in the tibial or foot muscles then this will be enhanced by achilles tenotomy and the patient will derive little benefit. The results are most satisfactory in patients with severe claudication (less than 50 yards) and in limbs with good skin nutrition. Boyd et al. (1949) claimed good results in 22 of the 24 patients they subjected to this procedure while Schwartz et al. (1952) reported good results in 8 out of 10 patients.

This procedure does nothing to improve the blood supply to the ischaemic limb and does not therefore favourably influence its long-term prognosis.

Contra-indications

Rest pain or gross nutritional changes, such as ulceration, are definite contra-indications to the procedure. The temporary paralysis of the gastrosoleus following tenotomy without doubt causes venous stasis in the muscle bellies and thus may precipitate thrombophlebitis, particularly in patients with a history of phlebitis or swollen ankles. This can be partly guarded against by supporting the lower leg with elastic stockings in the first two postoperative weeks.

Although the operation has on many occasions been performed bilaterally the results are much superior with unilateral claudication. If bilateral tenotomy is contemplated it is preferable to carry out the procedure in two stages with sufficient interval for the patient to readjust himself to the new flat-footed gait.

If the above criteria are rigorously adopted achilles tenotomy will be found to be indicated in only a small percentage of the patients suffering from intermittent claudication.

THE OPERATION

1

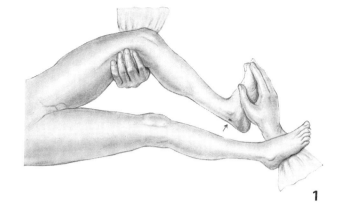

Position of patient

The patient lies on his back. The leg is held by an assistant, with the hip moderately flexed, abducted and externally rotated, knee flexed to 60° and the foot fully dorsiflexed. The tendo achillis is thus kept as a tight band by the assistant throughout the manoeuvre. The area is infiltrated with lignocaine.

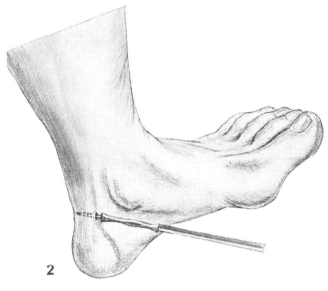

2

Insertion of tenotomy knife

The tenotomy knife is pushed along the deep surface of the tendon from within out, with its cutting edge facing the tendon. The fibres of the tendon are cut through about 1·5—2 inches (3·8—5 cm) above their insertion, care being taken not to incise skin other than at the puncture hole.

3

Division of tendon

At the final division of the tendon the foot is felt to suddenly dorsiflex an additional 15—20°. No sutures are required and crepe bandage pressure controls any bleeding. The patient is encouraged to walk the following day.

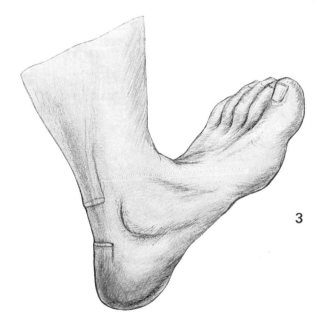

SPECIAL POSTOPERATIVE CARE AND COMPLICATIONS

The paralysis of the gastrocnemius and gastrosoleus muscles may result in a postoperative deep phlebitis. This may be controlled by supportive bandaging throughout the first few postoperative weeks.

When the patient begins to walk he tends to come down hard on the heel, which may become bruised and tender. This common complication may be minimized by fitting a sponge rubber pad inside the heel of the shoe. If both sides are tenotomized at the same session the patient will need the help of sticks for some time to maintain his balance.

References

Boyd, A.M., Ratcliffe, A.H., Jepson, R.P. and James, G.W.H. (1949). *J. Bone Jt Surg.* **31-B,** 325
Schwartz, D.I., Pennock, L.L., Pessolano, C.J. and Littman, D.S. (1952). *J. Bone Jt Surg.* **34-A,** 619

[*The illustrations for this Chapter on Achilles Tenotomy were drawn by Miss D. Davison.*]

Meralgia Paraesthetica

Charles Rob, *M.C.,* M.D., M.Chir., F.R.C.S.
Professor and Chairman of the Department of Surgery,
University of Rochester School of Medicine and
Dentistry, Rochester, New York

and

James A. DeWeese, M.D., F.A.C.S.
Chairman of the Division of Cardiothoracic Surgery,
University of Rochester Medical Centre, and
Professor and Surgeon, Strong Memorial Hospital,
Rochester, New York

PRE-OPERATIVE

Meralgia paraesthetica is an irritative neuritis of the lateral cutaneous nerve of the thigh. The symptoms are worse after hard exercise and when lying in bed and consist of numbness, paraesthesia or pain in the distribution of the lateral cutaneous nerve of the thigh. It is characteristic that flexion of the hip relieves the symptoms and so the patient may soon learn that they are relieved by sitting on the side of the bed or in an upright chair.

These symptoms are caused by compression of the lateral cutaneous nerve of the thigh as it passes through the inguinal ligament. The normal situation is for this nerve to pass behind the inguinal ligament. In patients with meralgia paraesthetica it passes through the inguinal ligament and is compressed and stretched over the deep fasciculus of this ligament.

It is important to stress that these symptoms are not relieved by division of the nerve. They are relieved, however, by removal of the compression of the nerve. The responsible agent is the deep fasciculus of the inguinal ligament which lies behind the nerve. Division of the band frees and preserves the nerve, and cures the patient. Division of the superficial fasciculus of the inguinal ligament which lies in front of the nerve does not free the nerve from compression and does not relieve the symptoms.

Anaesthesia

General anaesthesia is preferred, but local anaesthesia is satisfactory.

THE OPERATION

1

Exposure of nerve

The lateral cutaneous nerve of the thigh normally passes behind the inguinal ligament but in patients with meralgia paraesthetica it passes through this ligament, so that in these patients a portion of the ligament lies posterior to the nerve. The incision commences 0·5 cm below the anterior superior spine of the ileum, it then follows the line of the inguinal ligament for a distance of 4–6 cm. It is carried down so that the lateral portion of this ligament is exposed. The lateral cutaneous nerve of the thigh is then identified just below the inguinal ligament.

2

Division of posterior fasciculus of inguinal ligament

The surgeon now follows the lateral cutaneous nerve of the thigh to the inguinal ligament. If the nerve passes through this ligament the diagnosis is confirmed. If it passes behind the inguinal ligament the diagnosis probably has been mistaken. The surgeon mobilizes and divides all of the inguinal ligament which lies behind the nerve, after which the deep fascia and skin are closed in the usual manner.

POSTOPERATIVE CARE

The patient may get up from bed as soon as he has recovered from the anaesthetic. He may leave the hospital the next day, and 1 week later the sutures should be removed.

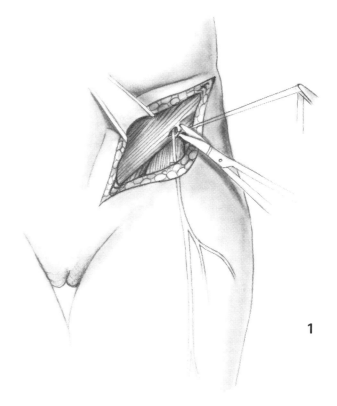

1

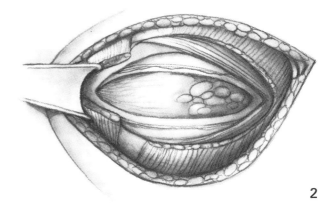

2

References

Ecker, A. D. and Woltman, H. W. (1938). 'Meralgia paraesthetica, a report of 150 cases.' *J. Am. med. Ass.* **110**, 1650
Stevens, H. (1957). 'Meralgia paraesthetica.' *Archs Neurol. Psychiat.* **77**, 557

[*The illustrations for this Chapter on Meralgia Paraesthetica were drawn by Mr. R. Wabnitz.*]

The Thoracic Outlet Syndrome

G. W. Taylor, M.S., F.R.C.S.
Professor of Surgery and Director,
Surgical Professorial Unit,
St. Bartholomew's Hospital, London

and

J. S. P. Lumley, F.R.C.S.
Assistant Director,
Surgical Professorial Unit,
St. Bartholomew's Hospital, London

The thoracic outlet syndrome is a collective term given to various anatomical anomalies which can compress the nerves and vessels of the upper limb in the root of the neck. The term embraces other conditions such as the anterior scalene, the costoclavicular and the hyperabduction syndromes.

The bony abnormalities encountered are: (*a*) a partial or complete cervical rib; (*b*) a prominent seventh cervical transverse process; (*c*) callus from a healed fracture of the first rib or clavicle and (*d*) a high or congenitally abnormal first rib.

The possible sites of compression are between the first rib and (*a*) the clavicle, (*b*) the coracoid process, (*c*) the pectoralis minor tendon, (*d*) the scalenus anterior, (*e*) the seventh cervical transverse process, and (*f*) an incomplete cervical rib; and between the scalenus anterior and the scalenus medius. Also described are fibrous bands, prominent bellies of the above muscles and an abnormally developed scalenus minimus muscle.

The presence of these anomalies is not invariably accompanied by symptoms, and symptoms are very rare in childhood. Often they are precipitated by abnormal posture, particularly in positions of prolonged abduction (painters, truck drivers) or downward traction (carrying heavy loads). Symptoms may be vascular or neurological, or occasionally, both. Arterial symptoms range from Raynaud's phenomena to frank digital ischaemia. The more severe syndromes are usually secondary to recurrent emboli arising from a poststenotic dilatation of the subclavian artery in association with a complete bony cervical rib. Neurological symptoms are predominantly nocturnal pain and minor sensory changes, particularly along the medial border of the hand and forearm. Motor weakness sometimes occurs and is most marked in the hand. Venous compression is manifested by pain, swelling and cyanosis of the limb.

The diagnosis is aided by a diminished or absent radial pulse, the presence of a subclavian bruit and delayed hand flushing. Various manoeuvres have been described to make the radial pulse disappear, but they may also do so in a normal person. These manoeuvres sometimes reproduce the patient's pain. Plain x-rays of the thoracic inlet and chest are important and arteriographic assessment is sometimes warranted in the case of aneurysm or arterial occlusion. Nerve conduction studies, although rarely diagnostic, may be useful in comparing the pre- and postoperative status. In the differential diagnosis, cord lesions and pressure on nerve roots from cervical spondylosis must be excluded as well as peripheral neuropathy and proximal arterial disease.

Operative treatment is directed at removal of a cervical rib (if present) or the first rib. Occasionally division of pectoralis minor tendon may also be necessary.

Complete excision of a cervical rib is best undertaken through a supraclavicular approach, whereas the transaxillary approach is preferred for removal of the first rib. Infraclavicular resection of the first rib may be done but does not allow such an extensive posterior clearance. A posterior, thoracoplasty-type approach to the first rib has been described but is not recommended.

SUPRACLAVICULAR APPROACH FOR REMOVAL OF A CERVICAL RIB

1

The operation is undertaken under general anaesthesia using endotracheal intubation. The patient lies supine with a sandbag between the shoulders and the head rotated laterally away from the side of operation. The diagram shows the relative position of the abnormal cervical rib to the anatomy of the root of the neck. Note the position of the subclavian artery and the T1 root of the brachial plexus.

The incision is 10 cm long situated 2 cm above and parallel to the clavicle and centred over the junction of its medial and middle thirds.

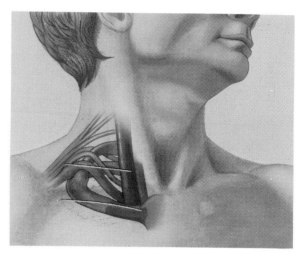

1

2

The subcutaneous tissue and platysma muscle are divided in the line of the incision. The clavicular head of sternomastoid is isolated and also divided in the line of the incision as is the posterior belly of the omohyoid muscle. The external jugular vein may require ligation and division. The internal jugular vein, and the scalene pad of fat (containing the supra-scapular and transverse cervical vessels) are now encountered.

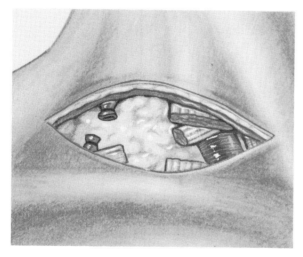

2

3

The fat pad is best divided between ligatures exposing the underlying scalenus anterior muscle over which runs the phrenic nerve (passing downwards from lateral to medial). The nerve is carefully mobilized and retracted medially, the muscle being then divided transversely near its attachment to the first rib. The posterior aspect of the muscle can be identified by a distinct thin aponeurosis, which gives a characteristic 'fish belly' appearance.

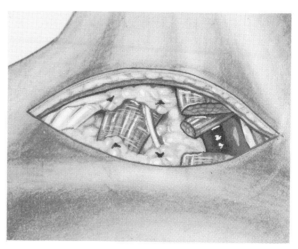

3

4

The trunks of the brachial plexus pass laterally, deep to the scalenus anterior muscle, and the abnormal cervical rib with the subclavian artery and the T1 branch of the brachial plexus are now seen.

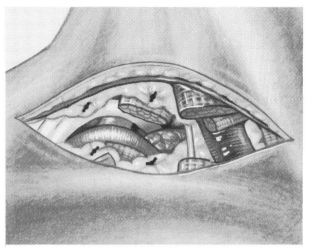

4

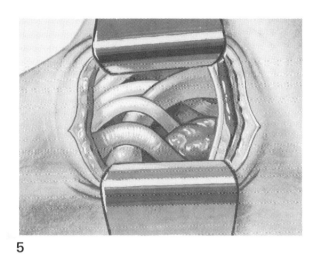

5

5

The artery arches over the prominent boss that marks the articulation of the cervical rib with the first thoracic rib. The artery and the 1st thoracic nerve root are carefully mobilized, and the margins of the cervical rib identified by a combination of sharp and blunt dissection.

6

The rib is transected and then nibbled away, care being taken to ensure that its rough cut surfaces do not come into contact with the artery or any nerve roots.

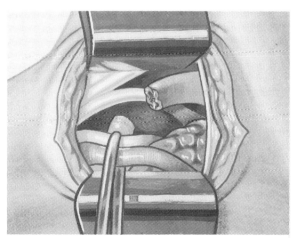

6

7

The rib is removed posteriorly as far as the transverse process of the seventh cervical vertebra and anteriorly, the articulation with the first rib is removed completely by sharp dissection. Following this procedure the artery and the T1 nerve root will lie without tension over the dome of the pleura with its covering suprapleural membrane.

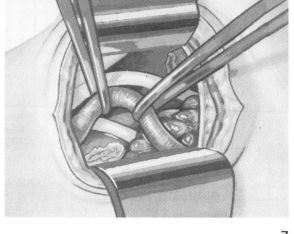

7

8

At this point any poststenotic dilatation of the artery may be explored through a longitudinal arteriotomy. Excess aneurysm wall and any thrombus are removed and the artery closed by direct suture. Only rarely is patching, replacement or bypass of the vessel, with vein or Dacron, necessary. If prior arteriography has shown distal arterial occlusion Fogarty catheterization should be undertaken and any recent thrombus extracted.

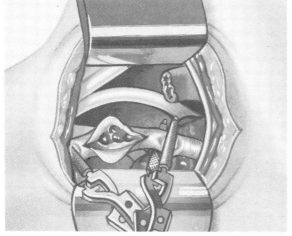

8

9

If there has been significant arterial insufficiency in the periphery of the limb, thoracodorsal ganglionectomy should be undertaken. The dome of the pleura is depressed and any residual fibres of the suprapleural membrane are divided radially towards the first rib. The sympathetic chain is identified extrapleurally over the neck of the first rib firstly by palpation, and then by visualization. At this stage it is not always possible to preserve a thin or adherent pleura intact. A lighted retractor is used to identify the chain as it passes into the superior mediastinum. The chain is divided below the third or fourth thoracic ganglion, and the rami communicantes to the fourth, third and second ganglion are divided. The chain is turned superiorly and stitched to the cut end of the scalenus anterior or any adjacent tissue.

The sternomastoid and the platysma muscles are re-approximated with a continuous suture line. If the pleura has been opened a small catheter is left in the pleural space until the subcutaneous suture line has been completed, and is withdrawn after the lung has been fully expanded with application of positive pressure by the anaesthetist.

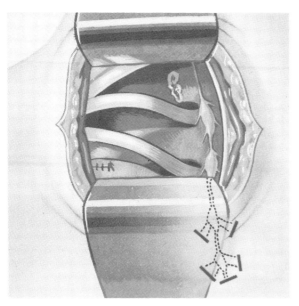

9

TRANSAXILLARY RESECTION OF THE FIRST RIB

10

Prior to the operation the upper arm, axilla and the upper trunk are shaved as far as the mid-line anteriorly and posteriorly. The patient is placed supine on the operating table with the operative side slightly raised. The lower arm is draped separately to allow manoeuvrability. With the arm in the abducted position a 10-cm transverse incision is made over the third rib just below the axillary hairline.

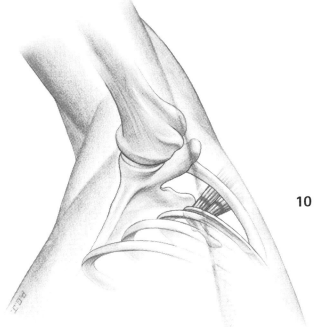

10

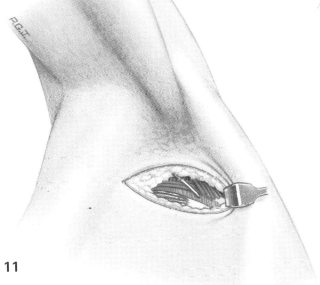

11

11

This incision is carried down to the fascia over serratus anterior and the chest wall. The dissection is now carried upward over the chest wall to the first rib, the intercostobrachial nerve being located and usually requiring division. The lateral thoracic nerve is identified and preserved.

12

The arm is now raised vertically and by further dissection the axillary vessels and the cords of the brachial plexus can be freed from the first rib. During the rib exposure particular attention must be paid to minimize the degree of traction which is put on the brachial plexus and its branches, and to this end the arm must be replaced by the side at 10-min intervals during the procedure. The hammerlock hold provides the assistant with the best method for maintaining the raised position.

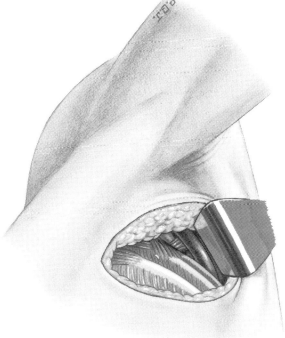

12

13

The attachments of scalenus anterior and medius and the subclavius muscle, to the superior surface of the rib are now divided and the surface cleared from the costal cartilage to the transverse process, care being taken to visualize the brachial plexus and axillary vessels throughout the procedure. The periosteum over the inferior surface and attached intercostal muscles are now cleared with a periosteal elevator over the same length of rib, particular attention being given to preserving adherent pleura. Once the rib has been freed from the costal cartilage to within 1 cm of the transverse process, it is divided with a rib shears and removed. Again all adjacent important structures must be visualized throughout the procedure. Fibrous bands and the attachment of a cervical rib to the first rib are divided under direct vision but incomplete cervical ribs are best left intact since their removal may endanger adjacent nerve roots. If the pectoralis minor tendon appears to be impinging on the neurovascular complex it is divided.

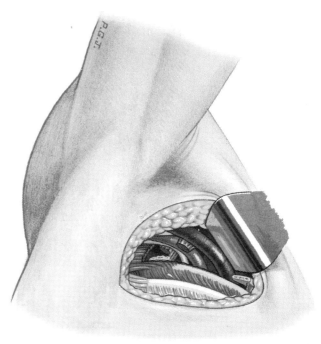

13

14

On completion of the dissection the lung must be inflated and any pleural leak identified. These do not usually require special drainage, though a suction drain to the axilla is desirable. After suturing the wound, the arm is bandaged to the side for 24 hr after which time progressive mobilization is encouraged.

14

INFRACLAVICULAR APPROACH TO THE FIRST RIB

15

The patient is positioned as for the supraclavicular approach, but the arm is abducted and the incision placed 2 cm below the clavicle.

The first rib is exposed by splitting the fibres of pectoralis major, usually between the sternal and clavicular heads. Clearing of the superior and inferior surfaces of the rib is carried out as in the trans-axillary approach, particular care being taken of the axillary vein. The nerves and vessels should again be visualized throughout the dissection. The rib can usually be resected to within 3 cm of the transverse process.

The anterior part of a cervical rib may be excised and the incision may be extended laterally to allow division of the pectoralis minor tendon.

Closure of the wound should follow the technique described for the supraclavicular approach.

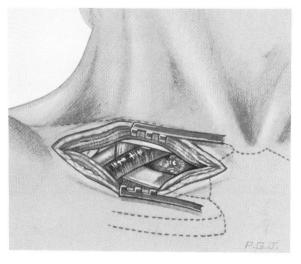

15

[The illustrations for this Chapter on The Thoracic Outlet Syndrome were drawn by Mr. P. G. Jack.]

Operation for Cervical Rib

Jere W. Lord, Jr., M.D., F.A.C.S.
Clinical Professor of Surgery,
New York University School of Medicine

and

Jefferson Ray, III, M.D., F.A.C.S.
Attending, Thoracic Surgery,
St. Joseph's Hospital, Marshfield, Wisconsin

PRE-OPERATIVE

Symptoms

The cervical rib syndrome typically produces more than one of the following upper extremity symptoms and signs: pain, paraesthesia, numbness, weakness, discolouration, swelling and ulceration. Pain is usually of ulnar nerve distribution but may be referred along the radial aspect of the arm or down the centre.

These findings, however, are not restricted to the cervical rib syndrome but are common to all neurovascular compression syndromes of the upper extremity. This group of syndromes has been called alternatively 'shoulder girdle syndromes' and 'thoracic outlet syndromes'. Moreover, other pathological processes may be confused with these syndromes, although none classically has elements of both neural and vascular compression.

Aetiology and anatomy

The causative mechanism in all neurovascular compression syndromes is mechanical compression of the brachial plexus and the subclavian vessels. The site of compression varies in each particular syndrome and may be multiple. The triangle of pressure in the cervical rib syndrome, through which the neuro-

vascular bundle passes, is formed by the anterior border of the cervical rib (or its fibrous attachment to the first rib), the superior border of the first rib, and the posterior aspect of the anterior scalene muscle. In addition, pressure may be exerted by the clavicle, costocoracoid ligament and subclavius muscle.

Diagnosis

The five basic considerations in formulating a diagnosis of the neurovascular compression syndrome are as follows:

(1) A history of neurovascular symptoms associated with certain postural attitudes such as hyperabduction of the arm, extension of the neck or retraction of the shoulder.

(2) Signs of compression of the subclavian-axillary vessels and/or brachial plexus.

(3) Demonstration of dampening or obliteration of the pulse with reproduction of the aggravating postures. The three manoeuvres used to elicit a pulse dampening are called: (a) the 'Adson' (the patient takes a deep breath, extends his neck fully, turns his chin towards right and then left); (b) costo-

clavicular (the patient assumes exaggerated military position, shoulders drawn downward and backward); (c) hyperabduction (the patient's arm is abducted by examiner to 180°).

(4) Exclusion of other conditions characterized by neurological or vascular symptoms in the upper extremity (such as herniated cervical disc, cervical arthritis, and bursitis).

(5) Finally, the relief of symptoms by appropriate therapy.

Many patients have asymptomatic cervical ribs, diagnosed incidentally at x-ray examination. If x-rays demonstrate a cervical rib in a patient with the neurovascular compression syndrome, a presumptive diagnosis of cervical rib syndrome may be made. The presence of a proved anomaly, however, does not rule out the concomitant presence of other causes of abnormal pressure. At operation a thorough exploration of all other possible sites of compression is made routinely.

Indications

The rationale of medical therapy for patients with the cervical rib syndrome stems from an appreciation of the factor of posture of the neck and shoulders, and the important part that correction of posture may play in alleviating symptoms. If symptoms are mild and there is no evidence of arterial insufficiency or oedema from venous occlusion, a trial of exercise therapy with the aid of an experienced physical therapist is warranted.

Surgical intervention is strongly advocated for patients with evidence of vascular compression. Too often, temporizing with conservative therapy has allowed progression of the compression to frank arterial or venous thrombosis. Stenosis of the subclavian artery, caught in the vice formed by the cervical rib and the scalenus anticus muscles, may lead to poststenotic dilatation or even aneurysmal formation. In some patients thrombotic material in the aneurysm may embolize to the hand, presenting a variety of ischaemic symptoms and signs. Correction of the stenosis by excision of the cervical rib and excision of the aneurysm with the interposition of a vein graft may be required for cure. Another strong operative indication is severe neurological symptoms. A lesser indication is failure of the patient with moderately severe symptoms to respond to medical exercise therapy.

Choice of approach

Historically, many portions of the cervicobrachial region bordering on the neurovascular supply have been subjected to surgical procedures. At present we use three different approaches to relieve neuro-

vascular compression caused by the cervical rib syndrome.

SUPRACLAVICULAR APPROACH

For the patient with vascular involvement or with vascular and neurological involvement in the absence of costoclavicular compression a supraclavicular approach is employed. Pressure is relieved on the vessels by sectioning the anterior scalene muscle. If there is a neurological component to the signs and symptoms, the cervical rib is also resected.

AXILLARY APPROACH

We reserve the axillary approach for those patients in whom there is evidence of costoclavicular compression. Operation here consists of resection of the first thoracic rib and the cervical rib.

Resection of clavicle

If a definitive vascular operation is necessary, as is the case after arterial thrombosis, or aneurysm, then the clavicle is resected with its periosteum to permit exposure of the subclavian-axillary artery.

Complications encountered in the supraclavicular approach are infrequent but can also be serious. Sectioning of the anterior scalene muscle too close to the first thoracic rib can result in subclavian vein bleeding with disastrous results. Should this occur, a period of compression of the vein should be attempted before efforts to visualize the vessel are made. The only effective approach to the vessel involves mobilizing the clavicle. Another complication is a painful postoperative neuritis. This stems from too forceful retraction of the brachial plexus after the Penrose drain has been placed around it.

Complications encountered in the axillary approach include inadvertent injury to the subclavian vessels while resecting the first thoracic rib with bone clippers, and the not infrequent production of a pneumothorax. Aspiration of air through a catheter during the closure usually suffices. Postoperative needle thoracentesis to extract the air may, however, be necessary.

Results of operation have been favourable: 90 per cent of patients without established arterial thrombosis will have relief of symptoms and be freed of the possibility of vascular occlusion. Operations for relief of the cervical rib syndrome where arterial thrombosis has occurred are, of course, less successful but should be attempted. If feasible, arterial reconstruction may be added.

THE OPERATION

SUPRACLAVICULAR APPROACH

The supraclavicular approach is used for vascular and neurological symptoms in the absence of costo-clavicular compression.

1

The incision

The incision is made 1 inch (2·5 cm) above the clavicle and extends for 3 inches (7·5 cm) towards the point of the shoulder, curving slightly backwards toward the scapula. Dissection is carried down to the anterior scalene muscle.

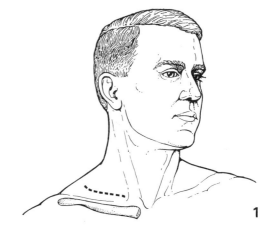

1

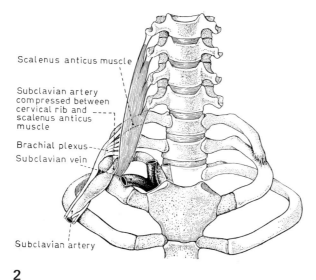

Scalenus anticus muscle

Subclavian artery compressed between cervical rib and scalenus anticus muscle

Brachial plexus

Subclavian vein

Subclavian artery

2

2

Sectioning of anterior scalene muscle

After exposing the anterior scalene muscle this is sectioned from its attachment to the first rib, great care being taken to avoid injury to the subclavian vein. Frequently, there is a tight fascial band at the posterior aspect of the muscle. When cut, this releases vessel compression.

3

Mobilization of brachial plexus and resection of cervical rib (for cases with a neurological component)

The brachial plexus is mobilized by passing a Penrose rubber drain behind it and using gentle retraction while freeing the rib from its bed. When the brachial plexus is adequately mobilized, the cervical rib can be resected easily.

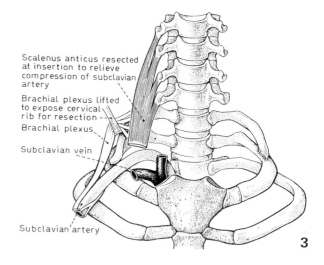

Scalenus anticus resected at insertion to relieve compression of subclavian artery

Brachial plexus lifted to expose cervical rib for resection

Brachial plexus

Subclavian vein

Subclavian artery

3

AXILLARY APPROACH

The axillary approach is used for vascular and neurological symptoms combined with costoclavicular compression.

4

Position of patient

The patient is placed in a 90° lateral position with a sandbag supporting the spine. The arm is elevated by an assistant.

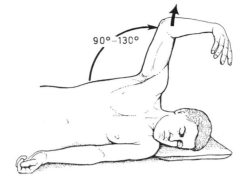

4

5

The incision

A 2·5—4-inch (6·3—9-cm) incision is made transversely with a slight downward curve across the lower aspect of the axilla below the axillary hairline. The incision is carried to the rib cage, halting at the tissue plane just above the anterior serratus.

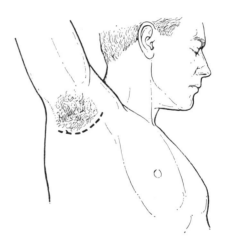

5

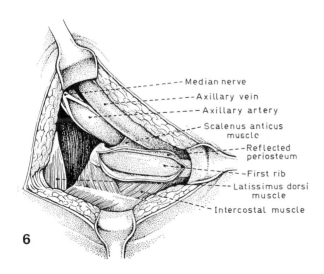

Median nerve
Axillary vein
Axillary artery
Scalenus anticus muscle
Reflected periosteum
First rib
Latissimus dorsi muscle
Intercostal muscle

6

6

Resection of first thoracic and cervical ribs

The first thoracic rib is exposed by carrying the dissection upwards in the same tissue plane. The intercostobrachial cutaneous nerve is retracted. Now the arm and shoulder are retracted vertically, opening the axillary tunnel. The scalenus anticus and medius muscles are divided at their insertion to the first rib. An incision is made along the periosteum of the first thoracic rib and the periosteum is elevated. The first thoracic rib is resected subperiosteally from the costochondral junction anteriorly to 1—1·5 inches (2·5—3·8 cm) from its posterior attachment. Some surgeons prefer extraperiosteal resection of the first rib although in our experience regeneration has not been a serious problem. The cervical rib is then resected throughout its length.

References

Eastcott, H. H. G. (1969). *Arterial Surgery,* p. 216. Philadelphia: J. B. Lippincott
Lord, J. W., Jr. and Rosati, L. M. (1971). *Thoracic Outlet Syndrome.* Ciba Clinical Symposia, No. 23.
Roos, D. B. (1966). 'Transaxillary approach for first rib resection to relieve thoracic outlet syndrome.' *Ann. Surg.* **163,** 354
Roos, D. B. and Owens, J. C. (1966). 'Thoracic outlet syndrome.' *Archs Surg.* **93,** 71
Rosati, L. M. and Lord, J. W., Jr. (1961). *Neurovascular Compression Syndromes of the Shoulder Girdle (Modern Surgical Monographs).* New York and London: Grune and Stratton

[*The illustrations for this Chapter on Operation for Cervical Rib were drawn by Mr. N. O. Hardy.*]

Excision of Carotid Body Tumours

Charles Rob, *M.C.*, M.D., M.Chir., F.R.C.S.
Professor and Chairman of the Department of Surgery,
University of Rochester School of Medicine and
Dentistry, Rochester, New York

PRE-OPERATIVE

Carotid body tumours present unusual technical problems, largely due to their anatomical position and to the fact that many are very vascular. Similar tumours may occur in other areas, notably the jugular body tumour (or glomus jugulare), the vagal body tumour and those which occur on the aortic arch.

Carotid body tumours grow slowly; they are rarely malignant and of a personal series of 62 such tumours, only three were malignant with metastases in the cervical lymph nodes. The reason for recommending removal is that, as they enlarge, they become unsightly and may cause symptoms due to their size and vascularity. Because these tumours rarely threaten life, operation must be safe to be justified. Unfortunately, the mortality and morbidity of many published series has been high (Lecompte, 1951). The reason for this has been the high incidence of hemiplegia which may follow this operation. One purpose of this chapter will be to discuss our views of the best ways of preventing this.

The diagnosis can usually be made clinically, but when a doubt exists an arteriogram produces a diagnostic picture, the arborization of the vessels in the vascular tumour being characteristic.

There is no special pre-operative preparation and general anaesthesia with an endotracheal tube is preferred.

THE OPERATION

1

Anatomy

Carotid body tumours lie on the bifurcation of the common carotid artery. They are densely adherent to the arteries at this point but can be removed if the dissection is carried out in the adventitia of the common carotid artery and of its branches. The carotid sinus nerve will be divided during the operation. It is important to preserve the hypoglossal and vagus nerves.

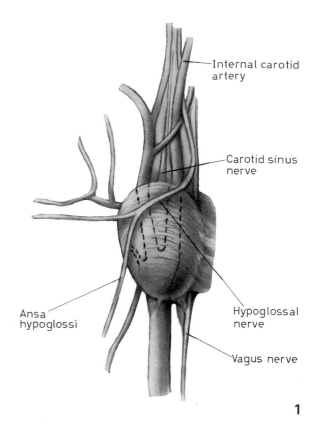

Internal carotid artery

Carotid sinus nerve

Ansa hypoglossi

Hypoglossal nerve

Vagus nerve

1

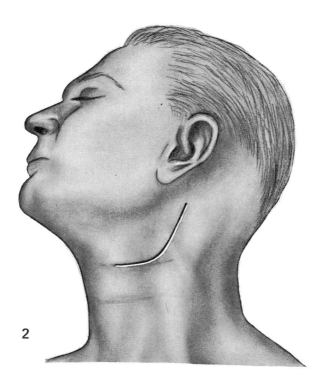

2

2

The incision

For most tumours a curved incision following one of the skin folds of the neck and centred over the bifurcation of the common carotid artery is satisfactory. It is wise to carry the posterior part of the incision upwards just in front of the anterior margin of the sternomastoid muscle. The platysma muscle is divided in the line of the incision. The great auricular nerve should be preserved if possible. For a very large tumour or the occasional tumour with cervical lymph node metastases, an incision in the line of the anterior edge of the sternomastoid muscle gives wider exposure.

3

Isolation of common and internal carotid arteries

This is an important step and should precede the mobilization of the tumour. The common carotid artery is isolated first and a tape placed around it. The hypoglossal (XIIth) nerve is next identified and followed towards the skull. This nerve is then displaced forwards and upwards. The ansa hypoglossi is divided. The internal carotid artery is then identified and freed just above the tumour and a tape passed around it.

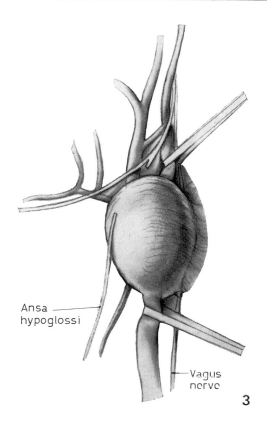

Ansa hypoglossi

Vagus nerve

3

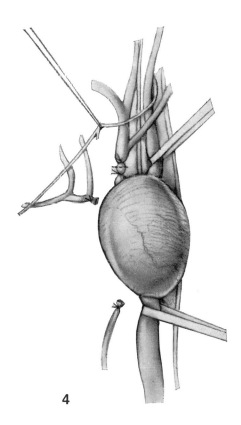

4

4

Mobilization of tumour

The tumour is freed first anteriorly, laterally and posteriorly, then medially. At this time brisk bleeding may occur from the vascular tumour. Although these tumours are sponge-like, firm compression by the surgeon during the dissection will control all but the most severe haemorrhage. It is of great importance to avoid rotating the carotid vessels through more than 90° during this dissection. In our opinion, twisting the internal artery is an important and avoidable cause of thrombosis and hemiplegia. Preservation of at least some of the branches of the external carotid artery until the completion of this phase of the operation helps to prevent excessive twisting of the internal carotid artery.

5

Removal of tumour

The surgeon now enters the adventitia of the common carotid artery and frees the tumour as much as possible from the arteries. He next divides the remaining branches of the external carotid artery. Clamps are now applied to the common and internal carotid arteries. The dissection in the adventitial plane is now continued and the tumour is split longitudinally and removed. The defect in the artery produced by the divided external carotid artery is now inspected. The presence of good blood flow from both the common and internal carotid arteries is confirmed by momentary removal of each arterial clamp. The vessels are flushed with saline and the external carotid opening oversewn with 5/0 arterial silk. If it appears that this part of the operation will take a long time a Javid type of arterial shunt may be inserted (*see* Chapter on 'Occlusions of the Carotid and Vertebral Arteries', pages 53–62). If the common or internal carotid arteries have been injured the defect may be repaired with a saphenous vein patch graft.

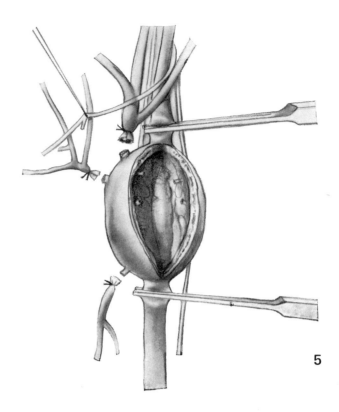

5

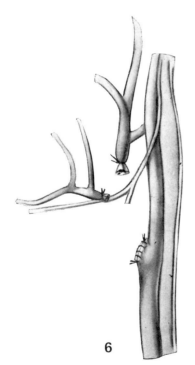

6

6

Closure

The internal and then the common carotid clamps are removed in this sequence, and light pressure applied to the arterial suture line until it is dry, extra sutures being inserted if necessary. The wound is then closed in layers and it is usually wise to insert a small drain. Heparin may be injected during the period of arterial clamping. Because local heparin rapidly enters the systemic circulation, we give 75–100 mg of heparin intravenously just before the arteries are clamped and counteract it with protamine sulphate (75–100 mg) given intravenously at the time the clamps are removed.

POSTOPERATIVE CARE

The drain is removed after 24 hr and the sutures a few days later depending upon the type of incision used. In most patients the procedure is benign and the patient can leave the hospital before the sutures are removed.

Should a cerebral deficit develop, the key investigation is early ophthalmodynamometry. An acute occlusion of the internal carotid artery can be diagnosed by a fall in intra-ocular pressure. The test makes no demands on the patient: if it is positive, urgent re-operation (usually before the patient has left the recovery and operating room areas) will often permit a satisfactory restoration of the carotid flow. If ophthalmodynamometry is negative, then the cause of the cerebral deficit is likely to be occlusion of a small intracranial vessel and, under these circumstances, the treatment is not surgical.

Reference

Lecompte, P. M. (1951). *Tumours of the Carotid Body and Related Structures.* Washington, D. C.; Armed Forces Institute of Pathology

[*The illustrations for this Chapter on Excision of Carotid Body Tumours were drawn by Miss D. Elliott.*]

Shunts and Fistulae for Haemodialysis

Allyn G. May, M.D.
Associate Professor of Surgery,
University of Rochester and
Strong Memorial Hospital,
Rochester, New York

and

Carl H. Andrus, M.D.
Assistant Professor of Surgery,
University of Rochester Medical Centre
and Strong Memorial Hospital,
Rochester, New York

Achievement of good vascular access for chronic intermittent haemodialysis requires planning and attention to detail. The simplest and most effective approach should be used, sacrificing in the process as few vessels as possible, so that subsequent vascular access procedures, should they prove necessary, will more likely be successful.

The upper extremities provide the best sites of access. The radial artery and cephalic vein at the wrist level are preferable. However, the ulnar artery and the basilic vein of the forearm can also be used. Chronic renal failure patients, who have been subjected to numerous venupunctures during the course of their disease, may have thrombosis of all of the superficial forearm veins of adequate size. In these patients the greater saphenous vein and posterior tibial artery or dorsalis pedis artery can be used.

For short-term dialysis and for severely uraemic patients who require immediate haemodialysis, external shunts, such as the Scribner (Scribner *et al.,* 1960) or Allen-Brown (Thomas, 1969), are indicated. Before choosing the vessels to be used, the Allen Test should demonstrate that interruption of the artery does not compromise the circulation of any portion of the hand. To do this test, the patient is asked to elevate the extremity over his head. Then the ulnar and radial arteries are both occluded at the wrist by compression, and the patient is asked to make a tight fist. With the arteries still occluded, the hand is brought down and the patient opens the hand, palm up. Finally the artery *not* to be used for the shunt is opened, and the collateral circulation provided by that artery is judged by the rapidity of flushing of all of the palmar surface of the hand. If the test suggests that a significant part of the hand is supplied by the artery still occluded (i.e. the artery proposed for the shunt), then an alternate artery must be selected.

Insertion of a Scribner shunt into the cephalic vein and radial artery

1

Local anaesthesia is used. A 3–4 cm transverse skin incision is made on the radial aspect of the wrist and a 1-cm segment of the cephalic vein is mobilized and encircled with in 4/0 silk.

Care should be taken not to injure the radial nerve which lies in the medial part of this incision on the fascia.

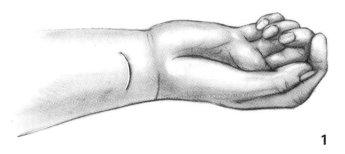

1

2

By palpation the radial artery is located beneath the fascia which is opened by means of a longitudinal incision. The artery is encircled with a 4/0 silk. Sometimes a branch or two must be ligated to avoid troublesome retrograde bleeding after insertion of the cannula.

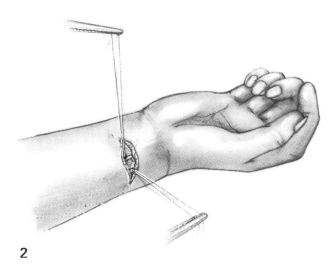

2

3

Teflon vascular cannulae are then chosen on the basis of vessel size, and tied snugly into the silastic arterial and venous tubes by means of 4/0 silks with the ends left long. The cannula and tube assemblies are filled with sterile heparinized saline and clamped. Various shapes of silastic tubes are available for use in different shunt configurations. It is important to choose tubes of configurations that will not interfere mechanically with each other and to construct adequate subcutaneous spaces in which these tubes can smoothly course without causing angulation of the cannulae in the respective vessels.

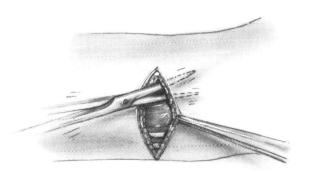

3

4

The vein is tied distally and another 4/0 silk is passed about the proximal part of the mobilized segment. Tension is placed on each silk and a longitudinal venotomy is made. The venous cannula is inserted through the venotomy and the proximal silk tied. One end of this silk is then tied to the long end of the silk holding the silastic tube into the cannula, thus fixing the assembly in position. The incision edges are brought together temporarily in order to demonstrate the best location for the skin stab wound through which the curved silastic tube will be brought. The stab wound must be placed with care to avoid angulation of the assembly in the vein and obstruction to its outflow.

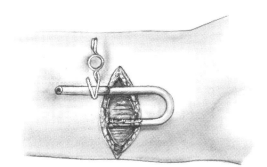

4

The artery is similarly tied distally and encircled by a proximal fine silk. Proximal control of the arterial flow can be achieved by tension on the proximal silk or, better, by a small bulldog clamp. A longitudinal arteriotomy is made and the arterial cannula introduced, and tied in place as before. In atherosclerotic patients the intima can easily be damaged during cannula insertion so that an obstructing intimal flap covers the cannula tip. The arterial assembly should be tested for this complication by momentary release of all arterial clamps once it is tied in place. Absence of pulsatile flow from the silastic tube will require more extensive proximal exposure and lengthening of the arteriotomy to deal with the intimal dissection.

5

Once again the wound edges are approximated temporarily to determine the sites of egress for the arterial tubing. When both tubes have been brought out through stab wounds, they are immediately connected with a Teflon connector and all camps are removed to allow flow. Observation of the velocity of blood flow through the shunt at this time is an opportunity to estimate the quality, durability, and usefulness of the shunt. The faster the flow the better the shunt. Lastly, the incision is closed in one layer with continuous or interrupted vertical mattress skin sutures. Dressings should be very loose to avoid compression of the vein and slowing of blood flow which would promote clotting and failure of the shunt. The sutures should not be removed for 2 weeks.

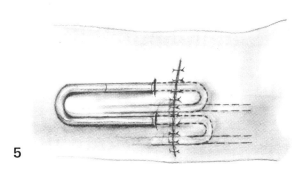

5

Construction of an arteriovenous fistula using radial artery and cephalic vein (Brescia *et al.*, 1966)

A tourniquet is placed on the arm so that the incision can be located at the point the vessels are closest together. Local anaesthesia is used and a 3—4-cm transverse incision is made. It is important for success that the vessels be brought together without sharp angulations. Thus, an adequate subcutaneous plane must be developed between the vessels and adequate lengths of vessels mobilized by tying and dividing branches to allow easy approximation. If the vessels lie unusually far apart, then it is best to tie the vein distally, spatulate its proximal end, and to construct an end-to-side arteriovenous anastomosis.

Ideally the side-to-side arteriovenous anastomosis is made as it produces a more extensive and useful dilatation of the superficial venous system. Tiny bulldog clamps are placed on the two vessels and longitudinal incisions are made in the vessel walls which will be contiguous. All blood is flushed from the vessel lumen with heparinized saline. Most incisions are made between 7 and 10 mm in length. Smaller incisions may be necessary with very small vessels. At this distal location in the extremity these arteriovenous fistulae rarely increase cardiac output excessively or result in steal syndromes.

6

The anastomosis is made with 6/0 arterial suture using continuous technique between stays placed at the end of the incision. The 'back wall' suture line is sewn from the inside of the anastomosis, using two lateral stays to provide good exposure. Immediately after completion of the anastomosis the vascular clamps are removed and the presence of a venous pulse and thrill sought as a sign of a successful fistula. The wound is closed in one layer. Sutures are left in 2 weeks and a simple, non-compression dressing is applied. The arterialized vein should be allowed to mature for 2 weeks before use for haemodialysis.

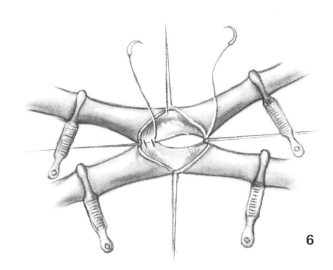

6

Use of the Allen-Brown prosthesis for arteriovenous shunts

In patients in whom it is impossible to construct an arteriovenous fistula and in whom it is undesirable to interrupt an artery for risk of ischaemia, the Allen-Brown prosthesis may provide excellent vascular access.

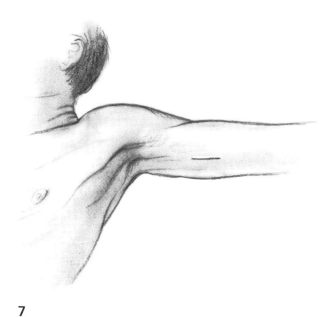

7

7

The operation may be done under local anaesthesia. An 8-cm longitudinal incision is made on the medial aspect of the arm over the pulsations of the distal brachial artery. A segment of this artery is mobilized without ligation of any branches. A segment of the basilic vein or one of the venae commitantes of the brachial artery is also mobilized. The venous portion of the shunt is constructed first. In our experience the Allen-Brown prosthesis for the venous portion of the shunt frequently fails because of clotting. Consequently we use a Scribner cannula, such as described above, rather than an Allen-Brown prosthesis. The vein is tied distally and the assembly inserted through a longitudinal venotomy and tied in place. It is kept clamped and filled with heparinized saline.

Arterial access is next acquired. The knitted Dacron cuff of the Allen-Brown prosthesis is stretched and divided about 6 mm from its bond with the silastic tube. The Dacron cuff is spatulated almost to the silastic tube, leaving only enough cuff at the apex of the spatulation to allow insertion of a vascular suture. The cuff is clotted by stretching it in freshly drawn, non-anticoagulated blood from the patient in order to minimize blood loss through the fabric after completion of the anastomosis and removal of the vascular clamps. The chosen arterial segment is isolated by vascular clamps. A longitudinal arteriotomy is made and the lumen is irrigated with heparinized saline.

8

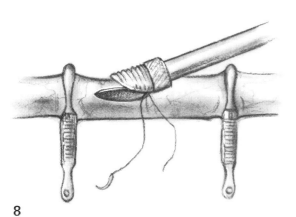

8

An end-to-side anastomosis is made with 5/0 arterial suture. The anastomosis should be located at a site on the artery so that the skin stab wound for egress of the silastic tubing is not too near the elbow joint. A flange on the prosthesis near the anastomosis is designed to prevent twisting. Adequate space in the subcutaneous tissue should be prepared for it. The wound of egress should be at least 4 cm from the arterial anastomosis. When both halves of the shunt have been inserted, they should be connected and flow established without delay. The wound is closed in layers without drainage. A loose dressing is applied. This sort of shunt can be used immediately.

Alternate means of vascular access for haemodialysis

In patients who lack satisfactory superficial veins in the upper extremities and who require long-term vascular access, it is possible to construct an arteriovenous fistula using bovine arterial xenografts (Haimov *et al.*, 1974) (heterografts) or, preferably, venous autografts if a greater saphenous vein is available (May *et al.*, 1969). The graft may be placed between the distal radial artery and the median cubital vein of the forearm. Both anastomoses may be end-to-side and the tunnel should be made quite superficial in the subdermal plane. If an adequate length of greater saphenous vein is available, a loop fistula can be constructed with anastomoses to the brachial artery and median cubital vein. The course of the venous autograft then should describe a course from the brachial artery down the anteromedial aspect of the forearm, gently curving distally to the anterolateral aspect, and ascending to the venous anastomosis in the antecubital fossa. Multiple small incisions should be made to ensure a subdermal tunnel without sharp angles. These vascular grafts should be allowed to heal for several weeks before use.

In case of clotting

The Allen-Brown shunt can be easily declotted by means of the small Fogarty thrombectomy catheter because there are no reverse curves in the silastic tubes of such shunts. Consequently the Fogarty catheter can be introduced throughout the entire lengths of the arterial and venous assemblies. However, the Scribner shunts cannot be declotted with this technique if the configuration of the silastic tube used in the shunt possesses a reverse curve because the Fogarty catheter cannot negotiate the curve. Therefore, Scribner shunts must be declotted by other techniques. First, the clct should be removed from the external part of the shunt by clamping the silastic tube at skin level and milking out the clot. A syringe is then applied and the air exhausted and replaced with sterile saline. Next, alternate suction and gentle pressure is exerted with the syringe to loosen and, if possible, to retrieve the remaining clot in the syringe. A syringe of small volume should be used on the arterial assembly to avoid retrograde embolization of the clot into the cerebral circulation. If the clot is not removed at the first attempt, it may be successfully removed at another time when the clot has contracted and thus freed itself from the walls of the vessel and prosthesis.

References

Scribner, B. H., Caner, J. E. Z., Buri, R. and Quinton, W. (1960). 'Technique of continuous hemodialysis.' *Trans. Am. Soc. artif. internal Organs* **6**, 88

Thomas, G. I. (1969). 'A large vessel applique A–V shunt for hemodialysis.' *Trans. Am. Soc. artif. internal Organs* **15**, 288

Brescia, M. J., Cimino, J. E., Appel, K. and Hurwich, B. J. (1966). 'Chronic hemodialysis using venipuncture and a surgically created arteriovenous fistula.' *New Engl. J. Med.* **275**, 1089

May, J. Tiller, D., Johnson, J., Stewart, J., Sheil, A. G. Ross (1969). 'Saphenous vein arteriovenous fistula in regular dialysis treatment.' *New Engl. J. Med.* **280**, 770

Haimov, M., Burrows, L., Baez, A., Neff, M. and Slifkin, R. (1974). 'Alternatives for vascular access for hemodialysis: Experience with autogenous saphenous vein autografts and Bovine heterografts.' *Surgery* **75**, 447

[The illustrations for this Chapter on Shunts and Fistulae for Haemodialysis were drawn by Mr. R. Howe.]

Arterial Infusion Chemotherapy

Edwin D. Savlov, M. D.
Associate Professor of Surgery,
University of Rochester School of Medicine and
Dentistry, and Director of Surgical Oncology,
Highland Hospital, Rochester, New York

and

Charles D. Sherman, Jr., M. D.
Clinical Professor of Surgery,
University of Rochester School of Medicine and
Dentistry, Rochester, New York

PRE-OPERATIVE

General considerations

Although surgery and radiation therapy are the primary methods of treatment of cancer at the present time, they are limited to treatment of a local area. Chemotherapy on the other hand, when given intravenously or orally, is carried throughout the body and is systemic therapy. Increasingly this type of approach is being considered in association with primary surgical or radiation treatment as an adjuvant.

Because of the problems of systemic toxicity of the known chemotherapeutic agents, techniques have been devised to deliver high concentrations of the drugs to tumour-bearing areas in an attempt to lessen toxic effects on the bone marrow and gastro-intestinal tract. These techniques are most useful when the tumour is localized to an area of the body with a single arterial supply. Two main methods, *arterial infusion* and *isolation perfusion*, have been utilized, making use of drugs appropriate to the duration of exposure of the tumour to the drug and the tumour type. Isolation perfusion chemotherapy is discussed on pages 342–345.

In arterial infusion therapy the arterial supply of a tumour is infused continuously with an appropriate drug, usually an antimetabolite, for a prolonged period of time, weeks or even months, in order to expose cells to the drug during vulnerable phases of the cell cycle.

Indications

Patients with localized advanced malignancy fed by a single accessible artery are most suitable for infusion.

(*1*) Head and neck cancer without distant metastases, confined to distribution of the external carotid artery, unilateral or bilateral.

(*2*) Primary or metastatic hepatic tumours may be treated by way of the hepatic artery.

(*3*) Extremities containing a neoplasm can be treated by way of the axillary or femoral arteries. Isolation perfusion may be preferred in these cases.

(*4*) Advanced local cancer arising from the pelvic organs can be treated by way of the internal iliac arteries.

(*5*) Local areas of melanoma can be infused with expectancy of 50 per cent response rate and complete remission of over 33 per cent of patients using dimethyl triazeno imidazole carboxamide (NSC 45388) (Savlov, Hall and Oberfield, 1971).

Contra-indications and precautions

(1) Blood counts, including platelet counts should be adequate.

(2) Since methotrexate is excreted by the kidneys, impaired renal function will result in unusually high blood levels of the drug, increasing toxic effects.

(3) Previous radiation therapy and poor nutritional state will increase the hazards of antimetabolite therapy.

(4) Full co-operation by the patient is essential in infusion therapy. Not only should written consent be obtained, but the patient should understand as completely as possible the aims, techniques and possible side-effects of therapy.

(5) Tissue diagnosis of malignancy is mandatory before undertaking any chemotherapy, particularly long-term infusion therapy.

(6) Hepatic arteriograms via the aorta prior to cannulation are necessary in revealing the variations in hepatic vascular anatomy which are so common.

Apparatus required

Teflon tubing is used, a size which fits a No. 20-gauge blunt cannula. This is connected by Venotube (Abbott), with a one-way valve (B–D) in the system to prevent reflux, to an infusion set adapted for use with an infusion pump.

A number of satisfactory pumps are available. We have used: Sigmamotor kinetic clamp pump No. AL-2, pre-set to deliver 500 ml per 24 hr; Sigmamotor variable flow pump No. TM-11; Sigma-motor portable pump with rechargeable battery, model No. ML-5 or the Watkins USC1 Chronofusor. The position of the catheter is checked during placement by injection of fluorescein dye ('Fluorescite') and observation under ultraviolet light. Further visualization may be obtained by arteriography, although this is not usually needed.

THE OPERATIONS

EXTERNAL CAROTID ARTERY CANNULATION VIA THE SUPERFICIAL TEMPORAL ARTERY

1

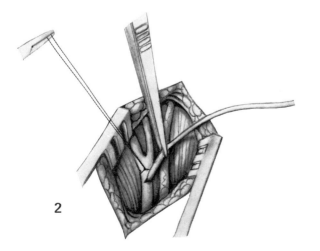

The incision

A vertical incision is made under local anaesthesia anterior to the tragus. The vessel is isolated, and is usually somewhat tortuous, especially in older patients.

2

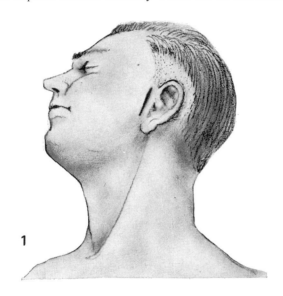

Isolation of artery and retrograde insertion of catheter

After distal ligation, a fine catheter can be passed downward into the neck, using moderate traction to aid in negotiation of curves, usually a distance of 6–8 cm. Five millilitres of fluorescein dye is injected and the area of the tumour is observed with an ultraviolet light to assure perfusion of the diseased area.

3

Closure

The catheter is doubly ligated in the vessel with fine silk and brought out through a stab wound above the incision. The catheter can be brought above the ear and taped to the postauricular region, using a tongue depressor as a splint. Dilute heparin is injected into the catheter to prevent clotting within it prior to onset of infusion.

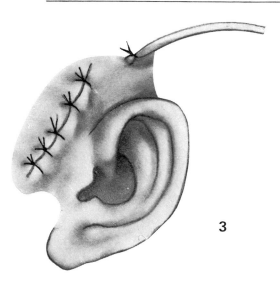

3

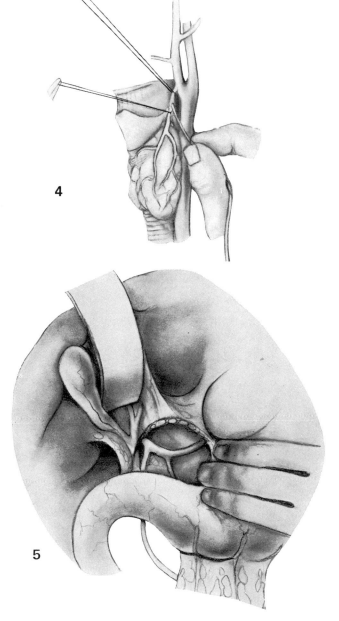

4

ALTERNATE CANNULATION OF EXTERNAL CAROTID ARTERY VIA SUPERIOR THYROID ARTERY

4

If the superficial temporal artery cannot be used, the superior thyroid artery can be approached through the neck. Use of branches to cannulate a large artery is preferred, rather than direct intubation into the main artery. Insertion of the catheter through a long length of the superior thyroid artery helps further to diminish the chance of extrusion of the catheter.

INFUSION OF LIVER THROUGH HEPATIC ARTERY

5

The incision, and isolation of the gastroduodenal artery

At laparotomy the gastroduodenal artery is isolated.

5

6

Placement of catheter

The tip of the catheter is inserted through the gastro-duodenal artery into the hepatic. Holding ligatures are placed around the catheter. Other branches of the hepatic artery are ligated to restrict the infusion to the liver alone.

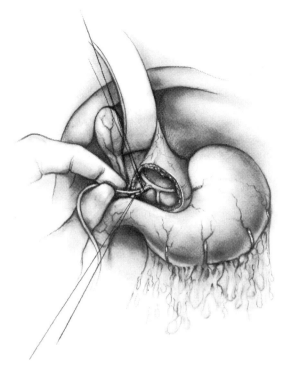

6

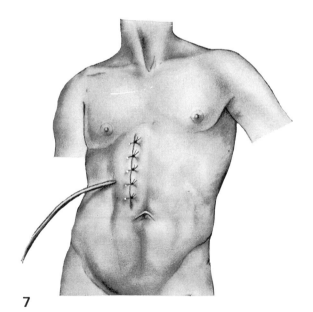

7

7

Closure

The position of the catheter is checked with fluorescein dye injection. It is then brought through a small stab wound in the abdominal wall and the wound closed. The catheter is filled with heparin to prevent clotting.

Similar techniques are used for the other sites.

POSTOPERATIVE CARE

Drug dose schedules

(*1*) In head and neck cancers, the drug of choice is methotrexate 50 mg per 24 hr by continuous infusion, with concomitant intramuscular administration of citrovorum factor (Leucovorin) 6 mg every 6 hr. Therapy is discontinued with the onset of local toxicity in the area of infusion (mucositis, skin erythema) or systemic toxicity. If systemic toxicity appears before the local reaction, the dosage of citrovorum factor should be increased in order to achieve some degree of local toxicity—the indication of maximal antimetabolic effect in the infused region. Repeated courses of methotrexate can be given until maximal clinical response is noted, with recovery periods between toxic episodes. The catheter may be left in for several months as long as it is filled with heparin between treatments.

(*2*) Malignancies in the liver are best treated with FUDR infusion using 20–25 mg per 24 hr. Dosage is reduced when hepatic function studies reveal impairment. Infusion may be continued, with interruptions as indicated by hepatic or systemic toxicity, for 2 months or more.

Precautions and complications

White cell counts and differential counts are obtained daily during the first week of therapy, and twice or three times weekly subsequently. Haemoglobin and platelet counts are done two or three times weekly. Suitable serum chemistries are obtained once or twice weekly.

Care must be taken to keep the catheter in its proper position. Repeat fluorescein studies should be done if slippage is suspected. Other potential complications include air emboli, clotting in the catheter and haemorrhage, although the latter is uncommon in the absence of gross infection. Hemiparesis has been seen after internal carotid artery infusion, due to either arterial spasm by drug irritation or thrombosis. Since leucopenia frequently occurs, antibiotics should be given if there is any significant risk of infection.

References

Savlov, E. D., Hall, T. C. and Oberfield, R. A. (1971). 'Intra-arterial therapy of melanoma with dimethyl triazeno imidazole carboxamide (NSC 45388).' *Cancer* 28, 1161
Watkins, E. and Sullivan, R. D. (1964). *Surgery Gynec. Obstet.* 118, 3

[*The illustrations for this Chapter on Arterial Infusion Chemotherapy were drawn by Mr. R. Wabnitz.*]

Isolation Perfusion Chemotherapy

Edwin D. Savlov, M. D.
Associate Professor of Surgery,
University of Rochester School of Medicine and
Dentistry, and Director of Surgical Oncology,
Highland Hospital, Rochester, New York

and

Charles D. Sherman, Jr., M.D.
Clinical Professor of Surgery,
University of Rochester School of Medicine and
Dentistry, Rochester, New York

PRE-OPERATIVE

Indications

Isolation perfusion of an extremity is performed for two main reasons.

(*1*) To control advanced malignant disease confined to an extremity, in an attempt to destroy all tumour tissue and avoid amputation.

(*2*) As an adjunct to radical surgical excision of a primary melanoma or sarcoma in an extremity, with the purpose of eliminating residual tumour which may persist in tissue planes, lymphatics or blood vessels.

High local concentrations of cytotoxic agents, usually alkylating agents or rapidly-acting antibiotics, can be achieved without excessive systemic toxicity.

Contra-indications

Contra-indications include the presence of disseminated disease outside the perfused field, and severe vascular disease.

Drugs used

In melanoma, phenylalanine mustard is usually employed. Rochlin favours the addition of actinomycin D in sarcomas.

Apparatus

Disposable oxygenator; pumps; heater unit; tourniquet; availability of monitoring equipment.

Pre-operative preparation

Clinical evaluation of the patient should include complete haematological assessment. The pumps are calibrated to assure 150–500 ml/min flow rate. Antibiotics are started pre-operatively.

THE OPERATION

LOWER EXTREMITY PERFUSION VIA THE EXTERNAL ILIAC VESSELS

1

Draping and tourniquet

Either general or spinal anaesthesia is satisfactory. The extremity is prepared and draped from the mid-abdomen, with a sterile tourniquet placed beneath the upper thigh. A Steinmann pin is inserted into the iliac crest to anchor the tourniquet when it is tightened.

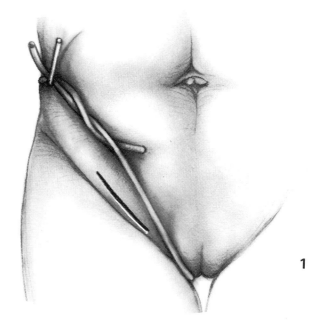

1

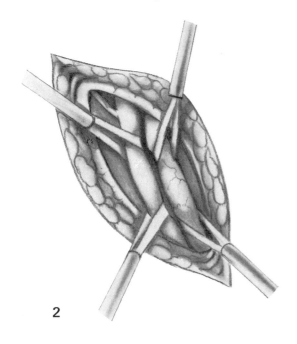

2

2

The incision, and exposure of vessels

Incision is made above and parallel to the inguinal ligament. Peritoneum is reflected medially to expose the iliac vessels. Sampling of lymph nodes is obtained from the peri-iliac and obturator regions. If these are involved, perfusion is contra-indicated. Branches and tributaries are carefully clamped or ligated to prevent collateral circulation. Control tapes are passed around the main vessels above and below the sites elected for cannulation.

3

Insertion of cannulae

Heparin, 1·5 mg/kg body weight is administered intravenously and allowed to take effect. The artery is then occluded proximally, and a suitable arterial cannula is passed distally through a small arteriotomy and ligated into position with the tip of the cannula just below the inguinal ligament in the common femoral artery. The vein is similarly cannulated. A long fine polyethylene catheter may be passed upward into the vena cava through the same venotomy for sampling. The tourniquet is then tightened above the wound and held in place by the previously-placed Steinmann pin.

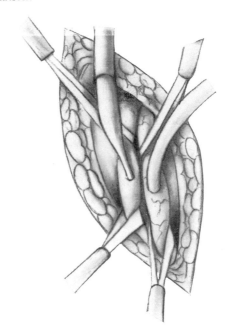

3

4

Pump management, monitoring, and drugs

The disposable oxygenator is primed with 500 mg of dextrose solution. Cannulae are connected to the pump-oxygenator and perfusion is maintained at 150–200 ml/min. Arterial line is passed through a heat exchanger maintaining a temperature of 37–39°C. Radio-iodinated human serum albumin (RISA) is injected into an arterial side-arm, and specimens are obtained at 5- to 10-min intervals simultaneously from the vena cava and from the extracorporeal circuit. These are counted at once. Systemic leak is calculated using the known volume of the extracorporeal system, and estimated volume of the perfused limb and of the systemic circulation.

The drug dose and exposure time should be reduced if leakage will be more than 20 per cent in 45 min. Papaverine, 100–200 mg, is usually injected just before administration of the drug. Phenylalanine mustard 1·0–1·4 mg/kg of ideal body weight is given in three or four divided doses at 4-min intervals with maximum dosage of 100 mg to any patient. Isolation perfusion is then maintained for 30–45 min after the last dose.

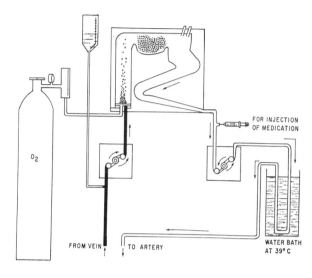

4

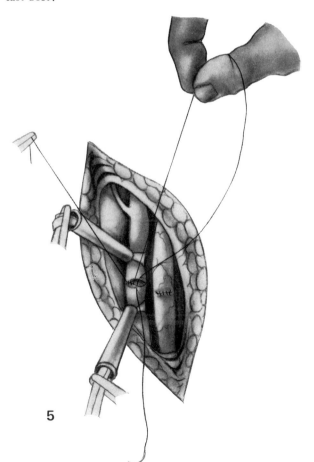

5

5

Withdrawal of catheters and closure of vessels

Dextran, 500 ml, followed by heparinized blood, 500 ml, is then washed through the limb, after which the arterial and then the venous cannulae are removed. The vessels are repaired and then tapes and tourniquets are released. Protamine, 1·0 mg/kg is given intravenously.

Wound closure

The wound is then closed without drainage, unless large skin flaps have been developed in which case, Hemovac suction catheters are used.

SPECIAL POSTOPERATIVE CARE

All patients are given broad-spectrum antibiotics postoperatively. The limb pulses, temperature and colour are observed frequently. Blood counts may be expected to reach a nadir on the tenth to fourteenth postoperative day, usually with a white cell count of 3000 if leakage has been 15–20 per cent. The limb may be mildly oedematous and erythematous for several days after perfusion. Haemovac tubes are removed in 2–4 days, when drainage has ceased.

Complications

Complications such as severe leucopenia, infection of the wound, and haemorrhage from femoral vessels are infrequent. Prolonged leg oedema and nerve damage have not been a problem when PAM is used.

[*The illustrations for this Chapter on Isolation Perfusion Chemotherapy were drawn by Mr. R. Wabnitz.*]

Index